OCCUPATIONAL HEALTH
FOR THE NURSE AND OTHER
HEALTH WORKERS

OCCUPATIONAL HEALTH

FOR THE NURSE AND OTHER HEALTH WORKERS

Edited by

A. J. KOTZE

M Cur (Pret), B Cur I et A (Pret), RGN, RM, OTT, Int.Care, N Adm., N Ed., CHN

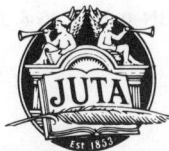

Juta & Co, Ltd

CAPE TOWN   WETTON   JOHANNESBURG

First Edition 1992

© Juta & Co, Ltd 1992

PO Box 14373, Kenwyn 7790

ISBN 0 7021 2668 3

SET, PRINTED AND BOUND IN THE REPUBLIC OF SOUTH AFRICA
BY THE RUSTICA PRESS (PTY) LTD, NDABENI, CAPE

D352

Foreword to First Edition

During the past decades, the clinical practice of occupational health as a field of study, became increasingly important in South Africa. A great increase in work-related health problems, with their resultant impact on family and community life, has created the need for a book which provides for the learning needs of the nurse and other health workers in the field of occupational health.

The topics for this book have been carefully selected and are designed to meet the educational needs of nursing students in a variety of nursing courses such as the basic, post-basic and graduate training programmes.

The student is guided through events in the history of occupational health chronologically. The local occupational scene is described in a way that should enable the reader to grasp the complexities inherent in the administration of health services in Southern Africa.

Essential information (basic concepts; occupational hygiene; occupational safety; the nurse in occupational health services; and selected elements of emergency planning) provides a background to specialized topics such as occupational medicine and industrial psychology.

A. J. KOTZE
Pretoria
1992

Authors

My sincere thanks to all the contributors, whose support never failed.

Acutt, Jenny
B.A.Cur., R.G.N., R.M., C.H.N., N.Ed., O.H.N.

Bergh, Ziel C.
M.A. Psych. (Counselling and Industrial Psychology). Senior Lecturer, University of South Africa. Practising Counselling and Industrial Psychologist.

Campbell, Yvonne
R.N., R.M., O.H.N., Occupational health Adviser.

Hattingh, Susan
B.A.Cur Hons., B.Cur(I et A), R.N., R.M., Psych., O.T.T., Lecturer, University of South Africa.

Kotze, A. J.
M.Cur (Pret), B.Cur(I et A) (Pret), R.G.N., R.M., O.T.T., Int.Care, C.H.N., N.Adm., N.Ed.

Mets, Johann T.
M.B. Ch.B. (Leiden), M.R.C.S (Eng), L.R.C.P. (Lon), D.O.M. (Stell), M.F.O.M. (Eng), M.D. (Pret), F.A.O.M.A. (U.S.A).

A special word of thanks to our language editor, Rodger Loveday.

Authors

My sincere thanks to all the contributors whose support never failed.

Contents

Contents

Chapter 1: A Historical Overview of the Development of Occupational Health

by A. J. Kotze

1.1 INTRODUCTION

'Strange is God's behaviour, I think, that he makes mountains of iron, ochre, brimstone and gold; then says: "Now sort that out. Fight over it, dig it, stamp misery on the faces of the poor with it, make the rich richer . . . and put it back into the soil again"' (Cordell, 1983:7).

The appalling conditions in the Welsh copper mines between 1826 and 1913 moved many a writer to expose the squalid conditions and human suffering which preceded the Welsh Industrial Revolution.

Employers felt little or no concern for the environment or for the personal health of their employees. Human life was held cheap, and mine bosses failed to exhibit any real interest in the health and welfare of their workers. Cordell writes: 'And in that consuming of tree and land, I heard the protests of my people; the groans and breathlessness of worked-out colliers, the shrieks of entombed children, the screams of women trapped in machines' (1983:295).

As human beings progressed technologically, they became increasingly exposed to the hazards generated by each new technology. The earliest developments in technology were manifested in the manufacture of tools: first in stone, then in bronze, and later in iron. These

1

ages lasted for many thousands of years. But in the last two centuries, technology has developed more and more rapidly. So rapidly, in fact, has technology developed since the middle of the 18th Century, that it now seems as though human beings are increasingly overwhelmed and disorientated by technological innovations. This disorientation has resulted in a failure of the natural ability of human beings to adapt and acclimatize themselves. But, in ancient times, even the craft of tool-making exposed people to numerous injuries such as those caused by fire, fumes and festering wounds. (Ffrench:2).

Classical Greek literature records the clinical observations of the most celebrated physician of the ancient world, Hippocrates (5th Century B.C.). Hippocrates was a pioneer of clinical observation in medicine, and he took due note of the appalling work conditions of the time. He urged students of medicine to take into account those factors in the environment which might influence people's health.

Although varying degrees of awareness of occupational hazards existed throughout history, it is only in modern times that occupational health has become a recognized discipline in the health sciences. Unfortunately, in many communities, this recognition is not yet legally enforceable because of the lack of appropriate legislation and because, in many countries, there exists no infrastructure of health services concerned with the welfare of workers.

The role of the occupational health nurse is inseparable from the history of occupational health. She has a central function in any effective health service in the workplace.

1.2 LEARNING OBJECTIVES

At the end of this section the reader should be able to:
- relate the history of the development of occupational health services
- analyse and describe the significance of certain crucial developments in the development of occupational health services
- identify some important people and groups which contributed to the development of services

1.3 DEVELOPMENTS DURING SPECIFIC PERIODS IN HISTORY

1.3.1 The Ages of Antiquity History reveals that both modern and ancient societies have been slow to recognize and act upon the hazards to which people are exposed in working environments.

Many examples are known of how people protected themselves from hazardous situations in ancient times. These measures were often ineffective, and neither the employer nor society accepted responsibility for human health in such conditions.

Teleky mentions protective equipment such as arm-protecting plates which were worn by the archers to protect their wrists against the recoil of the bow string, and tubes worn on the fingers of the right hand which grasped the bow string. Other such examples are the leather rings which women placed on their heads when they carried water vessels, and the strips of tape worn on the cheeks and lips by the flute players (Teleky, 1948:3).

Mining is one of mankind's oldest industries. Many years passed before anything was done to counteract the dangerous conditions which claimed many lives. The hazardous nature of the mining industry was recognized even in antiquity. But the total disregard for the miner's health and safety may be ascribed to the fact that a miner in those times was often a slave, prisoner or criminal, and it therefore never occurred to anyone to improve working conditions. Such miners often made futile attempts to protect themselves by wrapping themselves in bags and sacks, and by using animal bladders to cover their mouths as a protection against the inhalation of the dust which occurs in mines (Schilling, 1973:1).

1.3.2   The Middle Ages   Economically and scientifically, the early middle ages was a period characterized by retrogression. The earliest workers' guilds were developed in Europe and England. These guilds were organizations of employers in particular trades who made regulations to protect guild masters and consumers. Mention was made of provisions for sick, disabled and aged workers, but still no protective health measures were enforced. When measures *were* enforced which incidentally benefited the health of workers, the health or welfare of workers was never the primary reason for such regulations. Such measures were designed to regulate competition, and concerned themselves, for example, with age restrictions and the length of the working day.

In medieval times, medicine in Western Europe deteriorated to an all-time low, although it flourished in the Moslem world. In Europe, medical science failed to take into account all the threats to human health inherent in working conditions, and the environment causes of many occupational hazards.

1.3.3   Modern Times   The Renaissance was followed by increased activity in the mining industry, in metal work and in many other trades (sixteenth and seventeenth centuries). It was also during this time that the transition from feudalism to capitalism was accelerated. In 1524, there appeared the first known monograph to deal with the topic of industrial hygiene. The author, Ulrich Ellenbog, intended his book to be used by goldsmiths and other metal workers. It suggested guidelines for protecting workers against the noxious effects of silver, mercury and lead fumes.

Agricola (1494–1555) was the first person to gather observations about miners and their diseases. These observations were then published by Hoover and Paracelsus (Schilling, 1973:2). Agricola was the official town physician in a flourishing mining centre in Bohemia. Mining in central Europe during this period was characterized by rapid growth, and the need for skilled labourers. The demand for gold and silver was increasing all the time. As demand increased, conditions in mines worsened as the mines got deeper. Paracelsus writes: '(I)n the mines of the Carpathian mountains, women are found who have married seven husbands, all of whom this terrible consumption has carried off to a premature death' (Schilling, 1973:2).

Both Agricola and Paracelsus were and are, even now, considered physicians of genius. It was because of their work as physicians in Eastern European mining towns that the recognition of occupational diseases began to gain momentum.

Agricola made many suggestions to miners as to how they might maximize their personal protection. 'He also gives a very fine description and excellent pictures of the devices for the intake and outlet of air in the mines' (Teleky, 1948:8). Paracelsus suggested the ingestion of certain drugs which, he believed, would be effective against the harmful effects of substances inhaled in mines. This treatment was, however, questioned by Stockhausen, a physician for the miners of the Lüneberg mines. He wrote that prophylaxis is better than cure, and that measures should be taken to prevent the inhalation of fogs, fumes, vapours and metal dust. Stockhausen wrote accurate descriptions of conditions such as silicosis, and lead colic.

1.3.4   The 18th Century Bernado Ramazzini (1633–1714), a physician and professor of medicine in Modena and Padua, is considered to be the father of occupational medicine. It was said of this physician that he showed an unusual sympathy for the less fortunate members of society—a quality practically unique for a physician of that time. Schilling (1973:4) says that 'neither his medical colleagues, nor the influential people of society had any strong humanitarian sense to inspire them to heed his words, nor at that time was there any economic necessity to protect the life and health of workmen'.

Ramazzini published the first systematic study of occupational diseases. In this book he collated his predecessors' and his own observations. His conclusions were also based directly on first-hand observations of conditions in workshops in Modena. His book contains many suggestions for personal prophylaxis, but very little mention is made of hygiene in the workplace, or of the potential hazards created by using tools. This may be accounted for by the fact that, as physician, he was more interested in the clinical aspects of disease, and in the conditions which led to disease. In describing the working conditions of certain trades, and the hazards which they generated, he laid the foundations for occupational hygiene.

The importance of this work may be gauged from the fact that his book was reprinted numerous times and translated into a variety of languages. Some translators even added observations of their own.

Ackermann's adaptation of Ramazzini's book is well known, and almost three times longer than the original. The section on mines and smelting works contains many suggestions for hygiene based on adequate machinery. He mentions ventilation systems which, for those times, were unusually elaborate.

In this century, there have been great advances in technology. It is also in this century that the modern factory, with all its design factors and various precautions, made its first appearance.

1.3.5   The 19th Century Towards the end of the 18th century, a great ferment in spiritual, scientific, political and economic ideas took place in Europe (Teleky, 1948:15). Great advances had already taken place in the 18th century in the natural sciences and technological development. The latter years of the 18th century witnessed political revolution and economic evolution (the French Revolution beginning in 1789).

The cotton and textile industry originally flourished in India. It was introduced by the Moors into Spain and later spread to Europe. Towards the end of the 16th century, spinning and weaving thrived in England as a cottage industry. With the advent of water-driven and then, later, steam-driven machines, factories spread all over the countryside. It is said that, by 1810, there were already about 5 000 steam engines in England.

The science of chemical analysis laid the foundations for the development of organic chemistry, and, consequently, the chemical industry. The first analysis was made by Lavoisier (1743–1794). It was during this time that the chemical industry grew. Its growth posed many health problems for communities because of its processing and production of poisonous substances.

Changes in method of manufacturing—from 'cottage industries' to factories—so unsettled traditional patterns of family and community life that this period became known eventually as the Industrial Revolution. Schilling writes that forces not dissimilar from those preceding the Industrial Revolution have enabled rapid industrialization to take place in developing countries (1973:4).

The wealthy and powerful middle classes, which owned factories and all kinds of enterprises, and which influenced governments, lived lives which were in sharp contrast with those of the working class. The development of cities dependent on industry caused workers to realize that their labour conferred on them powerful bargaining capabilities. The appalling misery and degradation caused by the living conditions of the working classes were gradually admitted by physicians. These conditions were investigated and opposed by pioneers and reformers, many of whom came from privileged backgrounds. These reformers sought to bring pressure to bear on governments, pressure to eliminate the unacceptable conditions in which most members of the working classes laboured. The influence of these men and women on governments gradually resulted in legislation which effected the improvements in working conditions. Thus the economic, educational, moral and living standards of workers slowly improved. Workers organized themselves into trade unions and learnt to make use of the processes of bargaining to obtain various advantages and facilities. It was, however, a long and slow process which took many decades before real progress was achieved.

The initial effects of industrialization on community and individual health may be summarized as follows:

- a disruption of family life because of migrant labour
- a high incidence of social and physical ills such as prostitution, disease, alcoholism, overpopulation, child abuse, crime, and vagrancy
- the appearance of epidemics in overcrowded, insanitary dwellings
- malnutrition caused by failure to adapt from an established rural life to life in towns and cities
- poverty and unemployment caused by changing conditions of supply and demand, and by an over-supplied labour pool
- misery and confusion caused by the migration of working people from the established certainties of rural life to the ugliness, degradation and squalor of new industrial towns

- exposure to specific hazards of occupational diseases and injury
- exposure to the adverse effects of excessively long working hours;
- exposure to increasingly more dangerous technology in the form of newly developed machines
- prolonged hours of exposure to the toxical hazards of chemical substances
- exposure to the pressure of continuous work at a rate totally unsuited to the well-being of the worker and often beyond the limits of his or her physical and psychological capacities.

Schilling says that problems arising from industrial progress in tropical countries today are, in many respects, similar to those that prevailed in the West during the period of industrialization. In addition, these countries have to cope with the additional burdens of pandemic non-industrial diseases. Such situations demand an approach which takes into account the health of the whole community in relation to the changed modes of employment and the changing environment (1973:5).

1.4 FACTORS WHICH CONTRIBUTED TO THE AMELIORATION OF CONDITIONS IN FACTORIES AND MINES

These factors may be summarized as follows:
- the efforts of liberals, humanists and reformers such as Rousseau, Voltaire, Kant, Thomas Jefferson, Howard, Tuke, Wilberforce and the Seventh Earl of Shaftesbury
- the fact that public opinion influenced governments to intervene where adverse conditions existed
- the fact that enlightened employers such as Sir Robert Peel, Robert Owen, and Michael Sadler, influenced the British parliament to introduce legislation to control hours of work
- the influence exerted by physicians such as Percival Pott, Thomas Percival, Sir Robert Peel, and Charles Thackrah resulted in legislation which regulated conditions in factories in England. Soon after this, public health legislation was passed to control environmental conditions in towns.
- the early influence of the trade unions exerted to obtain improvements in working conditions (health conditions excluded—this came much later).

1.5 THE DEVELOPMENT OF OCCUPATIONAL HEALTH SERVICES IN VARIOUS PARTS OF THE WORLD

1.5.1 Great Britain Isolated examples of occupational health services existed in Britain during the 18th and 19th centuries. Thus, for example:
- Crowley Iron Works, in Sussex, employed a doctor, clergyman and schoolmaster.
- John Wood, a Bradford mill owner, also employed a doctor, and sent the children who worked for him to health resorts when they were overworked. On the premises of his factory there were baths and the hygiene of the plant was of a high standard.

The first Workmen's Compensation Act was promulgated in 1897, and this act made the provision of personal occupational health services mandatory. Larger firms appointed physicians in order to protect themselves against workmen's compensation claims. This naturally was out of line with the real purpose of occupational medicine, which is to promote the health of the worker.

World War I aroused a new interest in occupational health as nations strove to cope and survive. Shortage in munitions resulted in a sudden increase in activities in munitions factories and the adoption of very long working hours. A committee was appointed in England to examine the effects which working in these factories had on the health of their workers. The toxic effects of substances which were used in these factories were also studied.

The gradual development of occupational medicine after the economic slump caused by the war, was further hampered by deficiencies in the systematic training of doctors in occupational medicine (Schilling, 1973:14).

1.5.2 United States of America The Industrial Revolution only began in America after it was already well under way in Britain and Europe. Each state in the USA was free to adopt its own occupational health policy. The first state to pass legislation relating to occupational health was Massachusetts, with the Child Labour Law (1836). A Bureau of Labour Statistics was established in Massachusetts and this encouraged other states to follow suit. These Bureaus eventually became the state Departments of Labour.

The United States Federal Government could only control the working conditions of people working for the federal government, and each individual state could create its own policy with regard to the health of workers. The result today is that standards of health and safety vary considerably from state to state.

Various structures were created by the federal government to promote occupational health and safety, for example, a Bureau of Labour (1884); a Bureau of Mines (1910); the Office for Industrial Hygiene (1914). Federal funds were made available to states for instituting programmes. This system was eventually discontinued and federal activities decreased in the early 1950s.

Schilling writes that federal encouragement and funding created a body of occupational hygienists which enabled the United States to lead the world in the field of environmental measurement and control in the workplace (1973:15).

Among the first industries to set up industrial medical services in the USA, were railroad, steel and mining companies. These services developed along very similar lines to those in the United Kingdom, with large firms employing full-time medical or nursing personnel. Various acts were passed between 1960 and 1970. Each of these helped to raise standards of occupational health and safety.

Alice Hamilton, who spent 40 years of her life searching for and identifying occupational hazards which had been overlooked by industry and plant physicians, ranks among the great pioneers in this field (Schilling, 1973:16).

1.5.3   USSR In Eastern Europe, the first important phase in the development of Occupational health began after the October Revolution of 1917. But it was only after World War II that developments took place in countries such as Bulgaria, Rumania, Czechoslovakia and Yugoslavia. The recent liberation of Eastern European countries such as Rumania and East Germany again revealed appalling working standards and environmental pollution.

Occupational health services in general was not a field of study which interested many members of the medical profession in the USSR. An exception proved to be F. F. Erisman, who was one of the founders of the science of hygiene in Russia.

The first Commissar of Health in the Russian Soviet Federative Socialist Republic, Alexander Semashko, helped to formulate a policy for health which was based on two main principles, namely that health services should be free, and that they should concentrate on prevention. The activities of Semashko led to the establishment of the first Chair of Hygiene of Labour, and later a Research Institute in Occupational Health and Safety in Moscow.

The health services in the USSR are separated into therapeutic medicine and prophylactic medicine. Therapeutic services are provided by hospitals, polyclinics, and medical departments in large plants. Prophylactic services are the responsibility of sanitary and epidemiological stations in towns, rural areas, and in large plants (Schilling, 1973:18).

1.6 THE INFLUENCE OF WORLD WAR II ON OCCUPATIONAL HEALTH

The war, and the economic expansion which followed World War II, stimulated the development of occupational health in various parts of the world. This was mainly due to the following factors:

- The increased demand for manpower during wartime led to the employment of the disabled as well as the fit. Greater emphasis was placed by occupational health services on assessing degrees of *ability* to work.
- The development of military equipment, which was adapted to suit the soldier, sailor and airman, so that his fighting efficiency was increased, contributed to the development of the science of ergonomics.
- The great need for war manpower led to substantial improvements in the rehabilitation of sick and injured soldiers.
- The care of the worker became an economic necessity, because of the manpower shortages.
- Countries which developed quickly because of rapid industrialization gave a high priority to the health of the worker and to safe and hygienic working environments. This contributed to the overall national prosperity of such countries.
- Other factors, such as the realization that a service at the worksite reduces time taken off from work, also influenced the expansion of occupational health services.

1.7 THE INFLUENCE OF TRADE UNIONS

During the twentieth century, a much stronger influence was exerted by trade unions in the interests of obtaining legislation and compensation laws to cover occupational diseases and injuries (Schilling, 1973:20):

- In the USSR, trade unions have extensive responsibilities for health and safety through their factory inspectors.
- Trade unions in the United Kingdom contributed towards an Institute of Occupational Health in the University of London.
- The Kupat Holim in Israel provides comprehensive medical care for its members who comprise 90 % of the working population. It also opened its first Department of Industrial Medicine in Tel Aviv in 1945.

1.8 THE EUROPEAN ECONOMIC COMMUNITY

The International Labour Conference of 1959 compiled a blueprint for health services in all places of employment. All the countries of the European Common Market, who have political systems similar to those of the USA and Great Britain, adhere to the basic recommendations made by the ILO, namely to provide occupational health services in all industrial, non-industrial and agricultural undertakings and for public services.

The European Economic Commission in 1962 recommended that:

- services must be based on statutory requirements, and not voluntary efforts.
- larger undertakings with 200 or more workers should have the services of a full-time physician.

This Commission based its recommendations on the principle of employers voluntarily providing their own health services, in addition to those which are enforced by law or which are provided by the government.

1.9 CONCLUSION

It took many centuries before employers accepted the full responsibility for the prevention of health hazards in the workplace. Social and legal constraints and structures to protect the health of the worker are still being developed today. In many countries, well-established services exist, but, in some areas of the world, formal structures are still inadequate, with the result that workers are still exposed to conditions which are detrimental to their health.

1.10 BIBLIOGRAPHY

Brown, M. L. 1981. *Occupational Health Nursing*. New York: Springer Publishing Company.

Cralley, L. J. and Cralley, L. V. 1985. *Patty's industrial hygiene and toxicology*. Volume III. Second Edition 3A, USA: John Wiley & Sons, Inc.

Currer C. and Stacey, M. 1986. *Concepts of Health, Illness and Disease: A comparative perspective*. Leamington: Berg Publishers Ltd.

Ffrench, G. *Occupational Health*. Great Britain: Medical and Technical Publishing Co. Ltd.

Gardner, W. and Taylor, P. 1975. *Health at Work*. London: Associated Business Programmes Ltd.

Girdano, D. A. 1986. *Occupational Health Promotion*. New York: Macmillan Publishing Company.

Schilling, R. S. F. 1973. *Occupational health practice*. Great Britain: Butterworths & Co (publishers) Ltd.

Teleky, L. 1948. *History of factory and mine hygiene*. New York: Columbia University Press.

Chapter 2: Concepts Related to Occupational Health

by A. J. Kotze

2.1 INTRODUCTION

Ramazzini was the first physician to emphasize the importance of enquiring into the type of occupation of the patient (1713). The influence of man's occupation on his health cannot be overlooked because one half of a person's non-sleeping life is taken up by employment. This period of a person's life may continue for as long as forty years. In the Middle Ages, man's working life was much shorter because of the devastating effects of poor working conditions on the worker's health, and because the average life span of people was much, much shorter than today.

There are other factors which also play an important role in determining a person's total state of health. These are:

- hereditary
- environmental
- health care
- lifestyle

Work constitutes an essential element in the lifestyle of people. Understanding the interaction of the various factors which influence man's health will facilitate a philosophy for health care which is balanced in its approach to total health and welfare. The working environment influences not only the worker. It may also have a harmful influence on the family of the worker and on the community, e.g. exposure by family members to the asbestos dust accumulated on the clothing of the asbestos worker may lead to the development of malignant mesothelioma of the pleura of the lung.

Schilling says that the occupational physician's responsibility does not end at the factory gates. An industry may have adverse effects on the health of neighbouring communities because of the discharge of toxic waste products into the atmosphere, into the water, or onto the land (1973:24). The last decade has proved yet again how much of this is happening in modern times.

On a psychological level, many perceptions developed around the concept of work-related illness. In earlier years the worker accepted the inevitability of diseases caused by working environments. It was only after the industrial revolution and the success of militant social and political protest and reform that the health and welfare of the worker was regarded as a matter of any importance. Other harmful conditions in our lives and environments are not necessarily always attributable to our working conditions, but may be factors such as emotional agitation, stress and overwork in general.

An occupational health service should therefore incorporate into its design a holistic health programme, a programme which will anticipate physiological, psychological and community manifestations of disease. Comprehensive measures must be instituted to decrease the threat to health in all spheres of activity. No one group of health workers can do this alone, and a multidisciplinary approach must be followed.

An essential part of this kind of programme is that workers accept responsibility for participating in decision-making about their own health care needs (Cralley and Cralley, 1985:68).

2.2 LEARNING OBJECTIVES

At the end of this section, the reader should be able to:
* define and describe concepts such as
  — occupational health and medicine
  — occupational health services
  — occupational health nursing
  — occupational hygiene
* analyse the interdisciplinary approach in occupational health

2.3 WHAT IS OCCUPATIONAL HEALTH?

Ffrench writes:

'Occupational health can be said to be the creation of a state of physical and mental well-being, within the occupational environment, while taking into consideration factors relating to the social and domestic life of each individual' (as:6).

Today, great emphasis is placed upon the preventive aspects of occupational health. It is believed that the primary goal should be to keep people at work, and to prevent them from becoming ill—whether through causes originating at work or at home.

Prevention of disease goes hand in hand with the promotion of good health. The work site may be a natural and effective setting for health promotion programmes, because large numbers of people can be involved in such programmes while they are at work.

The World Health Organization describes occupational health as:
* the promotion and maintenance of the highest degree of physical, mental and social well-being of workers in all occupations

- the prevention among workers of departures from health caused by their working conditions
- the protection of workers in their employment from risks resulting from factors which are inimical to health
- the placing and maintenance of the worker in an occupational environment adapted to his physiological and psychological condition.

2.4 DESCRIBING OCCUPATIONAL HEALTH SERVICES (see also pp. 88–89)

Ideally, occupational health services should make provision for the following components:

TABLE 1

The components of occupational health		
Occupational Safety	Occupational Hygiene	Occupational medicine & nursing
Environmental control: Analysis Legislation Organization Safety systems	Hazard: Identification Monitoring Control	Administration Screening Surveillance Primary health care Health education Health promotion & supervision Emergency care Treatment of diseases Rehabilitation Epidemiology & research

The scope of occupational health services: Company policy is directly responsible for the scope of services offered in industry. Gardner and Taylor say that the objectives and responsibilities of an occupational health service can only be as good or as bad as the company policy allows (1975:20). Successful health programmes require a commitment from management. A high quality health care programme should be based on the philosophy of health promotion, on the needs of the organization, and on the needs of the employees and their families.

Each company should strive towards the goal of establishing a healthy and safe working environment, but each worker must also be motivated to accept responsibility for their own and their family's health, by working safely and maintaining a healthy lifestyle. With this policy in mind, the *aims of an occupational health service* should be:

- to protect and maintain the physical and mental health of all people at work

- to assist management to implement company policy
- to identify, assess and advise management on the control of any health hazard which may affect the employee or public, hazards arising from the company's activities
- to advise on the effects of ill health on the working capacity of all staff at the recruitment stage, during employment, and on retirement
- to provide an individual health service based upon company policy to each person in the organization, the purpose of which is to supply primary and secondary treatment of illness and injury;
- to respect the confidentiality of personal medical information, and to act in accordance with the highest ethical standards of the professions concerned (Gardner and Taylor, 1975:20).

2.5 OCCUPATIONAL HEALTH NURSING

In occupational health nursing, the nurse's client is not a patient, in the usual sense, but a worker who is exposed to a work environment which may be hazardous to his health.

The role of the occupational nurse is extensively concerned with the prevention of illness and the promotion of health, with a lesser emphasis on the curative aspects of health care.

It may be said that the primary goal of the occupational health nurse is to assist the worker to maintain the optimal state of physical and psychological well-being.

The nurse is required to care for many groups of workers from different age, sex, socio-economic, educational and cultural backgrounds.

- She is required to solve health problems which extend along the entire continuum of health and illness.
- The tasks she is called upon to perform may cover a wide range of skills, varying from the very simple to clinically advanced operational tasks.
- The nurse lives and works in a matrix of interpersonal relationships between the worker and herself. Problems are identified, and solutions are sought which are compatible with the work environment, management policy and the health system on the one hand, and the special health, social and environmental needs of the worker on the other.

2.6 OCCUPATIONAL MEDICINE

This specialization within the occupational health is concerned mainly with people and with the causal relationships between work and health (Gardner and Taylor, 1975:17).

This branch of medicine deals with the worker and occupationally related diseases. Its objective is the protection of the worker against hazards in the working environment, and the treatment of emergency conditions sustained during worktime (Schröder and Schoeman, 1989:3). This definition can be extended to include many more aspects of occupational medicine included in the field, e.g. the treatment of the worker with chronic disease, primary health care, and rehabilitation.

2.7 OCCUPATIONAL HYGIENE

This is the science and art which is devoted to the recognition, evaluation and control of those environmental factors which arise in the workplace, and which may cause sickness, impaired health, or discomfort and inefficiency among workers or among the citizens of a community (this is according to the definition of The American Industrial Hygiene Association).

Occupational hygiene is also an applied science encompassing the application of information from various other sciences, e.g. chemistry, engineering, biology, mathematics, medicine, physics, toxicology.

2.8 AN INTERDISCIPLINARY TEAM APPROACH TO OCCUPATIONAL HEALTH

Occupational health may be described as a unique discipline, because it requires an interdisciplinary team effort in order to have an effective health promotion programme.

Related disciplines, such as nursing, medicine, industrial hygiene; and safety organizations and management, must all communicate and liaise in such a way that a total health care programme will develop which will best serve the needs of industry, the worker, the community and the consumer.

Members of an occupational health team all contribute unique skills to the assessment, planning, implementation and evaluation of the total health programme.

2.9 BIBLIOGRAPHY

Baker, M. and Coetzee A. C. 1983. *An Introducton to Occupational Health Nursing in South Africa*. Johannesburg: Witwatersrand University Press.

Brown, M. L. 1981. *Occupational Health Nursing*. New York: Springer Publishing Company.

Cralley, L. J. & Cralley, L. V. 1985. *Patty's Industrial Hygiene and Toxicology*. Volume III. Second edition 3A. U.S.A: John Wiley & Sons Inc.

Currer C. and Stacey, M. 1986. *Concepts of Health, Illness and Disease. A Comparative Perspective*. Leamington: Berg Publishers Ltd.

Ffrench, G. *Occupational Health*. Great Britain: Medical and Technical Publishing Co. Ltd.

Gardner, W. and Taylor, P. 1975. *Health at Work*. London: Associated Business Programmes Ltd.

Girdano, D. A. 1986. *Occupational Health Promotion*. New York: Macmillan Publishing Company.

Schilling, R. S. F. 1973. *Occupational Health Practice*. Great Britain: Butterworths & Co (publishers) Ltd.

Searle, C., Brink, H. I. L., and Grobbelaar, W. C. 1989. *Aspects of Community Health*. Cape Town: King Edward Trust.

Schröder, H. H. E. en Schoeman, J. J. 1989. *Inleiding tot Beroepshigiëne*. Goodwood: Nasionale Boekdrukkery.

Chapter 3: The Development and Structure of Occupational Health Services in South Africa

by A. J. Kotze

THE DEVELOPMENT OF OCCUPATIONAL HEALTH SERVICES IN SOUTH AFRICA

3.1 INTRODUCTION

The history of the development of occupational health in South Africa is as complex as the development of general health services. Because of major socio-economic and political changes over the last two centuries, occupational health services are currently dispersed, fragmented and diffused, with numerous departments and organizations responsible for rendering services and executing control.

The development of occupational health services is closely linked to socio-economic development. After the discovery of diamonds and gold in the late nineteenth and early twentieth century, many small towns were transformed from predominantly rural agricultural communities into industrial towns. There were large-scale migrations from rural to urban areas, and extensive immigration from neighbouring states to South Africa. This caused upheavals and dislocation in family life, and all the problems associated with rapidly but randomly developing industrial towns. Shortages in housing, schools and health services quickly developed. Criminal and anti-social activities increased in urban areas. The complex ethnic structure of the country is still today characterized in some areas by problems similar to those experienced in overseas countries during the earlier part of the Industrial Revolution. This is mainly caused by the fact that, in Africa, we find first- and third-world conditions existing side by side in many areas. Our heterogeneous society, with densely populated urban areas and under-developed rural areas, generates unique problems and challenges for any health care service.

3.2 LEARNING OBJECTIVES

At the end of this section the reader should be able to:
- give an overview of the development of occupational health in South Africa
- identify and describe the structures and legislation relevant to occupational health in South Africa
- discuss the history of the development of occupational health nursing and training in South Africa

3.3 SOME MILESTONES IN THE OCCUPATIONAL HEALTH HISTORY IN SOUTH AFRICA

3.3.1 Development of the mining industry The discovery of gold and diamonds resulted in a period of economic growth which was unprecedented in the history of this country. Mining activities exposed large numbers of workers to the dangers of high concentrations of silicone dust.

During the period between 1886 and the outbreak of the Anglo-Boer War in 1899, ignorance about the dangers of dust inhalation led to the early death of many mine workers. Towards the end of 1901, the government mining engineer reported that, out of 1 377 white miners employed before the war, 255 had died.

3.3.2 Commissions of enquiry The *first commission of enquiry* into phthisis was appointed by Lord Milner in 1902. The report of this commission showed that the average period for the development of advanced phthisis was less than six years. True occupational health services were now established for the first time:

- Dust suppression methods were prescribed and legally enforced.
- Health examinations were introduced.
- Compensation measures for silicosis were introduced.

The *Mining Regulations Commission* was appointed in 1907 to further investigate the whole problem of dust control in mines. In 1911, a *third commission* consisting mainly of medical practitioners was appointed to inquire into the incidence of miner's phthisis and tuberculosis on the mines.

The *first legislation* was published in 1911. This was The Miners Phthisis Act, which made compensation for phthisis compulsory. The general health of mineworkers received little or no attention at this time. Although large numbers of mineworkers were imported from neighbouring African countries, health conditions on the mines and in the hostels were critical. Facilities, utterly primitive and inadequate and the diet of workers was inadequate, resulting in conditions such as scurvy, pneumonia and meningitis (Baker and Coetzee, 1983:11).

Finally, due to public pressure, conditions were improved and the Chamber of Mines invited an overseas expert to visit South Africa. This expert was Colonel W. C. Gorgas from the U.S.A. On his recommendation, the pioneer of occupational medicine in South Africa, Dr A. J. Orenstein was appointed by the Rand Mines Group. He also acted as Surgeon General for the S.A. Army in World War I. Baker and Coetzee are of the opinion that Dr Orenstein played a leading role in the development of occupational health services (1983:12).

Many more acts were subsequently promulgated—these were all finally consolidated into the Occupational Diseases in Mines and Works Act, Act 78 of 1973.

The Erasmus Commission

Research into occupational diseases revealed that conditions in industry left much to be desired, and that an in-depth investigation was necessary. In 1975, the Erasmus Commission of Enquiry was appointed to report on

- the nature, incidence and extent of occupational diseases in the RSA;
- statutory measures and facilities and their effectiveness;
- the manpower situation, with specific referral to occupational health;
- health control in the workplace;
- the establishment of health services in the workplace;
- the protection of the community against environmental pollution resulting from industries;

This report was extremely comprehensive and many recommendations were made by the Commission. It was stated by the Commission that a certain measure of confusion existed in the field of occupational health in South Africa, due mainly to the fact that legislation relating to occupational diseases had been replicated in many places. This, in turn, had led to the *duplication* of services in the different government departments responsible for the implementation of such legislation (Erasmus 1976:8).

Now, more than a decade later (1991), not all of the recommendations made by this Commission have been implemented, and so it would be pointless to discuss them here. Rather the very fact that a commission was appointed and that a report was presented, shows that there still exists today a great need for the rationalization of all occupational health services. Most departments concerned with implementing legislation concerning the worker are well aware of specific problem areas, but because legislation has not been rationalized or consolidated, and because no one controlling authority exists, many of the most serious problems still continue to exist today.

The Wiehahn Commission

Labour relations have gradually developed over the years in South Africa, and have become a specialized field of study. In 1977 the government appointed the Wiehahn Commission to examine labour relations and legislation. The findings of the Commission were published in six separate reports. The key role played by employers in labour relations was emphasized, and practical guidelines were given to employers by the Commission. It was also recommended that the Department of Manpower be responsible for the overall implementation of the government's manpower policy (Searle, Brink and Grobbelaar, 1988:500).

3.3.3 Lung diseases on the mines

Miner's phthisis

This term was first used to describe the condition, often accompanied by tuberculosis, caused by dust in the mines.

Silicosis

It gradually became clear that the majority of dust-related diseases occurring in or near mines were caused by silica dust. The term 'silicosis' was coined to describe this condition in 1946. During this period, legislation was passed which required other kinds of mines to implement controlled working and safety conditions—mines which mined, for example, asbestos, coal, chrome, tin, etc. Various other kinds of dust-related diseases, such as asbestosis and pneumoconiosis were also identified.

Pneumoconiosis

This generic term was coined in 1956 to include *all* forms of dust-related diseases. Subsequent experience has, however, shown that there are many occupational diseases that may occur as a result of conditions in mines. Provision was made for these in the Occupational Diseases in Mines and Works Act, Act 78 of 1973.

In 1956 the Pneumoconiosis Research Unit was established. This research unit was later expanded to become the National Research Institute for Occupational Diseases.

3.3.4 Occupational health in industry World War II played an important role in the stimulation of the development of industries in South Africa, and, in more recent times, sanctions applied against this country have had a similar effect. Industries developed to provide for the internal needs of the country.

During the war, equipment for troops had to be manufactured, and the mines experienced problems in obtaining the necessary machines and equipment. After the war, South Africa, with its reserves of raw materials, offered attractive opportunities to many overseas investors, and this led to escalation in industrial development.

It is noticeable that the manufacturing industry has developed extensively during the past 40 years. Control over these industries is exercised by the *Department of Manpower*.

The first legislation to control conditions in the industry was the Factories, Machinery and Building Works Act, Act 22 of 1941, today known as the Machinery and Occupational Safety Act, Act 6 of 1983.

3.4 GOVERNMENT DEPARTMENTS, AND STATUTORY BODIES CONCERNED WITH OCCUPATIONAL HEALTH AND LEGISLATION

In the following section we will present an outline of organizations and the legislation which concern occupational health and matters related to the worker and the workplace.

3.4.1 The Department of National Health and Population Development This Department regulates and coordinates general health policy. It administers the following legislation:

The Health Act, Act 63 of 1977

This act stipulates measures for the implementation of health services by relevant organizations in the country. The following are the specific provisions of The Health Act which relate to occupational health:

— reference to preventive and promotive health measures, measures which obviously also apply to workers;

— The Minister may declare certain medical conditions as notifiable (after consultation with the Ministers of Mineral and Energy Affairs and Manpower). This provides for the notification of conditions, the closing of premises, and the disinfection and evacuation of certain buildings or areas.

— Local authorities are designated as responsible for environmental health services within their own areas. Their responsibilities include general hygiene; the prevention of nuisances, unhygienic or offensive conditions (these may include factories, industrial or business premises); the prevention of the pollution of water or the atmosphere.

Table 2.
* Structure and Legislation for Occupational Health Services in South Africa, 1991

Department of National Health & Population Development	Department of Manpower	Department of Mineral & Energy Affairs
Legislation	Legislation	Legislation
• The Health Act • The Nursing Act • The Medicine and Related Substances Act • The Pharmacy Act • The Atmospheric Pollution Prevention Act • The Hazardous Substances Act • The Mental Health Act	• The Workman's Compensation Act • Labour Relations Act • The Wage Act • Unemployment Insurance Act • Machinery & Occupational Safety Act • Basic Conditions of Employment Act • Manpower Training Act	• The Occupational Diseases in Mines and Works Act
Research Services	Statutory Structures	Departmental Services
• Medical Bureau for Occupational Diseases • National Centre for Occupational Health	• The Workman's Compensation Commissioner • Industrial Courts • Wage Board • Unemployment Commissioner • Advisory Council for Occupational Safety • National Manpower Commission • National Training Board	• Government Mining Engineer

* This is a list of only the most important acts and services.

Statutory councils

A lot of other legislation is also administered by the Health Department, and for this purpose several Statutory Councils were instituted. Among these are: The Medical Research Council, The Medicine Control Council, the Pharmacy Council, The National Air Pollution Advisory Committee, The South African Medical and Dental Council, and The South African Nursing Council.

These Councils are responsible for the implementation of legislation which is also applicable in the field of occupational health. This legislation comprises:

• The Nursing Act, Act 50 of 1978
• The Medical, Dental and Supplementary Health Service Professions Act, Act 56 of 1974

- The Medicines and Related Substances Control Act, Act 101 of 1965
- The Pharmacy Act, Act 53 of 1974
- The Atmospheric Pollution Prevention Act, Act 45 of 1965

The Hazardous Substances Act, Act 15 of 1973

This act empowers the Minister of National Health and Population Development to categorize substances into different groups, according to the degree of danger they pose to human health. Any substance or mixture of substances which may be toxic, corrosive, irritant, strongly sensitizing or flammable, because they generate pressure, or when they are handled or ingested, or which may cause injury, ill-health or death, may be declared to be Group I or Group II hazardous substances.

Electronic products may be declared Group III hazardous substances (e.g. X-ray units and electron accelerators).

Radio-active material may be declared to be a Group IV substance (subject to the approval of the Minister of Mineral and Energy Affairs).

The selling of substances and the operation of hazardous substances must be subject to licensing or registration by the Director-General.

The Medicines and Related Substances Control Act, Act 101 of 1965, and The Abuse of Dependence-producing Substances and Rehabilitation Centres Act, Act 41 of 1971

These are the two most important acts governing the control of medicines and drugs. The latter act is mainly a penal measure dealing with illicit situations such as drug possession and trafficking, and rehabilitation measures.

Occupational health centres must apply for a permit authorizing the handling of medicine to the Director-General of the Department of National Health and Population Development.

The Mental Health Act, Act 18 of 1973

This Act provides for the reception, detention and treatment of mentally ill persons in institutions.

Special procedures, to be followed in cases of emergency, where it is expedient for the welfare of the patient or the public to place a person under care and treatment in an institution, are defined.

Departmental Research Services for Occupational Health and Diseases
Medical Bureau for Occupational Diseases (MBOD)

The Bureau was established in 1973 under the Occupational Diseases in Mines and Works Act, Act 78 of 1973. Its main function is the surveillance of the health of at-risk workers in and at controlled mines and works. To enable the Bureau to fulfil this function, a system of certification has been developed:

Certification Committee

This committee considers all applications for certification and deals with cases individually. A complete medical and labour history and the result of special investigations are presented. Applicants are notified of the committee's finding in writing, and may appeal against the finding to:

The Reviewing Authority

This authority reviews the case and may confirm the finding of the committee or may disagree with it. In the latter event, a joint sitting of the two bodies will decide by majority vote on the outcome of the case. These two bodies deal with diseases which are compensatable according to scales laid down by legislation.

Other functions performed by the Bureau:

- Medical services. Over the years the Bureau has built up an experienced team of medical specialists who carry out examinations.
- A data-base has been built up which provides unique opportunities for research into various aspects of occupational diseases.
- X-rays are taken for screening and diagnostic purposes for all dust-related occupational lung diseases.
- The lung function laboratory is one of the most sophisticated in the country, and workers are put through a battery of tests.
- Routine audiometric screening is carried out in an attempt to build up a data-base for the development of standards, as noise-induced hearing loss still remains a widespread problem in the mining industry.
- The inspectorate of this department represents the Bureau for a wide range of matters in controlled mines and works; they visit mines and works at least once a year.
- An epidemiology research unit conducts research into dust-related diseases.

The National Centre for Occupational Health (NCOH)

This centre functions under the aegis of the Department of National Health and Population Development. It is well equipped with scientists in a variety of disciplines and provides facilities for the following research, service and teaching functions:

Pathology

Research is a vital function of this section, and relates mostly to the effect of mine dusts and gases on the respiratory systems. The Centre carries out post mortem heart and lung examinations on deceased miners on behalf of the Medical Bureau for Occupational Diseases.

Biochemistry

This department does analytical work for any industry on request. A data-base is being built up and the results should be useful for research into metal toxicity. Blood and urine samples are analysed to detect levels of toxic substances such as lead.

Immunology and Microbiology

Advanced and sophisticated tests are currently available which help researchers to better understand immunological mechanisms and their relationship to other factors in microbiology. The field of occupational asthmas in factories processing organic and inorganic material, is studied extensively.

Occupational medicine and epidemiology

Major themes in the research programme of this unit are occupational health services; occupational mortality; social aspects of occupational diseases, such as compensation and other consequences of accidents; recognition and epidemiological measurement of asbestos-related diseases, and biological measurements.

Occupational Hygiene

The work is divided into three main sections, namely:

- Service. This consists mainly of ad hoc investigations into environmental conditions in different types of factories. A report with concomitant advice is usually offered after the investigation.
- Teaching. Formal and informal training are provided by members of the Institute.
- Research. This is pursued as and when other commitments permit it.

3.4.2 The Department of Manpower and Legislation and its jurisdiction over occupations This department is responsible for the implementation of the government's manpower policy. Thus the department administers all labour legislation and regulations which include the following:

The Workman's Compensation Act, Act 30 of 1941

This act is designed to compensate workmen for accidents and industrial diseases sustained as a result of their work, excluding mining operations, which is covered under different legislation (Occupational Diseases in Mines and Works Act, Act 78 of 1973).

To facilitate the administration of the act, every employer (as defined in the act), must register with the Workmen's Compensation Commissioner and pay assessments to a fund called *the accident fund*.

Should an incident occur, a claim may be put to the compensation commissioner. A large part of the administration of the occupational health nurse revolves around these claims and the procedures involved. She must be familiar with the implementation of the regulations of the Act.

The Workman's Compensation Commissioner

The Commissioner handles all claims under the Workman's Compensation Act.

The Labour Relations Act, Act 28 of 1956

This act forms the cornerstone of industrial legislation in South Africa, and provides for a formalized system of collective bargaining with the machinery for the resolution of industrial disputes. The Industrial and Appeal Courts instituted by the Department of Manpower deal with matters relating to industrial relations.

The Wage Act, Act 5 of 1957

The Act is designed to supplement the machinery created for collective bargaining by the Labour Relations Act. This act makes provision for a Wage Board, consisting of three members appointed by the Minister. This Board acts, when requested to do so, by the Minister, and investigates wage matters, and reports back to the Minister of Manpower. Specifically excluded from this Act are persons employed by:

- the state;
- farming operations;
- domestic services;
- universities, colleges, schools or educational institutions maintained wholly or partly with public funds.

The Unemployment Insurance Act, Act 30 of 1966

The aim of this act is to render financial assistance to workers during periods of unemployment, illness and pregnancy (under prescribed conditions).

The office of the Commissioner of Unemployment functions from departmental and magistrates' offices, and deals with the administration of this legislation.

The Machinery and Occupational Safety Act, Act 6 of 1983

This is important legislation for the employer and the occupational health nurse. It provides for the safety of persons at a workplace or in the course of their employment, or in connection with the use of machinery, or any incidental matter. This act does not apply to Mines and Works and workers in the explosives industry.

The Advisory Council for Occupational Safety

In 1983 this council was established by the Minister of Manpower under article 4 of the act. Employers, employees, and representatives of the government serve on this council of nine members. The function of the council is mainly:

- to gather technical information;
- to make recommendations and report to the Minister on matters relating to the act;
- to implement the act;
- to carry out any other work referred to it.

Various technical committees are appointed by the advisory council to investigate safety matters, and many regulations have been drawn up.

The Basic Conditions of Employment Act, Act 3 of 1983

The Mines and Works Act, the Wage Act and the Manpower Training Act take precedence over this act, but this act applies to employees covered by these statutes in so far as those statutes do not provide for matters regulated by this act (Strauss, 1987:235). The act makes provision for matters such as:

- maximum weekly and daily ordinary working hours;
- meal intervals;
- overtime and payment thereof;
- work on Sundays;
- annual and sick leave;
- termination of service procedures.

Training and Manpower Legislation

The Department is further responsible for the administration of the Manpower Training Act, Act 56 of 1981. This act regulates and promotes the training of manpower through The National Training Board and various administrative bodies.

Various other statutory commissions and councils exist which serve as extensions of the Department of Manpower in the administration of all the legislation relevant to the worksphere of this Department, e.g. The National Manpower Commission; the Wage Board; the Industrial Court, and the National Training Board. These do not play a direct role in occupational health, but may indirectly influence health matters.

3.4.3   The Department of Mineral and Energy Affairs

This Department and associated institutions are responsible for the administration of sections of the following legislation which relates to occupational health:

The Occupational Diseases in Mines and Works Act, Act 78 of 1973.

The Government Mining Engineer

This branch of the department performs important statutory obligations in respect of supervising mines and works.

The main purpose is to ensure the safety and health of mine workers and the public in the vicinity of mining operations. This is done through:

— a special emphasis on accident prevention and a decrease in the incidence of injuries on mines;
— investigating various safety hazards, e.g. ventilation and mining layouts in deeper gold mines, the removal of toxic products and the treatment of timber used in mines with special fire retardants;
— ensuring that all underground workers in coal mines receive equipment for self-rescuing; ensuring that refuge bays and other arrangements are made to safeguard workers against possible exposure to noxious fumes;
— giving attention to the problem of noise and radiation exposure.

3.4.4   Conclusion

It should by now be clear to the reader that occupational health services in this country are regulated by numerous structures and acts, which profit and serve the workers.

There have been two important commissions of enquiry into occupational health and related fields (those of Erasmus and Wiehahn) in this country. Many of the old acts have been updated to make provision for the changing scene and needs in the field. The most recent and most urgently needed legislation was circulated for comment in 1983, namely the Occupational Disease and the Occupational Compensation Bill. These bills will provide a consolidation of those matters covered in many separate acts at present. These bills have not been promulgated by Parliament.

3.5 OCCUPATIONAL HEALTH NURSING IN SOUTH AFRICA

3.5.1   Historical background Searle says that occupational health nursing in South Africa dates back to the establishment of the refreshment station and hospital at the Cape by the Dutch East India Company in 1652 (1965:359).

Although few occupational health services were established at the workplace, it is known that, during the last century, many hospitals were established by industrial concerns, with the specific purpose of caring for the ill worker. The various mining houses were primarily responsible for this development, as they made use of migratory labour and their workforces were very large. This development led to the establishment of services which were only of a curative nature, and were not preventive and promotive services as we see today. Many of these hospitals are still maintained today.

The primary function of the occupational health nurse in South Africa is a public health one aimed at protecting the health of the workers in industry, commerce or other types of services which employ large numbers of workers.

Factors which diminish the worker's ability to produce at an optimum level are vital, not only to the worker and the employer, but to the national welfare of the country. Due to the expanding South African economy and the relative shortage of skilled labour, the work of the occupational health nurse is of considerable economic significance to the community as a whole (Searle, 1965:381).

Very little is known about the pioneer nurses in the occupational health field of this country. Baker and Coetzee say that the first known industrial nurse in South Africa was a Matron Herron-Brown, who was employed by the United Tobacco Company Ltd, in Cape Town in 1923 (1983:15).

In the report of the Medical Officer of Health for the year ending June 1902, mention was made of the lady Sanitary Inspector, who was a trained nurse. Her duty was to visit the workrooms of milliners, dress-makers, and places where females were employed, to report on the sanitary conditions in these places. Although the main purpose of this was to decrease the high infant mortality rate in the city at the time, it may indirectly be regarded as an occupational health service.

3.5.2   The training of nurses for occupational health The occupational health nurse in South Africa is also a front-line community health nurse. Her sphere of activity extends beyond the care of the worker—she also works with the family of the worker within a given community. This approach led to the development of certain trends in the training of the nurse for occupational health in South Africa:

Health visitors and school nursing

Like many aspects of our South African system of health service organization, the concept of a health visitor was derived from Great Britain. The concept was later expanded to include the Sanitary Inspector. Both these categories of ladies were employed by local authorities or voluntary organizations to promote the general health of people and improve sanitary conditions in towns and workplaces. The training course for health visitors and school nurses was first introduced by the Witwatersrand Technical Institute (with the assistance of the S.A. Trained Nurses' Association) in 1926 for whites, and in 1935 for other population groups. The latter was offered at the training school for mission workers of the Vroue Sendingbond of the Nederduits Gereformeerde Kerk.

The course in public health nursing/community health nursing

When South Africa withdrew from the Commonwealth, it became necessary to establish a local examining body for the examination of health services personnel—this function was undertaken by the old department of Education, Arts and Science. In 1964 the first regulations and syllabus for a National Diploma in Public Health Nursing was drawn up.

This course made provision for the needs of the public health nurse of that period, and included aspects related to behavioural as well as public health sciences.

The examination of this course was taken over in 1977 by the South African Nursing Council. The year 1980 saw the development of the Diploma in Community Nursing.

Today courses in community health are offered by Universities (up to doctoral level); Technikons and Technical Colleges; and Nursing Colleges.

The change from the title *public health nursing* to *community nursing* broadened the scope of practice of the community nurse to encompass all aspects of the health care of the family—including that of the worker. It is for this reason that occupational health nursing is included in this training course. For the purposes of this course occupational health nursing is not seen as an entity on its own, but a comprehensive approach is used when planning health services for the worker. The worker is part of a community and a family, and each of these entities may influence the other.

It is, however, true that various fields of specialization have developed across the spectrum of community health nursing services, and this is a healthy trend—but only if fragmentation of health services is carefully avoided. Occupational health, per se, includes aspects of health care which are very specific to the occupational field, and for this purpose a more task-orientated course was developed by the leading nurses in this field.

3.5.3 The Occupational Health Nurses Discussion Group This group of nurses felt the need to get together and discuss problems common to their particular area of work. Thanks to the efforts of a Mary Ahlers, an industrial nurse of the United Tobacco Company Ltd in Johannesburg, the nurses in southern Transvaal were invited to form the first Industrial Nurses Discussion Group. This took place on the 20th of April, 1966. Membership of this group was limited to those registered nurses working in industry.

On the 11th of April, 1970, the name of the group was changed to THE OCCUPATIONAL HEALTH NURSES DISCUSSION GROUP (Southern Transvaal). The group now also included nurses from all kinds of occupations. Natal and Cape Town followed suit, and there are now eight occupational nursing discussion groups in the Republic.

3.5.4   **A South** This society was formed on the 30th of April, 1980. Its main aims are
          African to monitor the needs of the occupational health nurse, and promote
      Society of occupational health in industry.
   Occupational
          Health
          Nurses

3.5.5   **The** Ever since the formation of the first discussion groups, strenuous
   Certificate in efforts were made to establish a separate course for occupational
   Occupational nurses. The Board of the South African Nursing Association found
          Health that there were no authorities willing to finance such a course, and
         Nursing decided to take the initiative to start such a course.

The curriculum was developed by a group of senior occupational nurses and doctors. The first course was offered on the 2nd of June, 1976, in Johannesburg and was attended by 22 nurses. This course was based on occupational health nursing, and was offered over a period of six months.

The course was only recognized by the South African Nursing Council in 1981, when the necessary statutory recognition was given, and the regulations were published in the Government Gazette of 13th February, 1981.

The main objectives of this course are to equip the nurse in occupational health with the necessary knowledge and skills to function effectively and to promote the health of the worker in particular and the family in general.

3.6 BIBLIOGRAPHY

Annual reports, Republic of South Africa:
  Department of Manpower, 1988.
  Department of Mineral and Energy Affairs, 1989.
  Department of National Health and Population Development, 1989.
  Medical Bureau for Occupational Diseases, 1988.
  National Centre for Occupational Health, 1987.
Baker, M. and Coetzee, A. C. 1983. *An introduction to Occupational Health Nursing in South Africa*. Johannesburg: Witwatersrand University Press.
Erasmus, R. P. B. 1976. *Commission of Enquiry into Occupational Health*
Searle, C. Brink, H. I. L. and Grobbelaar, W. I. C. 1988. *Aspects of Community Health* Cape Town: King Edward VII Trust.
Searle, C. 1965. *The history of the development of Nursing in South Africa 1652–1960* Pretoria: The South African Nursing Association.
Strauss, S. A. 1987. *Legal handbook for Nurses and Health Personnel* Cape Town: King Edward VII Trust.

Chapter 4: Occupational Safety

by Susan Hattingh

With acknowledgement to the National Occupational Safety Association for personal assistance and literature

4.1 INTRODUCTION

Technical advances in machinery and the associate sophisticated procedures, complicated methods and unique material that are used, demand a greater understanding of safety and awareness of the potential risk that goes with it.

Comments such as those below often reflect management's attitudes: such negative attitudes in the work place can affect the entire organization adversely.

'I don't have money for this safety business'
'Accidents are caused by plain carelessness'
'Safety is not our business'
'We can't waste money on extra frills such as safety'
'Safety? I'm a man, not a sissy'
'Injuries are part of doing business'
'Taking risks is part of the job'
'Well, you must die of something, eventually!'

The safety of workers is best catered for when the greatest measure of safety precautions, of the best quality, can be provided at the lowest cost.

4.2 LEARNING OBJECTIVES

At the end of this section, the reader should be able to:
— discuss what is meant by safety
— define the following:
  • Accident
  • Serious physical harm
  • Injury
— classify the various types of accidents
— describe the factors that may cause accidents
— discuss how epidemiology can be applied to safety
— discuss the domino theory applied to accident causation
— describe what is meant by the iceberg effect of an accident
— list the reasons why costs escalate when an accident happens
— discuss how the nurse can contribute to a safety inspection
— write short notes on the responsibility of management to safety
— discuss the key activities for preventing accidents
— discuss the role and functions of safety committees
— write short notes on off the job safety
— define the following concepts:
  • ergonomics
  • anthropometrics
  • biomechanics
— discuss how ergonomics can contribute to safety
— write an essay on the role and functions of the National Occupational Safety Association
— discuss how safety is promoted by NOSA
— discuss how the occupational health nurse can actively be involved in accident prevention and control

4.3 DEFINITIONS

4.3.1   **What is** Few people seem to agree on the actual meaning of safety and
     safety numerous authors, researchers and organizations have attempted to define or describe it. Although definitions vary in length and complexity, there is a common bond which ties them together and involves accident prevention and/or mitigation.

Safety is described by Strasse, Aaron and Bohn (Bever 1984: 1) as 'a condition or state of being resulting from the modification of human behaviour, and/or designing of the physical environment to reduce the possibility of hazards, thereby reducing accidents'.

In the South African context of organized accident prevention, a simplified description of safety would be:
1. A work environment which contains no threat to safety and health (employer's responsibility in terms of the MOS Act and others).
2. A workforce with the necessary knowledge of work safety.
3. A workforce with a positive attitude to work safely.
4. A workforce which is physically and mentally healthy and correctly placed.

The implication of the above definition is that safety is to be understood as the prevention of accidents and the mitigation of personal injury or property damage which may result from accidents. In addition, the individual must be aware of the broad range of hazardous materials which may cause occupational diseases over a long period and cause physical or psychological harm or injury to the worker. Safety also involves precautions against hazards which are not seen or recognized as such.

Safety also involves personal security. It is legitimate to be concerned for one's safety in the face of criminal activity.

Violent crimes occur in the work place including murder, violence, rape, assault and robbery. There may also be property crimes such as burglary, vandalism and theft.

If all these above-mentioned factors are taken into consideration, safety appears to signify more than just accident prevention and/or mitigation. The individual is faced with an assortment of hazards and risks and there may be a variety of consequences either to the worker or to the management if safety is neglected.

Safety can therefore be defined as it is by Bever (1984:2) as 'a dynamic or ever-changing condition in which one attempts to minimize the risk of injury, illness, death or property damage from the hazards to which one may be exposed in order to maximize success'.

The co-ordination of the aforementioned measures to effect the results contemplated by Bever, would be done by management through the means of an organized accident prevention programme, such as the NOSA MBO-Safety and Health Management system.

4.3.2   **Accident/** There are numerous and varied definitions of an accident given by
incident different authors. An accident may be defined as a sudden uncontrollable, unplanned, undesirable happening which disrupts the normal functions of persons and causes or has the potential to produce or to cause unintended injury, death or property damage and/or business interruption.

Taking all the definitions into account an accident can be simply described as an undesired event that has caused or has the potential to cause injury/damage or to disrupt operations.

During an accident where injuries are sustained, there is physical contact or exposure of the body to some object (even another person), substance or any foreign object which is injurious.

Whereas the accident is unplanned and unintended, personal injury, property damage or criminal activity, such as violence, assault and robbery, is planned and deliberate.

Accidents/incidents could be said to happen because of poor or inadequate control.

4.3.3   **Serious** Serious physical harm is of such a nature that it may cause permanent
physical or prolonged impairment of the body in such a way that part of the
harm body is functionally useless or part of the internal bodily system is inhibited in its normal performance. Serious physical harm can also cause psychological and mental damage which may be irreversible.

4.3.4   **Injury** An injury is a harmful condition sustained by the body as the result of an accident and can take any form from less serious, e.g. an abrasion or bruise to a laceration or more serious such as a fracture, penetration of a foreign body, burns or electrical shock, all of which may or may not cause permanent deformation, malfunction and even fatal consequences.

4.4. BASIC CLASSIFICATION OF ACCIDENTS

In order to be able to effectively control accidents, one should be able to identify what classes of accidents form the major problem.

There are eleven basic types of accidents which may occur. These accidents may or may not occur independently.

4.4.1 Being struck These accidents occur when a person suffers a blow or impact from a
by falling moving object. Example: A person may be struck by a crane's chain,
objects a falling rock, material or equipment falling from above; also shooting accidents, in which one is struck by a bullet.

4.4.2 Stepping on, A person may sustain an injury when he walks into a solid object
striking which is stationary or moving. Example: A person may collide with a
against or moving vehicle such as a truck or forklift, machinery or equipment.
being struck
by objects

4.4.3 Caught in, on Here there are different accidents involved, but the basic principles
or between are the same. Example:
objects

- 'Caught in' accidents may occur when a person's arm, finger or foot is caught between moving machinery or a floor grate or wire mesh screen.
- 'Caught between' accidents occur when a tie, coat or ring is caught on a moving machine part, between a fan belt and the pulley.

4.4.4   Falls from Falls can take a variety of forms. Falls from above are also called
above 'falls from a different level'. Example: A person may fall from a ladder, catwalk, stairs or scaffold.

4.4.5   Falls at Falls at ground level are also called 'falls on same level'. Example: A
ground level person may slip on a wet or oily surface, trip while walking, or fall over undesired objects lying around.

4.4.6 Strain, over- These accidents occur when bad lifting habits are applied. Example:
exertion or picking up objects which are too heavy, pulling or pushing something
strenuous alone when it would have been better to have another person helping
movements or to use some form of mechanical aid such as a hoist, chain hoist, lift or forklift.

4.4.7   Electrical Contact with electricity may result in an accident. Example: Contact
contact or may be made to a live current or to improperly earthed or live
exposure equipment.

4.4.8 Exposure to Accidents caused by exposure may be the consequence of contact
or contact with too high or too low a temperature, as when working with dry ice,
with harmful cold storage, melting iron ore, or working in an environment where
substances one is exposed to ice or sun which may result in blindness or burns,
or radiation sunstroke, etc. Exposure to radiation, toxic agents, waste-products,
acid burns, and so on, may also cause accidents which fall into this
category.

4.4.9   Inhalation These accidents occur when working with noxious substances such as
gases, fumes or materials which may cause serious harm when
inhaled. Example: Petrol fumes, toxic wastes, asbestos, fibre, etc,
may be inhaled in working environments.

4.4.10   Ingestion Although one can choose what to eat, these accidents do occur.
Example: One may inadvertently eat or drink contaminated food by
eating in a contaminated environment. One may eat while working
with, for example, mercury, radio-active materials or salmonella
contaminated food.

4.4.11 Absorption The absorption through the skin of some toxic agents may result in
serious illness. Example: Organic phosphate products and some
vector and insect sprays handled by farm workers, may be absorbed
through the skin.
    There are other types of accidents not classifed here, including
accidents not classified for lack of sufficient data.

4.5 CATEGORY OF INJURY

There are basically three categories of injuries which the occupational health nurse may encounter. It is essential that every single
accident, however small, be recorded since minor accidents or
injuries may serve as a warning. With a slight change in circumstances
or conditions, minor accidents could result in fatal or serious injuries
and property damage.
- Minor injuries that require first aid treatment
- Injuries causing temporary total disablement (one shift or longer)
- Permanent disablement which may be partial, total or fatal.
    It is important to remember that the same events which cause
injuries also cause damage, disruption etc. The prevention of these
events would therefore be to the benefit of management as they all
cost money.

4.6 FACTORS THAT MAY CAUSE ACCIDENTS

The direct causes of occuptional accidents are the end product of
unsafe acts and unsafe conditions in the workplace. These unsafe acts
and unsafe conditions are controllable and so accidents can be
prevented. Accidents do not happen independently, but as a result of
a series of events which have taken place. The main factors in an
accident are:
- technical equipment
- working environment
- worker

These three factors in combination are the cause of accidents.

The equipment to perform a task, for example, may be inadequate or defective or safety equipment may have been tampered with or be entirely lacking. There may also have been an omission to inspect equipment.

The working environment may be unpleasant—noise levels may be too high so that it is impossible to hear safety signals; the lighting may be too poor or too bright to see properly; the temperature may be so high or low that workers cannot function well; inadequate ventilation may result in the building-up of toxic fumes and lead to drowsiness.

The worker may also be a contributory factor in that he may not have received adequate training, may have little experience of the task or his attitude may not be directed towards safety.

The aforementioned causes may lead to the performance of unsafe acts and/or the creation of unsafe conditions due to the fact that they develop as the result of no or inadequate control.

All occupational accidents are either directly or indirectly attributable to human failings. Man is unpredictable and makes mistakes. It can be concluded therefore, that most accidents are directly or indirectly attributed to humans.

It is important to realize that the causes of accidents are a complex chain of events and to ascribe the origin of accidents to the carelessness of the worker does nothing to identify the real cause of an accident.

Accidents do not just happen, they are caused by definite factors which can all be identified and eliminated. Negligence should never be given as the cause of an accident as negligence is unacceptable behaviour caused by some or all of the above-mentioned causes.

Accidents are classified according to their inherent characteristics, but almost every book written and each country has its own classification. The multiple classification system is perhaps one of the most useful. The essential types of accidents may be classified according to the following seven classes (according to the International Labour Office, Geneva, 1983: 13):

- nature of injury—identifies the injury in terms of its principal physical characteristics
- part of the body affected—directly affected part of the body is identified
- source of the injury—the object, substance, exposure or bodily motion which directly produced or inflicted the injury is identified
- accident type—here the event which directly resulted in the injury is identified
- hazardous condition—the hazardous physical condition or circumstance which permitted or occasioned the occurrence of accident is named and identified
- agency of accident—this identifies the object, substance or premises where a previously identified hazardous condition existed
- unsafe act—identifies the violation of a commonly accepted safe procedure

When analysing accidents the aforegoing would give a good indication of some of the causes leading up to an accident. However, more in-depth analyses of accidents are sometimes required to identify tenacious and repetitive causes. Examples are:
- sections of work place concerned
- equipment concerned

4.6.1 Fatigue and boredom Fatigue and boredom are important factors to consider when the causes of accidents are to be evaluated. Fatigue does increase the risk of accidents, but the relation between fatigue and accidents is complex.

Tiredness may be combined with emotional problems experienced at home and it is then termed as 'fatigue'. An extreme state of fatigue is termed 'exhaustion'.

The occupational health nurse and other health workers must be aware of the fact that shift workers may suffer from fatigue due to the disturbance in their twenty four cycles or biorhythms. These disturbances cause workers to make more mistakes.

Fatigue influences different people differently; workers who are interested in their jobs will give all their attention to them and will not feel fatigue as much as those workers who are bored or do not like their jobs. The latter tend to become inattentive and careless at times.

Accidents are related not only to physical fatigue, but to the mental attitude of workers. By correctly placing a worker and improving the general environment one can create interest and satisfaction amongst workers.

The worker must be recognized as a human being, given responsibility and appreciated by management; he should be kept informed of what goes on and be able to make proposals which are listened to; in general he should be well looked after. An enjoyable social setting alleviates boredom, but it is often not recognized nor is it encouraged by management.

There are some people who like to do monotonous work, but some find it intolerable; they could cause accidents as they are intellectually not fitted to do a particularly repetitive job. This aspect must be considered when selecting a new worker and when placing a worker.

4.6.2 Experience and inexperience It is difficult to observe a clear cut correlation between the length of service and experience of a worker and the accident rates. There are so many contributory factors leading to accidents. One cannot assume that inexperience leads to accidents but a new worker who is not familiar with the factory or work place may be easily distracted and this may lead to a relative frequency of accidents among newcomers.

It is therefore essential that new and inexperienced workers must go through a period of training and orientation before being given tasks which may cause accidents.

Although experienced workers are not unfamiliar with their surroundings or their jobs they take greater risks and are less careful.

If no serious accident occurs in a particular type of work for a considerable time, workers tend to become less careful because they think that the danger in what they are doing is not as serious as they have been told. They neglect safety measures until another accident occurs which shows them the importance of safety precautions.

Insufficient skill or attempting a skill beyond a person's ability is often a contributory factor in accidents. Physical limitations, for example size, strength, coordination, age and so on may also affect performance.

4.6.3 Physiological, psychological and social conditions
Some accidents can be attributed to the worker's physiological, psychological and/or social conditions and occupational health nurses should give special attention to these cases.

If these circumstantial handicaps cannot be eliminated then other more suitable work should be selected for the worker. The importance of giving a handicapped person a chance in life cannot be stressed enough; such handicapped people are as good and loyal as workers without disadvantages.

Physiological factors which are temporary in duration may influence a worker's ability to perform an activity. Reaction time is decreased if a person is dehydrated or has a low blood sugar as a result of not eating breakfast.

For the occupational health nurse the problem is not how to exclude such persons from work, but how to employ them in a useful way despite their physical, psychological and social defects or infirmities.

Physical impairments such as poor eyesight or hearing may cause the worker to miss written or verbal instructions—this may lead to accidents.

One of the most serious social problems that may occur in the work place is that of alcohol abuse and alcoholism. There are alarming figures of people who are dependent on alcohol.

The occupational health nurse must recognize an alcohol or drug problem and should become involved in taking steps to rectify it. Early recognition is unquestionably the key to a successful alcoholism or drug control programme and leads to effective accident prevention. The MOS Act and other industrial legislation makes special provision for workers dealing with alcohol and drug abuse.

Attitudes and emotions play an important role in determining and directing the behaviour of a person. The behaviour of a worker may be positive when his attitude is positively directed to safety, but negative if he acts in a reckless manner.

The supervisor should be assisted in the early identification and subsequent handling of the employee with an alcohol or drug problem. For the nurse it is valuable because she gains knowledge and can assist the employee and the employer in preventing loss, injury or death through accident.

If the language spoken in the work place is not understood, safety instructions may be misinterpreted. This may result in negative attitudes and frustration on the job.

To assist in this regard the SABS has evolved a system of symbolic safety signs. One of the unique features of this SABS publication is that it contains a training course to teach workers to interpret these signs.

The causes of accidents can be described in terms of the epidemiological triade:

Figure 1.

HUMAN (HOST)
- physiological
- psychological
- sociological

OPERATIONS
(AGENT)
- standards
- procedures
- equipment

ENVIRONMENT
- physical
- psychological

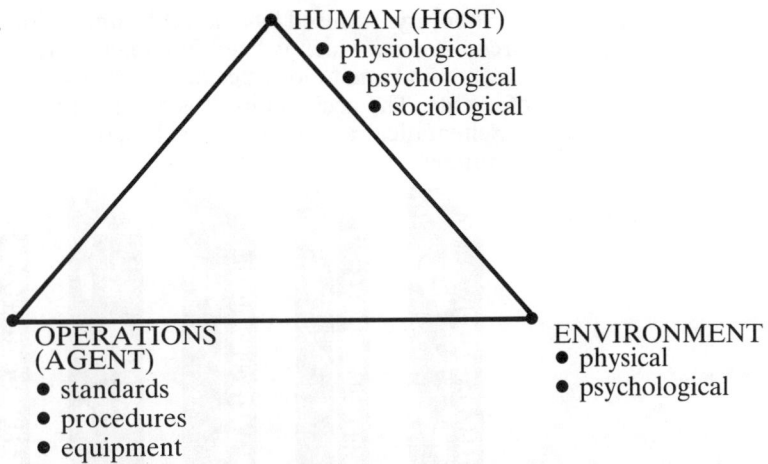

The interaction between the human as host, the operations as agent and the environment in which the operation takes place, indicate the close relationship between a state of wellbeing or illness. This also applies to safety. If one of these three factors (host, agent or environment) causes a problem, accidents may occur.

For example, if the human (host) has a physical problem such as poor eyesight, the agent is affected in such a way that operations cannot be carried out, procedures cannot be followed and the safety of a worker is threatened.

This also applies to the environment. If there is poor lighting, the worker (host) cannot see and procedures cannot be performed, equipment cannot be used according to standards and this may result in accidents.

More recently, in view of the concept of multiple causation, the agent is seen as a part of the environment rather as a separate factor. This results in an epidemiological dyade consisting of host and environment. In the case of occupational safety, the host is seen as the worker affected by a particular problem such as a physical, psychological or social problem. The environment comprises all the other factors that influence the safety of the worker.

The epidemiological dyade is depicted in the following figure:

Figure 2.

MAN (WORKER)

↑ ↓

ENVIRONMENT

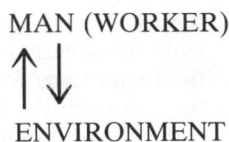

4.7 THE DOMINO CAUSE AND CONTROL SEQUENCE

Researchers who have studied the situational model of accident causation refer to the domino theory.

According to this theory there are six factors involved in the sequence of events which lead to an accident and its consequences. The injury and the consequences of the injury are the result of the cumulative action of the preceding factors.

An injury is caused by a natural culmination of a series of events or circumstances which is fixed in a logical order. One is dependent on another and one follows because of the other, constituting a sequence of events. The accident itself is one factor in the sequence of events.

Schematically this can be described in terms of a row of dominoes.

Figure 3.

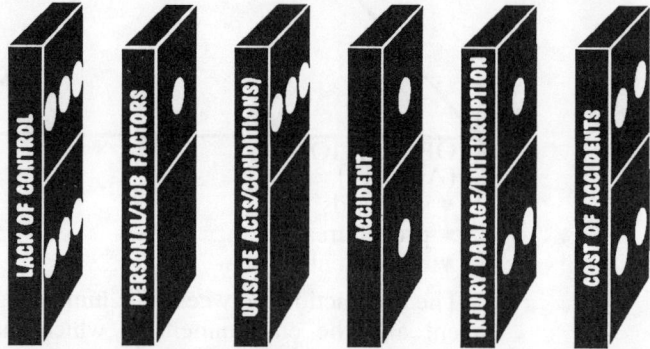

4.7.1   Lack of control Lack of control is defined as 'a lack of an organized system whereby all facets of an operation are subjected to control' (NOSA 1990: 1). These facets include:
- human
- environment
- equipment
- operations

The problems occurring with a lack of control include the following:
— there is no programme of work
— no set standards
— no responsibilities or accountabilities delegated or assigned
— no set measurement of expected performance
— no evaluation of deficiencies
— no organized programme for correcting deficiencies

All these problems lead to a lack of control—a lack of selfcontrol and/or a lack of supervisory control.

Control is aimed at adhering to strict standards. These standards include:
— rigid standards applied in selection of new workers
— rigid standards for identifying the needs for upgrading deficient workers already in employ
— rigid standards for identifying weaknesses such as substandard conditions in the environment, equipment etc.
— continuous monitoring of conditions and performances by workers
— corrective action through information gained by audits, inspections, investigations and reports.

Once the programme needs have been identified and the necessary standards or procedures drawn up, supervisors should be appointed as responsible for clearly defined control activities. This appointment is done in terms of the current industrial legislation (NOSA 1990: 4).

4.7.2 Personal/job factors Personal and job factors are defined by NOSA (1990: 5) as the human, environmental, mechanical, equipment, procedural and standards inadequacies which directly or indirectly cause the creation of unsafe conditions.

4.7.2.1   *Personal* This is seen as anything lacking in the human being which could cause
             factors him to perform an unsafe act or create an unsafe condition. These
factors include lack of knowledge and/or skill, physical and/or mental defects and improper attitude. In the modern management system taking note of these defects are not enough. The question that should be asked is WHY a person with the aforementioned defects is allowed to operate unchecked in any work situation or selected or placed in any work situation. The answer to this question lies in the weaknesses of the management system where there is a lack of specification; either task or job specification and/or man specification.

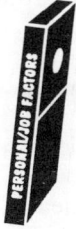

Human weaknesses can be controlled through the following measures:
— proper interviewing of prospective workers
— checking work records
— medical examination
— proper induction training
— task training with formalized follow-up
— retraining of old workers
— regular medical check-ups

4.7.2.2 Work or job- Work or job-related factors may include the following:
         related • anything lacking in the environment with regard to machines,
         factors   equipment etc which could cause an unsafe act to be committed or
                     an unsafe condition created
         • lack of task or job procedures, lack of performing inspections,
           lack of reporting, investigations, training, maintenance etc
         • lack of standards in housekeeping, layout, machine safeguarding,
           personal protective equipment etc
In many well-run companies all the essential programmes for upgrading the quality of the workers and the work-related aspects of an operation already exists. All that is needed is to put this into practice through the following measures:
— setting audits to comply to standards
— setting up an action plan to introduce controls on the conditions
  in the environment and the work quality
— evaluating personal needs through identifying skill requirements, training requirements and medical and welfare requirements
— identifying critical areas and/or tasks
— defining and assigning responsibilities and accountabilities

4.7.3 Unsafe acts/ Unsafe acts/conditions is defined as any deviation from standards
        conditions and/or procedures (NOSA 1990: 7).
                      Deviations from standards and/or procedures are caused by:
                      • lack of training
                      • lack of discipline
                      • lack of control such as job observation and spot checks
                      • no or inadequate procedures or standards
                      • ignorance or uninformed workers

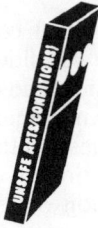

Unsafe conditions develop as a result of:
- natural deterioration of, e.g. equipment
- deterioration due to abuse
- poor design and planning
- no standards relating to physical conditions, machinery, equipment and tools.

The Machinery and Occupational Safety Act is very specific about what standards should be maintained regarding machinery, safeguarding, work place etc.

In order to prevent unsafe acts/conditions, the following should be done:
— training of all workers
— establishment of a standards (steering) committee
— inspection of standards
— establishing responsibilities and accountabilities
— introduce inspection and spot checking
— liaison between all departments such as health, operating, engineering, personnel etc.

4.7.4   Accident An accident is defined as an undesired event that has caused or has the potential to cause injury, damage and disruption of operations (NOSA 1990: 10).

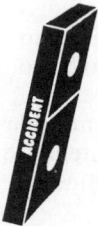

Most people associate the term 'accident' with injury. If no serious injury occurs, then they regard it as 'nothing serious' in the context of loss control, every unplanned event which adversely affects the operation is an accident. Even if the event (accident) does not show a potential to adversely affect an operation, it must be borne in mind that the existence of factors which combine to cause accidents could cause further accidents which could adversely affect the operation.

The control of the accidents include the following:
— education of all workers in the interpretation of the concept 'accident'
— proper reporting of all 'accidents'
— proper investigation of all 'accidents'
— proper follow-up to effect remedial action
— a committee to consider all reports and investigations as legally required.

4.7.5   Injury/ This is defined by NOSA (1990: 11) as any adverse effects or
damage/ potential adverse effects of accidents which could be minor, serious
interruption or catastrophic.

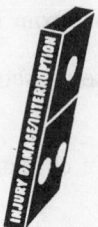

Many workers do not report an accident unless it is serious and there is usually very little reaction to accidents with a potential to cause adverse effects. A poor attitude is usually present regarding the entire problem of accidents as a counterproductive element in the operation.

It is important that all injuries, however small, are reported for the following reasons:
- complications
- acceptance of the case in case of complications, by the Workmen's Compensation Commissioner
- investigation

4.7.6 The costs of accidents— insured/ uninsured

Much has been written about the cost of accidents in the work place, but few attempts have been made to assess them accurately.

Occupational injuries and fatalities should be controlled like any other production costs and are a part of a company's operating costs such as raw materials, parts and labour.

It is important to calculate the costs arising from compensation for injuries as accurately as possible.

Categories of injuries include:

Medical-only cases which need first-aid treatment and take the form of cuts, scratches, bruises and minor strains that do not keep the injured worker off the job but for which medical expenses are incurred. It is estimated that these cases account for 67 per cent of all industrial injuries and only for seven per cent of the total cost of industrial injuries.

Temporary total disabilities which cause the worker to temporarily stay off the job. No permanent disability is incurred but the worker is prevented from performing his normal duties. These may be eye injuries, lacerations, strains, broken bones, effects of gas inhalation, skin rashes and so on.

It is estimated that this category accounts for 25 per cent of all injuries, but for 30 per cent of the total cost.

Permanent partial disabilities which may result in the worker staying off the job for a while and leaving some permanent damage to the injured worker's body, such as amputation. These cases account for only six per cent of all injuries, but for 50 per cent or more of the total costs.

Permanent total disability is an injury that prevents the worker from ever being gainfully employed again. For example loss of sight and limbs or mental disability such as brain damage.

These accidents account for $\frac{1}{8}$ of one per cent of all injuries and for four per cent of the total costs.

Fatalities which result in the death of a workman at any time subsequent to the accident, but as a result of an accident account for $\frac{1}{3}$ of one per cent of all injuries and for an estimated seven per cent of the total cost.

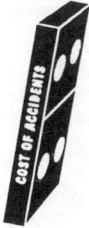

4.8 INSURED AND UNINSURED COSTS

The costs of an accident may be divided into two parts:
(1) Insured costs
(2) Uninsured costs
This can be understood in terms of an 'iceberg' metaphor.
(Source: Bird, F. E. 1974: 14.08).

Figure 4.

THE REAL COSTS OF ACCIDENTS CAN BE MEASURED AND CONTROLLED

INSURED COSTS
• Medical
• Compensation

1

5 TO 50
UNINSURED
PROPERTY DAMAGE
COSTS

UNINSURED COSTS
• Building damage
• Tool and equipment damage
• Product and material damage
• Production delays and interruptions

1 TO 3
UNINSURED
MISCELLANEOUS
COSTS

• Items such as hiring and training replacements, investigation time, etc.

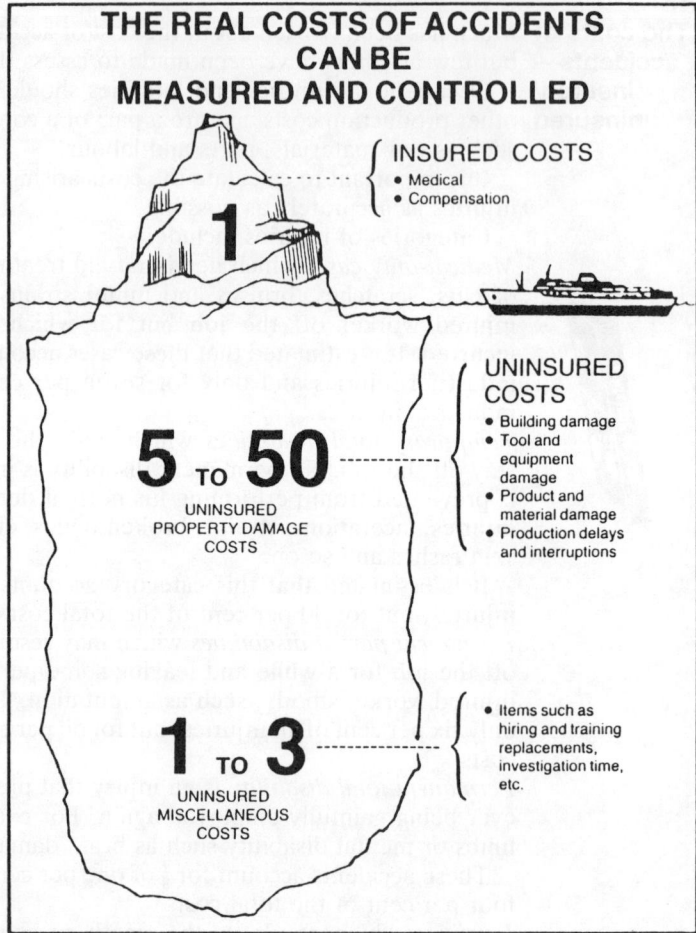

(Bird 1974: 14.08).

The insured costs are those above the waterline and are paid out to the company or worker: The uninsured costs are those under the waterline. These are hidden costs and are not covered by insurance. These hidden costs must be carried by the employer or the employee. These costs are up to 50 times greater than insured costs. This is reflected in the accident ratio as given by NOSA.

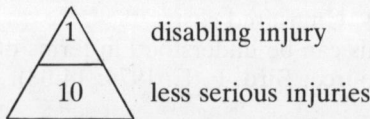

1 disabling injury

10 less serious injuries

Out of every one disabling injury there are ten less serious injuries which is mostly not reported as they are seen as unimportant.

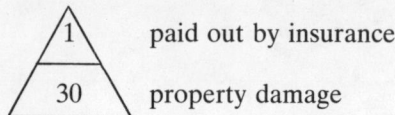

1 paid out by insurance

30 property damage

It is estimated that out of every one disabling injury, there are thirty cases of property damage. These are hidden costs and not covered by insurance and may cause delays and/or disruptions.

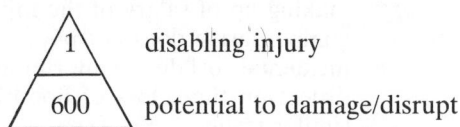

```
      /1\        disabling injury
     /────\
    / 600  \     potential to damage/disrupt
   /────────\
```

For every one disabling injury, there are 600 accidents or incidents with the potential to damage and/or to disrupt. These potential accidents are also called near-miss accidents.

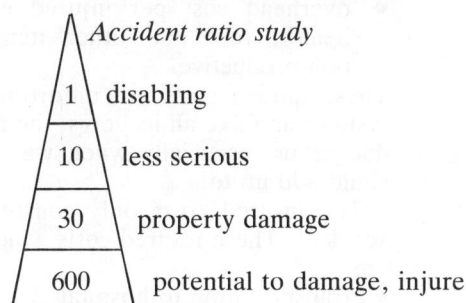

```
    /\  Accident ratio study
   / 1\  disabling
  /────\
 / 10   \  less serious
 /──────\
/  30     \  property damage
/─────────\
/ 600       \  potential to damage, injure
/───────────\
```

The money paid out by the Workman's Compensation Commissioner is only a fraction of the total cost of an accident.

It is essential for the occupational health worker to realize that there are uninsured 'hidden' costs (those under the waterline) which are paid by the employer himself and eventually felt by the community or country as a whole.

These uninsured or 'hidden costs' may take the form of:
- time lost by workers helping, watching, being curious or sympathizing with the injured worker
- time lost through injury to the worker
- time lost by foreman, supervisors and any other team members involved in investigating the accident to assist the injured worker, arranging for the injured employee's production to be continued by another worker
- time lost to training and selecting a new or other worker to take over the job
- writing accident reports or other official reports
- attending meetings or hearings on the case
- obsolescence of the machine before the accepted depreciated time
- decreased output when the employee returns to work and cannot go on with his activities because of the injury
- overtime may have to be worked in order to make up for the production loss
- first-aid staff spending time in treating accident rather than working on accident prevention and other health matters
- negligence of other work because of discussion of the accident
- equipment repairs, replacement of damaged equipment or cleaning due to fire or spoilage of material
- involvement of personnel and putting more tasks and strain on them

- lowered morale and consequences of the excitement of the workers due to the accident: strikes or unhappiness may occur which may result in further loss
- making up of salary of the injured worker where the workmen's compensation does not pay
- incidental cost due to interference with production, failure to fulfil orders on time, loss of bonuses, payment or forfeits and other similar results
- cost to employer under employee welfare and benefit systems
- cost due to the loss of profit on the injured worker's productivity and on idle machines
- overhead cost per injured employee—the expense of light, health, rent and other items while the injured worker is non-productive.

These hidden costs are unfortunately not reflected in accounting systems and like all icebergs, the mass below the surface is the most dangerous, especially when we consider what these hidden costs could add up to.

The insured costs only constitute half of the total cost of an accident. These insured costs which are partly covered by insurance are:

- transportation to hospital
- medical attention
- hospitalization
- rehabilitation
- compensation

Medical aids also have their limits, and the worker or employer has to pay the rest.

Other insured costs are sometimes covered by commercial insurers and could cover, to a certain extent,

- damage to property
- fire losses
- loss of profits due to some specified factors
- extra compensation with specified or state benefits

These insurance premiums are very expensive and cannot cover all the profits lost by the employer. They are a high price to pay for inadequate safety precautions.

4.9 ACCIDENT PREVENTION

When an accident happens the entire plant is affected. An accident involves the workers, machines and materials and therefore safe working conditions and procedures are of vital importance.

There is always a sequence of events that may lead to an accident. It is the interplay of these events or factors that may produce an accident and any alteration in this sequence or elimination of one of the factors in the accident chain, will usually prevent an accident.

If each domino in a series is within striking distance of the next one, all the dominoes will fall if the first is knocked over. But if one is removed, the subsequent dominoes will remain standing and so the accident will not take place.

This implies that accident prevention is simply the removal of one of these factors.

Accident prevention is not so simple but comprises a complex series of events.

The various means generally used at present to promote industrial safety are, according to the International Labour Office, Geneva (1983: 14–15), the following:

- Regulations

  These may include mandatory prescriptions concerning matters such as working conditions, maintenance, machine guarding, testing, duties of employers or employees, training, medical supervision and examination, and first aid.

- Standardization

  This includes laying down of official, semi-official or unofficial standards concerning the safe construction of certain types of industrial equipment, safe and hygienic practices, personal protective devices, set practices.

- Inspection

  Inspection is understood to mean that there may be a certain amount of enforcement of mandatory regulations concerning procedures performed, machines or environment.

During a safety inspection the following major categories of conditions and items should be considered:

- Personal protective equipment and clothing such as goggles, masks, safety shoes, respirators and so on, which should be worn at all times and should be clean, well fitted and of a high quality. (Personal protective equipment should protect to the maximum and cost should be the least concern when buying this equipment.)
- Machinery and parts thereof such as shields and guards of grinders, chain saws, pulleys, presses, drills, cutters and so on.
- Fire fighting equipment, such as extinguishers, hoses, hydrants, sprinkler systems, fire alarms, and so on.
- Vehicles such as motor cars, trucks, forklifts, cranes, railroad equipment.
- Structured openings and manholes such as shafts, pits, floor openings, trenches, drains and storm pipes.
- Electrical equipment conductors and procedures: their use, handling and maintenance; lockout systems, cables, wires, switchboxes and lamps.
- Hand tools: hammers, power tools, screwdrivers, sledges and files.
- Pressurized equipment: boilers, pots, tanks, pipes and hoses.
- Containers: gas cylinders, refuse bins and containers, barrels, solvents, acids and fuel tanks.
- Hazardous materials: flammables, explosives, gases, acids and other toxic materials.
- Waste: chemical, biological, solid or radiated.
- Atmospheric conditions: presence of dust, gases, fumes, vapours, radiation; also, illumination, noise level, oxygen flow.
- Building and construction: floors, windows, air-conditioning, stairs, roof, walls, rooms, showers, lockers and bathrooms.
- Storage: rooms, types of material stored together, ventilation and emergency actions.
- Elevators, escalators, lifts, crane cables, controls and safety devices.

- Conductors for lightning.
- Technical research: this includes matters such as investigation of properties by authorities and the setting of standards for what constitutes harmful materials, the study of machine guards and other safety devices, the testing and inspecting of personal protective equipment, the investigation of methods to prevent fires, explosions, inhalation of gas and fumes and other issues related to prevention.
- Medical and nursing research: medical or nursing research in the field of occupational health, includes the examination of the physiological and pathological effects of environmental and technological factors on workers and the physical circumstances which are conducive to accidents.
- Psychological research is performed to investigate the psychological patterns which are conducive to accidents, how the physical environment contributes to morale, for instance, and how low morale again contributes to accidents occurring in the work place.
- Statistical research: this is done to ascertain what kind of accident occurs, in what numbers and to which departments and people and in what particular operations. It also includes statistics of different diseases that may occur in the specific work place.
- Education: education and training is an important and integral part of accident prevention. Workers should be instructed in the safe use of tools, materials and equipment.

  Safety procedures should be taught in all courses, not only those in which machine use is taught. Every person should be educated in safety especially in road safety and home safety. Safety should be strictly enforced and learned as a daily routine, not only practised at work. It should become a firm habit at home, work or play.
- Training: all instructors should teach workers and especially new workers safety matters.
- Persuasion: there are various methods of publicity and there should be appeals to develop 'safety-mindedness'.
- Insurance: there should be provision of financial incentives to promote accident prevention in the form of reductions on premiums payable by factories, for example, where safety measures of a high standard are taken.
- Each person should take personal responsibility for implementing safety measures. These can also be any measures taken to make sure that no accident will occur which can cause injury or death to fellow workers. The people who should be most conscious and aware of safety include:
  - legislators
  - government bodies
  - technologists
  - physicians
  - nurses
  - hygienists
  - statisticians

4.10 ACCIDENT PREVENTION PROGRAMMES

Successful accident prevention programmes depend on three basic principles:
- leadership by the employer
- safe work habits and practices by employees
- safe and healthy working environment and conditions

An absence of any of these three principles may cause accidents on the job which may result in injuries, property damage, loss of production, escalation of costs, loss of worker morale and even death.

The responsibility for occupational safety and health must be willingly accepted by employers and employees alike and forms an integral part of the job of the occupational health nurse.

Together employers and employees should establish safety procedures and policies, stimulate awareness of safety in others and the environment and show interest in providing safe and healthy working conditions.

The responsibility for safe working conditions rests on the employer and that for safe work on the worker himself. The worker must develop and follow safe working habits at all times and must use safeguards and protective equipment properly. He should always be mindful of his fellow workers' safety.

Without the active and positive co-operation, interest and acceptance of responsibility for safety by management, an accident prevention programme will fail.

4.11 LEADERSHIP BY THE EMPLOYER

Representatives of both line and staff management must have a positive attitude and interest in safety.

The front-line supervisor is the person who deals most directly with the employee and thus bears the greatest responsibility for the implementation of safety and health matters. He should be given the appropriate authority, assistance and support to fulfil his responsibilities and should be highly trained in safety.

Top management cannot delegate responsibility in accident prevention and safety as they are the people who must establish safety policies, stimulate awareness of safety and establish measures to promote safe and healthy conditions in the work place.

Management has certain legal responsibilities towards its employers. It is especially the following three Acts which keep management responsible for its actions.
- The Machinery and Occupational Safety Act
- The Mines and Works Act
- The Workman's Compensation Act

The moral responsibility of management is directed not only towards the worker, but also to their families and to the public as a whole.

4.12 SAFE WORK HABITS AND PRACTICES BY EMPLOYERS

There are several factors that may play a major role in the safe performance of the worker's activity.

- understanding the difficulty of the activity
- ability level of the worker
- immediate state of the worker
- environmental factors
- knowledge
- skill
- experience

Understanding the difficulty of the activity

This is essential to perform any given task. It also involves the understanding of the risks associated with the task. Any task has its risks and benefits but inadequate knowledge may lead to failure to recognize and evaluate the risks or hazards associated with it.

Ability level of the worker

Skill is essential for most tasks performed by the worker. Insufficient skill or knowledge or the attempt to use a skill beyond one's ken often contribute to accidents.

There are also physical limitations that have to be considered when performing a task. Ergonomic factors must be taken into account. The physically handicapped or the older worker's limitations must especially be considered when performing a task; for example, hearing, vision, mobility, reaction time and so on can limit performances. Without adequate skill and knowledge one cannot perform safely. Fatigue and boredom must be prevented. The environment must be such that an enjoyable social setting can alleviate boredom. Boredom is sometimes the cause of a serious accident and not 'playing with the machine' as the findings of accident investigations sometimes state.

Immediate state of the worker

There is definite proof that physiological, sociological and psychological factors influence the performance and the state of mind of the worker. These factors are in constant flux and can be a threat to safety.

Alcohol abuse and social problems go hand in hand with accidents. Often those who are termed 'accident prone' are people whose attitudes, emotions and personal lives are not in order.

Attitude and emotions play an important role in the overall behaviour of a person, and also influence his or her way of thinking about safety. Habits develop because of attitudes which may be positive or negative and emotional states change. Bad habits are not easily broken or changed.

Strong emotions may sometimes disrupt normal behaviour patterns causing an individual who normally acts safely to act in a reckless manner, e.g. not wearing safety attire.

There are some aspects of behaviour to be considered which may also contribute to unsafe acts:

- Time and safety
  One of the most common reasons for taking risks at work is to save time—time for more leisure, time to enable one to do the job faster, to impress people such as supervisors, to enable one to

earn a bonus or more money, to win a competition, to prove
something or simply to save time. This wish to save time often
results in an unsafe act.

* Effort and safety
  This means to 'take the easy way out'. The safe way of doing the
  job may be demanding or seen as an effort either physically or
  mentally. A negative attitude to safety may result in an unsafe act
  where the worker takes a short cut.
* Group acceptance and safety
  Workers are often influenced by the negative attitude of the group
  and, not wishing to be outcasts, they join the group and ignore
  their own fears. Sometimes the consequences are dire. Often,
  therefore, it is new employers who are most at risk.

4.13 NOSA IDENTIFIES SIX KEY ACTIVITIES FOR PREVENTING ACCIDENTS

4.13.1 Engineering revision This includes improvements to the guarding of machines and tools in the working environment by qualified and authorized persons only. It also involves revision of work processes and procedures through participation of all concerned and with the consent of management.

4.13.2 Education and training There should be education and training for *all* people in the work situation—whether they are management, supervisors or workers.

Proper job descriptions lead to proper job instruction technique and to the improvement of skills and therefore to the improvement of relationships and attitudes.

General safety education should be included in the training and education programme of all employees so as to change or reinforce attitudes which are positive towards safety.

4.13.3 Employment practices The nurse's role in the selection of personnel will depend on her skill and ability to make an assessment of both the physical and mental ability of the worker and her position and attitude as an employee.

Selection of personnel depends on the physical and mental demands of the job, whether it is a new employee or one who has been moved from one job to another and has to be trained to perform a new job.

4.13.4 Example setting Safety rules do not exclude anyone—they also apply to the nurse. The nurse must therefore set an example for all to see by obeying safety rules.

4.13.5 Enthusiasm Enthusiasm, like negativism, is an infectious disease—people are affected by it. An enthusiastic leader is one who acknowledges the safety rules and safety achievements of others.

4.13.6 Enforcement This is the last resort if all else fails in order to enforce discipline on those who break safety rules. This must however be applied very carefully and only by those with authority.

Safety posters are an important aspect in accident prevention and are put on the walls at strategic places. These posters remind workers about possible dangers. In this way, the workforce is kept 'safety conscious' at all times.

4.14 SAFETY COMMITTEES

A safety committee is established as a practical means to promote safety by co-operation between management and worker.

Management often uses safety committees to explain safety policy and workers use the safety committee to bring certain views and suggestions on safety matters to the attention of management.

A safety committee helps to give workers confidence in the safety policy. Management can be confident that workers will appreciate and abide by the safety policy.

It is essential that the occupational health nurse is a member of this committee.

4.14.1 The functions of safety committees

4.14.1.1 Policy The members of safety committees have the general duty to promote the co-operation among all workers in an attempt to improve the safety standards. The committee should make sure that safety standards are set up and followed.

The members of the safety committees are chosen from the workers, not necessarily in authority themselves but certainly people who are respected and liked by the workers. Orders then do not carry the stigma of 'authority' or management. The greater the number of workers who can participate in setting safety policy, the more successful the committee will be. The members need not be experts in safety matters but should feel positive and competent to deal with safety issues.

The safety committee should prepare and adopt a constitution and should meet regularly. One item on every agenda should be to discuss any accident that has occurred since the last meeting. It should be clearly stressed that no blame should be put on a *person*. The discussion should rather be directed at determining the cause of the accident and new measures should be worked out to prevent a recurrence of those circumstances which led to it. Preparation of safety rules and regulations takes place in this safety committee and should be submitted for confirmation to and adoption by the proper authorities.

Everything possible must be done to keep the management and members interested in their work. The safety committee *must* be backed by the employer. Without management's approval, a safety committee cannot function.

The establishment of a safety programme and the evaluation, revision and testing of this programme is an important function of the safety committee. Every worker representative must feel free to express his opinion without the fear of criticism from superiors. All proposals for setting up a safety programme should be considered and should have the greatest possible support of both the employer and the workers. All the necessary information, such as statistics, should be available to the committee in order to develop new techniques, or revise those which already exist.

The trade unions are increasingly taking up safety issues at enterprise level. They seek improvements through negotiating health and safety agreements with employers. Participation by trade unions may bring about changes in policy on safety issues.

It is the function of the safety committee to implement and administer the company's statement of policy for a safe plant. This encompasses safety policies and practices, safety standards and industrial hygiene. NOSA emphasizes that no grievances or matters unconnected with safety should be discussed by the safety committee.

4.14.1.2 Executive The safety committee is involved in the investigations of all accidents. In some cases a worker who has had an accident is invited to tell the committee how the accident happened. These cases should be handled tactfully and objective criticism should be given.

All accidents are promptly reported to the safety engineer by the committee members. This is done so that hazardous conditions can be immediately removed. Where necessary other specialized members can be co-opted to the safety committee or subcommittees or inspection committees can be formed. Another of the duties of the safety committee is to do plant inspections and self-audits in order to investigate the conditions and procedures which may lead to accidents. It is important that constant auditing of all existing, planned and proposed installations, processes and procedures for unsafe conditions or acts should take place before injury or damage results. The testing and approval of all safety equipment and clothing is done by the committee. Equipment is checked for the necessary safety devices before it is bought.

A specific person or subcommittee is appointed who:
- records all minor and major accidents in an accident register
- sees to it that emergency planning has a means, plan and system to keep adequate watch on all sources of danger that can develop in a disaster
- ensures proper first aid and, if necessary, further medical treatment to anybody injured
- does the necessary paper work to notify the authorities concerned
- forwards the full particulars of an accident to all the members of the committee
- ensures that all the decisions, instructions and directives of the committee are implemented
- reports all near-accidents
- determines the frequency and severity of minor injuries
- determines the general and specific, actual and potential costs of accidents

4.14.1.3 Education It is not sufficient to give workers a booklet on safety instructions— the contents must be explained to them to ensure that they are understood. The safety committee has a responsibility towards the worker to inform him of new equipment, policy, procedures or any other changes that have taken place or are planned. This information can reach the worker by compiling, editing, publishing and distributing a monthly or bi-weekly safety publication. It must, however, be remembered that not all workers can read or understand the language the publication is written in. This can be overcome by lectures, safety talks, demonstrations or by obtaining audiovisual aids.

The introduction of safety competitions, contests, and safety weeks is also a step towards safety but care should be taken that accidents are not reported because of fear of being excluded from the competition.

The planning and supervision of the training of *all* employees or as many as possible should be a priority and should be conducted according to NOSA's training courses. The safety committee promotes safety training by reviewing all audiovisual materials for inclusion in the health and safety training programme for employees, by taking into account the following:

- nature of work
- culture of employees
- level of training
- age
- sex
- attitude
- relevance to work

The occupational health nurse has an important function within the safety committee and can contribute her knowledge and skill in health matters making individuals and their environment safe to work in.

The safety committee also has the important function of establishing appropriate relationships with professional and organizational groups outside the company.

4.14.1.4 Manage-
ment
involvement
Setting up a safety programme without the active interest, participation, involvement and approval of management is useless. The safety committee assists management in developing and operating a programme that will not only protect the worker by preventing accidents, but also by promoting productivity and preventing loss either of money or human life.

Management initiate participation and initiative in setting up a safety programme is essential. The acceptance by various levels of management both legal and internal, ensures greater management leadership in the programme.

The delegation of responsibilities, both legal and internal to supervisory and other staff, further helps to ensure good safety performance on all levels. Management involvement further extends to their insistence on the introduction of proper auditing systems.

4.15 OFF THE JOB SAFETY

Statistics have recently revealed a shocking number of accidents which are not related to the work place. NOSA states that the ratio of off the job accidents can be as high as ten to one compared to those happening in the work place. This may result in many lost man-hours. Off the job accident statistics are very difficult to obtain, but by being observant the occupational health nurse can detect evidence of the occurrence of such accidents.

An analysis of off the job accidents cannot be conclusive. The following areas are the likeliest for off the job accidents:

- *Assaults*—these may occur on the way home from work, at work or anywhere else.
- *Sport*—Injuries are often a result of unfitness.
- *Recreation*—These may take various forms; a person's own self management should act as a guideline as to whether recreational activities are safe, or could lead to injury and whether they are suited to one's physical build, age and ability.
- *Entertainment*—e.g. noise levels.
- *Home workshop*—such accidents happen in the workshop at home and can be in the line of building, metal- or woodworking, electronical and mechanical work.
- *Residence, garden*—e.g. tools, pesticides, swimming-pools. The safety measures taken in the work place should be maintained in the home. All electrical installations in the home should conform to wiring regulations and standards. One must respect electricity when it is working and when it is not. Only qualified people should modify or repair electrical equipment.

Other potentially hazardous equipment in the home should be handled, stored and treated correctly. The following are potential hazards:

- lawn mowers
- chemicals
- ladders
- tools
- gas cylinders
- flammables such as petrol, oil, etc.
- guns

4.16 ERGONOMICS

4.16.1 Definition Ergonomics is the study of the relation between man, the work he does and the environment in which this work is done. Ergonomics is concerned with design: work should be designed to match the man and his machine and to achieve optimal adjustment between man and his work environment so that the health and ability of man is enhanced.

The purpose of ergonomics is to ensure that a person's abilities are utilized efficiently and that the equipment being used will not endanger his health or safety.

Ergonomics also refers to the interaction between the work place, job practices, equipment and the employer's well-being. It is closely connected to safety—because if the job is ergonomically satisfactory, then the worker will work and apply safety measures. Therefore safety in the work place will be maintained. This will lead to work satisfaction among operators, a goal to be achieved by any standards of good management.

Ergonomic interventions in the work place lead not only to worker satisfaction, but also to increased productivity, minimum work-related morbidity and job-turnover and with this the recruiting and training of new workers. Work stoppages and maintenance problems are also limited if ergonomical factors are considered.

4.16.2 Anthropo-metrics Anthropometrics are concerned with the dimensions of the human body and its variations. The human body differs from person to person and it is therefore not economically possible to take each variation into account whenever the design of machines or related work environments is planned. An acceptable norm is derived from the majority and from that a design is ergonomically born. To accommodate the exceptions, special arrangements usually have to be made.

4.16.3 Bio-mechanics This is the discipline dedicated to the study of the human body as a structure which can function properly only within the confines of both the laws of Newtonian mechanics and the biological laws of life. Biomechanics relate to push, pull or support loads that can be exerted under varying conditions.

4.16.4 Ergonomics and accidents The occurrence of accidents is minimized through the application of ergonomic principles already outlined on the man-machine system. Wherever the prevalence and incidence rates of accidents are high or show signs of increasing, an investigation should be done. Information that should be gathered includes:
- job descriptions and demands on operators
- pre-employment data on medical examinations
- previous medical history
- epidemiological data on the prevalence of work-related symptoms
- records on injuries, absence, sick leave
- job turn over
- accident data
- environmental data
- productivity data
- occupational history of workers
- qualification, training and experience
- workload

4.16.5 Ergonomical self-assessment by the worker Workers who evaluate their own work places may contribute to valuable ergonomical changes that may benefit both the employee and the employer. If the work place is ergonomically more satisfactory and more comfortable for the worker, he can be much more efficient and productive in his work. Financially however, changes are not always possible, but if a number of options are considered, one can perhaps make changes at no great cost.
Ergonomic improvement should be:
- cost beneficial
- practical
- possible
- applicable to the majority

4.16.6 Conclusion Consideration should be given to the mental abilities of man when demands in the work place are made. Tasks should be constructed so that they do not require excessive mental and muscular effort, considering sex, age and state of health of the worker. But at the same time a task should not be so easy that boredom and inattention lead to unnecessary errors, poor materials and accidents.

4.17 THE NATIONAL OCCUPATIONAL SAFETY ASSOCIATION

The National Occupational Safety Association is an incorporated association not for gain which was established in 1951 through the instigation of the then Minister of Labour, the Honourable Ben Schoeman.

The recommendations of a committee appointed to investigate ways and means of slowing down the ever-increasing injury rate led to the formation of a company. This company, a joint venture of the workmen's compensation commissioner and employers was established through their employer organizations. NOSA claims that this could be considered as one of the very first examples of privatization.

NOSA is partially financed by the State Accident Fund in order to carry out occupational accident and disease prevention work. NOSA is therefore able to give employers a free or subsidized service by virtue of the fact that the employer's money is being fed back into accident prevention work.

The majority of employers fall under the jurisdiction of the Workmen's Compensation Commissioner which in terms of the Worker's Compensation Act must pay assessments to the State Accident Fund. According to the hazards in their industry and their claims experienced for each class of injury, this State Accident Fund meets hospitalization, compensation etc in a case where a workman is injured in the course of his employment.

There are, however, certain exempted employers who do not pay towards the State Accident Fund, but run their own insurance companies with the Workmen's Compensation Commissioner's permission. These employers include certain of the builders who pay their assessments to the Federated Employers' Mutual Co Ltd, gold mines pay to the Rand Mutual Assurance Co, and some of the larger municipalities and various government departments carry their own insurance.

NOSA involves employers by establishing regional groups in various areas where NOSA has offices in order to supply a service to employers. It serves as an excellent channel of communication between NOSA and employers.

The individual members of the regional group are volunteers who serve their employers and represent their employer organizations or firms within the framework of the objectives of NOSA. These objectives are:
- guidance
- education
- training
- motivation

The regional groups are situated in all the major centres of South Africa and industrial groups that cover mining and aviation have also been established.

The regional advisory groups have the following functions:

- They provide a forum where safety and safety-related problems are and can be discussed, in order to find possible solutions.
- They promote safety in general by:
  - talking to others (e.g. engineers, safety advisers)
  - bringing guests to the meetings
  - promoting safety amongst others (e.g. family, clubs)
  - setting an example to strive for safety in the work place
  - helping to persuade other employers to make use of NOSA training courses
  - selling safety to companies which have no safety programmes
  - giving NOSA feedback on its services in order to make services more effective.

They improve the committee members' own awareness of safety, building up their skills and experience by:

- assisting with specific safety elements
- bringing about positive steps in, e.g. inspection, plant operations
- previewing the latest video or film material on safety
- making members aware of training courses or giving feedback on courses on safety and self-development

4.17.1   NOSA's objectives The association's objectives are the guidance, education, training and motivation of various levels of management and the workforce alike in the techniques of accident and occupational disease prevention. Through the NOSA MBO system and using the NOSA 5 star objective—setting and recognition system as a framework they will ensure the highest degree of success in the prevention of injuries, damage to property and disruptions of business activities.

The modus operandi for achieving these objectives is by means of the NOSA Management by Objectives Safety System, training courses, publicity material and safety promotional activities.

To reach the GET'M-objectives (guidance, education training and motivation) there are formal and informal activities. The formal activities take place in the classroom where safety training courses are mounted for select candidates. These courses are offered throughout South Africa and after successful completion the candidate is presented with a certificate which licenses him/her to run certain of NOSA's courses. This licensed worker becomes a NOSA 'agent' to train workers. NOSA estimates that over 200 000 persons have been trained over the years.

The informal GET'M takes place through the NOSA staff who contact employers. The purpose of the visits to employers is to make them aware and to establish fully-fledged safety programmes. This is done by carrying out safety surveys, gradings and follow-up audits using the NOSA MBO Safety System as a framework.

4.17.2   **NOSA's mission**

> # MISSION STATEMENT
> To provide dynamic, proactive and cost effective consultative services in the fields of Loss Prevention, Occupational Safety and Health in the work environment to all industry and commerce.
>
> # CREDO
> ## OUR PROFILE
> To provide a comprehensive range of services and products in Occupational Safety and Health Management for all industry and commerce.
>
> ## OUR PURPOSE
> — To provide dynamic, proactive and cost effective consultative services in the fields of Occupational Safety and Health.
> — To strive for excellence in customer service by motivated employees.
> — To uplift our employees and ensure the continued growth of our business.
>
> ## OUR VALUES
> We are committed to providing:
> — Quality products and services
> — Outstanding customer service
> — Quality in everything we do.
> We believe in recognition and reward for our employees who contribute towards the Company's stated objective of providing quality in everything we do.
>
> ## OUR GOALS
> — To be the accepted authoritative consultancy in the field of Loss Prevention and Occupational Safety and Health.
> — To guide, educate and train all people in the techniques of Occupational Accident and Disease Prevention.
> — To continually strive for service excellence.
> — To create a work environment which is conducive to encouraging employees to participate in decisions that directly affect their daily work lives.
> (Source: NOSA, Pretoria 1991.)

4.18 THE ROLE AND FUNCTIONS OF THE OCCUPATIONAL HEALTH NURSE IN SAFETY AND ACCIDENT PREVENTION

In 1895 Florence Nightingale said: 'Nursing is not only a service to the sick, it is a service also to the well. We have to teach people how to live.'

The role of the occupational health nurse can never be ignored, nor should it be underestimated or regarded as inferior in any industry or work place. Most nurses working in industry are highly trained professionals who have the necessary skill, knowledge and motivation to participate actively in the safety and accident prevention programme in the work place. It is important that occupational health nurses must not take on duties for which they are not prepared. They must be involved and must accept every opportunity to learn more about the work environment and work practices. Occupational health nurses should not sit in a 'sterile' medical centre, waiting for an accident to happen.

The medical facility is much more than just a mere clinic, because the services rendered go beyond the therapeutic and prophylactic aspects of illness. The occupational health nurse is seen as the manager of this department. Medical officers are usually employed on a part-time basis and they see only those cases referred to them by the occupational health nurse. Where a company employs a full-time medical officer the managerial duties will have to be shared according to the needs and activities of the company concerned.

It is agreed that prevention is better than cure, and therefore the occupational health worker should and must work with management and other team members involved in safety, towards a safe environment for each worker in order to prevent injury and disease not only in the work place, but also in their private lives—safety must become a habit.

The functions of the occupational health nurse and other occupational health workers will depend on many factors. The most important are:
- how she/he is regarded by management
- what knowledge, skill, motivation she/he possesses
- what kind of industry she/he is working in
- what the job description is
- what team members are available
- the size of the industry
- the type of industry

The services rendered at the medical faculties go beyond therapeutic and prophylactic aspects of injury and illness. The occupational health worker must have a great awareness of the employee's needs, the legislation pertaining to the employee's welfare, disability and occupational hazards and the health and safety policy of the company.

It is absolutely essential that the occupational health nurse communicates with management and other departments in order to improve and strengthen the welfare of the employee. It is important to have good relationships and open communication channels between management and the workers. Through effective communication the occupational health worker can contribute to the improvement of job satisfaction, a happy and safe environment, loss, control and productivity.

It is important to realize that the employee must be seen and treated holistically. The occupational health worker must realize that each employee must be seen as a physical, social and psychological human being with his/her own identity, within a family which is a part of a community.

It is well known that there is interaction between the social, physical and psychological environment of the individual. When the chain between these factors is broken, the individual will become unbalanced. This may cause carelessness, demotivation, and other symptoms that can contribute to unsafe acts.

With extensive training the occupational health worker becomes sensitive to the problems of employees which can be related to social, physical or psychological factors.

The functions of the occupational health worker with regard to safety fall under the following main headings:

- health education and safety teaching to teach workers how they can protect their own health
- emergency planning
- accident recording and investigation
- records, claims, minor injuries, reports, statistics
- occupational diseases
- examinations and pre-employment tests to identify physiological, psychological and social problems
- communication—in order to work co-operatively with other team members of the occupational safety and health team
- co-ordination with other safety team members
- personal safeguarding, wearing of protective protection
- participation in the development of hazard control programmes geared to the nature and specifics of the work place. It must be strongly emphasized that the nurse, as with all the other safety team members, cannot work on her/his own. It is absolutely essential to perform these functions with the management's approval *and* together with the other team members, such as safety officers, security officers, loss control officers, hygienists, medical officers, etc
- participation in the selection, training and motivation of workers so that they learn how to follow safe work practices
- provision of primary care so that workers recover from injury and work compatibly with their therapeutic care plans
- collection and use of data to identify causes and make plans to correct both the situational and the behavioural problems
- counselling and/or providing crisis intervention and moral support to workers who are experiencing interpersonal, work or family problems that interfere with normal functioning and may be the cause of carelessness
- participation in environmental control programmes that aim to identify, eliminate and control health and safety hazards

4.19 CONCLUSION

An attempt has been made to show the importance of the role of the occupational health worker in accident prevention.

An accident happens as a result of a chain of events to which the occupational health worker should be observant.

Safety concerns ALL—it cannot be isolated as something that is only practised in the work situation. Safety involves not only the individual, but the whole community, the whole country and even the whole world. One serious accident may harm a whole nation.

It should be remembered that safety should be 'sold', but this is NEVER achieved by the YCNSSBSOYT formula (you cannot sell safety by sitting on your tail). Active involvement and participation by management, health workers and workers are the key factors to success for accident prevention.

4.20 BIBLIOGRAPHY

Arkles, R. S. 1985. *The social consequences of industrial accidents— dissertation series No. 7.* University of the Witwatersrand.

Bever, D. L. 1984 *Safety: a personal focus.* St Louis: Mosby.

Bird, F. J. 1976. *Management guide to loss control.* Atlanta: Institute Press.

Broder, J. F. 1984. *Risks analysis and the security survey.* Stoneham: Butterworths.

Brown, M. L. 1981. *Occupational health nursing.* New York: Springer.

Brune, D. K. and Edling, C. 1989. *Occupational hazards in the health professions.* Florida: C. R. C. Press.

Karvonen, M. (ed.) 1986. *Epidemiology of occupational health.* World Health Organizations, European Series.

McDonald, N. 1984. *Fatigue, safety and the truck driver.* London: Taylor and Francis.

Moore, C. J. and Allott, R. V. 1981. *Industrial safety.* London: Heinemann.

NOSADATA: 1991 of Samtrac Course.

Rogers, R. and Salvage, J. 1988. *Nurses at risk, a guide to health and safety at work.* London: Heinemann.

Schröder, H. H. E. and Schoeman, J. J. 1989. *Inleiding tot beroepshigiëne.* Johannesburg: OHASA.

Strauss, S. A. (6th ed.) 1987. *Legal handbook for nurses and health personnel.* Cape Town: King Edward VII Trust.

Chapter 5: Occupational Hygiene

by A. J. Kotze

5.1 INTRODUCTION

Although it is probable that the harmful effects of exposure to toxic substances in the workplace which can result in disease and death among workers, have been known for over two thousand years, means of controlling the hazards of the workplace were not available during the earlier periods of industrial development. Knowledge of the toxicity of materials is also late.

Cralley and Cralley say that the devotion of prime attention to the preventive aspects of worker health maintenance through controlling health hazards which are job-associated becomes evident if the best interest of the worker is to be served in the prevention of occupational diseases. Efforts towards an active recognition, measurement, evaluation, and pro-active control of workplace environmental health hazards did not develop until the turn of this century (1985:1).

5.2 LEARNING OBJECTIVES

At the end of this section the reader should be able to:
- define the concept of occupational hygiene
- identify the following:
  — basic components of occupational hygiene
  — cornerstones of an occupational hygiene programme
- recognize occupationally-related diseases
- classify and describe the occupational hazards and prevention thereof
- discuss the role and functions of the occupational health nurse in occupational hygiene

5.3 DEFINITION OF OCCUPATIONAL HYGIENE

Occupational hygiene is an applied science which encompasses the application of information from a variety of sciences such as chemistry, engineering, biology, mathematics, medicine, physics, and toxicology.

The American Industrial Hygiene Association defines industrial hygiene as:

The science and art devoted to
- the recognition, evaluation, and control of those environmental factors or stresses,
- arising in or from the workplace,
- which may cause sickness, impaired health and well-being, or
- significant discomfort and inefficiency among workers or among the citizens of a community (Cralley and Cralley, 1985:14).

5.4 THE RATIONALE OF OCCUPATIONAL HYGIENE

Occupational hygiene practice is based upon the following principles:
- environmental health hazards in the workplace can be measured quantitavely, and expressed in terms related to the degree of stress caused;
- hazards in the workplace usually show a dose-response relationship;
- the human body has an intricate mechanism for protection against invasion of hostile stresses into the body and deals with the stress agents when invasion has occurred;
- levels of exposure to specific stress agents should be kept within safe limits;
- continuous surveillance of the work environment and the worker should be carried out to ensure a healthy workplace.

5.5 THE BASIC COMPONENTS AND CORNERSTONES OF AN OCCUPATIONAL HYGIENE PROGRAMME

5.5.1 Components The main purpose of any occupational hygiene programme is to ensure a workplace which is safe for the worker. This requires a programme with a multidisciplinary approach. It must be designed around the nature of the operations, documented to preserve a sound retrospective record, and executed in a professional manner (Cralley and Cralley, 1985:16).

A basic programme should include the following:

- continuous data-collection for identifying and assessing the level of the hazards at the workplace;
- participation in a periodic review of worker exposure and health records to detect new hazards and assess old ones;
- a data storage system that will permit the retrieval of information to assess the long-term effect of exposures;
- assuring the relevancy of the data being collected;
- an integrated programme which will enhance the establishment of appropriate current control, and instituting new measures when indicated.

5.5.2 The cornerstones of an occupational hygiene programme

Various authors identify the following essential steps as cornerstones for such a programme:

- A first walk-through-survey of the workplace to recognize health hazards. During this survey a flow-diagram is drawn up which should contain the following information:
  — raw materials used and products made;
  — all by-products which are formed during the manufacturing process;
  — the manufacturing process, and associated dangers;
  — the general work environment.
- Proper identification of on-the-job health hazards, taking into consideration the following important factors:
  — threshold values of hazards;
  — results of over exposure to hazards;
  — available literature studies of similar hazards;
  Problem-areas are identified on the flow diagram (Schröder and Schoeman, 1989:9).
- Data evaluation, which should include the following information:
  — stress factors;
  — identification of dangerous areas;
  — monitoring to determine the extent of exposure;
  — indications of number of workers and the time spent in the area;
  — interpretation of results obtained.
- Environmental control must be applied and adhered to. Continuous control is necessary to ensure the success of control measures applied. General control measures such as the following can be applied:
  — the selection of workers through pre-employment examination;
  — control at the source;
  — control on the road of transfer;
  — control at the point where worker is placed;
  — improved working environment;
  — good housekeeping and education of workers (Schröder and Schoeman, 1989:11).

5.6 LEGISLATIVE CONTROL

It was only after the publication of the report of the Erasmus Commission in 1975, that occupational hygiene received the emphasis it deserves. This was made possible with the promulgation of The Machinery and Occupational Safety Act, No 6 of 1983 and a subsequent blue print.

In South Africa numerous other Acts indirectly contribute to the control of the environment e.g.:

• The Atmospheric Pollution Prevention Act, No 45 of 1965;
• The Hazardous Substances Act, No 15 of 1973;
• The Water Act, No 54 of 1956.

5.7 RECOGNIZING OCCUPATIONALLY-RELATED DISEASES

The causal or associative connection between a person's work and his ill-health, may be easily recognized in some cases, while in others it may present great difficulties. A short interval of time elapsing between cause and effect makes diagnosis less difficult but many occupationally-related diseases develop only after long periods of exposure, or the relationship between cause and effect may be chance.

The following *features* may be of help when trying to establish the nature of the relationship between the worker and hazards in the work environment:

• The strength of the association—do the observed features occur in everyone, in a large number of people, or only in a few of the people working with the substance?
• Consistency—how consistent have the findings been?
• Specificity—is the disease specific to a group of people, a worksite or type of work?
• Relationship in time—the time the disease takes to become manifest in a group of affected people may help to make the diagnosis clear.
• Biological gradient—the dose-response relationship gives important information in relation to the cause or association.
• Biological plausibility and coherence—all possibilities should be examined, even if they seem implausible.
• Experimental proof—it may be possible to prove causal connections.
• Argument by analogy—when investigating a problem it may be possible to draw an analogy between previously caused disease by a related substance and the one under scrutiny (Gardner and Taylor, 1975:63–4).

5.8 HOW SUBSTANCES CAN CAUSE HARMFUL EFFECTS TO THE HUMAN BODY

It seems ethically correct that every person should be told the truth about the hazards of the job he has to do, as well as the dangers of the substances he may be required to handle while doing his job. To conceal these facts may in the long-term be more harmful to the health of the worker and the worker-employer relationship. 'Men and women who are not told of the dangers in their working environment are deprived of information which they should use to protect themselves and become, as it were, children in unsafe environments. This is wrong.' (Gardner and Taylor, 1975:66.) In order to produce biological harm, a substance must gain access to, or be in contact with the body.

The *main routes of entry* into the body are:

- Inhalation: Vapour, gas, fumes, mist, spray, or dust can be breathed in.
- Ingestion: The swallowing of poisons by eating or smoking with unwashed hands which may be contaminated with a poisonous substance.
- Through the intact skin: Some chemical substances can gain access to the body even through an intact skin.
- Injection: This route is not very common in the work situation.

5.9 THE CLASSIFICATION AND DISCUSSION OF OCCUPATIONAL HAZARDS

An intimate knowledge of plant/occupational processes and procedures is essential in any meaningful control programme. The occupational hazards are generally classified into the following main groups: Chemical hazards; Physical hazards; Mechanical hazards; Biological hazards; Psychological hazards.

5.9.1 Chemical These are classified as arising from:
hazards

Dust   — which consists of solid particles, usually arising from processes such as crushing, grinding, detonation, impact, precipitation or drying. Inhalation of dust may lead to a variety of lung conditions, or general poisoning.

Fumes   — are finely particulate solids which arise by condensation from a vapour (often after a metal has become molten). The fumes are usually the oxide of a particular metal, and are highly toxic.

Gases   — which are a formless fluid which can occupy the space of enclosure. Gas can be changed to a liquid or solid by a combination of increased pressure and decreased temperature. Gases are usually irritating to the eyes, nose and mouth, and people will try to escape when exposed. (Carbon monoxide, however, has no smell and leads to loss of consciousness.)

Vapours— are the gases given off by a substance. Examples of vapours are solvent or petroleum vapours.

The *chemical hazards can also be classified* according to their *toxicological effects* on the human body, e.g.:

- *Irritants* affect different parts of the respiratory system
- *Asphyxiants* which obstruct the oxidation process in the tissues;
- *Narcotics* and analgesics which affect the central nervous system;
- *Carcinogenics* leading to a variety of malignant conditions;
- *Mutagenics* affecting the genetic structure in the body;
- *Teratogenics* which may cause abnormalities in the unborn foetus;
- *Systemic poisons* which may affect the body as a whole;

● *Dangerous dust* particles causing fibrosis, allergies and irritations.

Today, there are many thousands of *types of chemicals* on the market. The principles of dealing with any occupational hazard should be applied when dealing with these.

Manufacturer's literature can be a valuable source of information for the occupational nurse when examining these. It should specify the

— effects of exposure;
— chemical contents;
— precautions which must be observed when handling the substance;
— first aid treatment, should exposure occur.

The absorption of harmful substances in the body

The respiratory system

In the occupational situation, absorption via the respiratory system is probably the most important hazard.

Gaseous substances when inhaled are absorbed into the bloodstream, and spread through the body. The eventual dosage of gas absorbed and accumulated in the body will depend upon:

— air concentration;
— solubility of the substance;
— time of exposure;
— respiratory and circulatory tempo;
— biochemical reactivity of the substance.

Volatile substances absorbed via the respiratory system may also be absorbed into the digestive system if particles are swallowed when deposited in the nose and throat.

The skin

Substances may be absorbed through an intact skin. Absorption may take place through the epidermal layer or through the hair follicles.

Broken skin provides a direct route for substances to penetrate the body. Special mention is made when determining the Threshold Limit Values (TLV) to provide for substances which may be absorbed via the air and skin.

The digestive system

This method of contamination is not very common. It usually occurs when a substance is accidentally swallowed, or the worker drinks or smokes with contaminated hands. Should he cough up contaminated material and swallow it, it will be absorbed.

The result of the absorption of toxic materials

The toxicity of substances

This can be described as the inherent characteristic of a substance to cause harmful effects when coming in contact with or entering the body.

The toxicity of substances varies considerably, and for this purpose a standardized system was developed to measure and compare toxic levels of substances.

Schröder and Schoeman use the term median-lethal dose or LD_{50} and describe it as the statistically calculated amount of a substance needed to kill 50 % of a countable population, or a randomly selected sample of experimental animals (1989: 25).

The LD_{50} is usually expressed in the weight of the substance per unit of the body mass—the most commonly used unit is mg/kg. The smaller the mg value of the toxic substance, the higher the toxicity. The following generally applies to this rating:

- compounds with an LD of more than 5 000 mg/kg are non-poisonous;
- compounds with a slight toxicity have an LD of between 1 000 and 2 000 mg/kg;
- a moderately poisonous substance will have an LD of between 100 and 1 000 mg/kg;
- compounds with a high toxicity have an LD of below 100 mg/kg.

In South Africa a classification system is used to indicate the potential toxicity of a substance ranging from class I to IV, where class I indicates the highly toxic substances, and class IV those substances with no toxicity. Class I contains pesticides such as DDT, parathion and aldikarb (see The Hazardous Substances Act).

Measurement of chemical hazards

The measurement and assessment of chemical contaminants in industry is essential for the evaluation of such hazards. The following are standards used in industry for the evaluation of risks:

- Threshold Limit Values (TLVs)

  This is the average concentration in air of substances, which are normally harmless on prolonged exposure. The TLVs of a large number of industrial materials used in industry are known.

  The Threshold Limit Value should be regarded as a guide only to the control of risks, and is used as a communication tool between physicians, engineers and hygienists who design control equipment.

  These values represent a time-weighted average concentration above which excursions may usually be permitted, provided they are compensated for by equivalent excursions below the limit (Schilling 1973:290).

- Maximum Allowable Concentrations (MACs)

  These are used to indicate levels not to be exceeded. Both TLVs and MACs are based on the dose-response effects of human or animal exposure for each substance.

- Emergency Exposure Limits (EELs)

  These are used to calculate risks from large scale accidental air pollution. They are used in two ways:
  — to estimate risks to individual rescue workers;
  — to anticipate the risks to the community in the vicinity of the accident.

  (Use is made of reversible effects for short exposure to high concentrations.)

Please take note that very many more standards and measurements are used in the calculation of the exposure, toxicity and effects of substances which cannot be taken up in this publication, because of their specialized nature. The reader is advised to consult additional literature on occupational hygiene if further information is required.

5.9.2   **Physical** These are sometimes thought to be of less importance than the
         hazards chemical hazards, but this is not so. Physical hazards can cause severe injuries or disease, sometimes of a less tangible nature, but should not be underrated and overlooked.

The nature of physical hazards is varied, but the following are examples of those which are most common:

5.9.2.1   *Radiation* **Ionizing radiations**

These are divided into four main types:

- *Alpha* particles, which can only penetrate human tissue to the depth of one-tenth of a millimetre. Irradiation is limited to the immediate vicinity of the source.
- *Beta* rays exhibit various energies. They penetrate a few millimetres into human tissue before being absorbed.
- *Gamma and X-rays* are electromagnetic radiations of varying levels of energy. They often have a high penetration potential, and can irradiate all parts of the body uniformly.
- *Neutrons* are uncharged particles with a wide range of energy and power of penetration.

Radiation may take place from inside or outside the body. In industry, external radiation may occur, for example, from sealed sources, or from X-ray machines. Internal radiation can take place when breathing in or swallowing radio-active material.

The biological effect of exposure to radiation

The effect of the radiation on the human tissue is characterized by the following reaction phases:

- ionization (takes place very rapidly);
- physical-chemical reaction (as above);
- chemical reaction (may last for seconds);
- biological manifestation of the cell damage (this may last for minutes to years).

Cell damage may include:

- destruction of cells;
- delay in the cell division;
- alteration of the inherent cell structure (Schröder and Schoeman 1989:184).

Amount of cell/tissue damage will depend upon factors such as:

- the energy absorbed into the tissue;
- per unit mass of tissue;
- the dose and time of exposure (Gardner and Taylor 1975: 98–9).

The measurement of radiation exposure

The following are a few of the units used to describe radiation exposure:

RAD (radiation absorbed dose) 0.01J/kg

RBE (relative biological effectiveness)

1 for X-ray, gamma and beta sources
1 for X-ray, gamma and beta sources
2.5 for thermal neutrons
10 for alpha particles and fast neutrons

REM (radiation equivalent man) RAD × RBE

Ci (Curie) is the unit of source strength or activity of a radio-active substance, and is equivalent to 3.7×10^{10} disintegrations/sec. It is used in the evaluation of control requirements and in measurement of contaminants (Schilling 1978: 271).

Norms for radiation control

The following recommendations of The International Commission on Radiological Protection are internationally accepted as basic for protection:

— exposure of individuals to radiation must be in terms of the advantages of the work done;
— exposure must be optimized, and kept as low as possible;
— exposure limits may not be exceeded.

The measurement of radiation and radiation protection

Levels of radiation must be measured and recorded for individuals potentially exposed to radiation, so that the exposure dose can be compared with the recommended permissible doses. The common method used for recording doses of radiation is by means of individual film badges and dosimeters. These must be worn at all times, in an area of the body where most radiation is likely to occur. The records of radiation of an individual must go with him when changing jobs, otherwise his cumulative exposure will not be known (Gardner and Taylor, 1975:100).

The control of internal radiation can only take place by preventing the intake through:

— zoning and control of working areas;
— prevention of the spread of activities to uncontrolled areas;
— the provision of suitable handling facilities and environmental control;
— the use of protective clothing and equipment (Schröder and Schoeman 1989: 187).

National control of radiation in South Africa

Various semi and Government Departments are responsible for the application of Legislation in this regard:

the Atomic Energy Corporation for The Nuclear Energy Act, No 92 of 1982, (all the nuclear plants must be licensed with this department); the Department of National Health and Population Development, for The Hazardous Substances Act, No 15 of 1973, (licensing of all electronic equipment which emits radiation is done by this department).

Non-ionizing radiations

Many industrial processes make use of, or produce relatively intense radiant energy sources. Examples of these are welding, cutting, heating and wireless communication (Schilling 1973: 266). Non-ionizing radiation may be considered in four ranges of wave-length:

Ultraviolet radiation, and visible light

This can affect the skin, causing various degrees of sunburn. The incidence of skin cancer in the exposed areas of the skin is higher in people who are continuously exposed to the sun e.g. farmers, and labourers.

Conjunctivitis can also be caused by ultraviolet light—these conditions are commonly called arc eyes or welder's flash. All visible light sources, such as machines and electronic equipment, produce some infra-red emission.

Infra-red radiation

All hot bodies radiate heat. It is felt on the skin as heat, and will activate the normal mechanisms in the body to protect the skin from burning. This is, however, not the case in the eye, where damaging amounts of radiation can be suffered, without feeling the heat. Repeated exposure can cause cataracts, commonly known as glass blower's cataract. Various other types of eye injuries may also occur in severe and prolonged exposure e.g. retinal burns.

Laser beams

The name derives from light amplification by stimulated emission of radiation. It is a beam of light energy of one length, and uniform in phase, which travels together in step and in rhythm. The dangers of laser are inherent in the power or energy density of the beam. Even with a 1% reflectance from a dark surface, the light can be potentially hazardous to exposed skin or eyes (Schilling, 1973: 268).

Protection is based on avoidance of the beam and its reflection, which can be obtained by having non-reflective black surfaces to cut down on the reflection in rooms where these beams are used.

Microwaves and radiofrequency waves

Microwaves produce heat which is a great deal more penetrating than infra-red radiation. An internationally agreed upon safe exposure limit for microwaves is 10 milliwatts/square cm. Interlocks on oven doors are necessary to ensure that radiation ceases when the door is opened.

Waves shorter than 10 cm are absorbed within the skin (e.g. infra-red); 10–30 cm waves are absorbed mostly by subcutaneous fat, whilst the waves of 30 cm and longer penetrate into deeper muscular tissues. For this reason the longer waves provide the main risks as they are absorbed into deeper tissue, without giving the warning sensation of heat.

The cornea and the lens of the eye is again at risk due to the lack of blood supply to these tissues which can dissipate the heat of the waves.

5.9.2.2   Noise and hearing conservation   Noise is often accepted as inevitable in industry, but to the health worker this is an important hazard which may pose a threat to the health of the employees.

In order to understand the effect of sound/noise on the human body, the occupational nurse should be familiar with the following terms:

Sound

'Whenever a fluctuating disturbance is produced in an elastic medium, such as air, water, metal or plastic, there is a transfer of momentum from one molecule to the next and the disturbance spreads, usually in a spherical manner. As this momentum transfer takes a finite time, the disturbance travels through the medium at a given speed determined by the physical properties of the medium' (Harris, 1984:239–40). The disturbances caused by the displaced air produce sound waves, which, when transferred to the tympanic membrane of the ear, are observed by the sensory organ of the ear as sound.

Sound also displays various characteristics:

— *Soundwaves* vary in length. Generally, high-pitched sounds have short wavelengths, and low-pitched sounds long wavelengths.
— *Sound frequency* is the number of vibrations per second in the sound wave. Audible frequencies range between 15 to 20 000 Herz (Hz). Below 20 Hz frequencies is sensed as vibration in solid objects.
— *Sound speed* is determined by the transfer of momentum in a specific medium. In air, at a temperature of 21 °C, the speed of sound is 344 meter/second.
— *Sound pressure* is the departure of pressure from the normal ambient (surrounding) pressure in the atmosphere, and is expressed in Newtons/m^2.
— The *intensity of sound wave* transmission is related to the pressure changes in the medium. A large range of sound pressures is encountered in everyday life, and to measure this a decibel scale is used (dB). Exposure to sound intensities of 90dB and higher over prolonged periods can lead to permanent deafness (Harris, 1984:239).
— *Sound power* is emitted by any sound source, and this can be measured in watts. As the sound power is influenced by many external factors, it is a physical characteristic only used to compare sound sources.

Noise in industry

Sound waves usually spread out uniformly through the air. At a reasonable distance from the source, the average noise intensity is proportional to sound pressure squared, which gives us the familiar inverse square law. When applied, this law shows that the pressure in a sound wave reduces by six dB with each doubling of distance from the source to a receiver (Harris, 1984:243).

The application of various mathematical calculations show that:

— sound intensity decreases with the inverse square, proportional to the distance from the sound source;
— the sound pressure of a wavelength decreases in direct relation to the distance of the sound source.

The measurement of noise

Various instruments and techniques are available to measure noise. Although these devices may provide useful data on whether or not there is a possible risk of annoyance or hearing damage, the definition of hearing risk itself is dependent on a knowledge of how much acoustic energy has entered the ear.

The human ear responds in a non-uniform way to different sound-pressure levels—the perceived intensity/loudness may differ from person to person, and for this purpose a weighting curve has been constructed (A). Sound-pressure levels are then expressed in dB(A), which conforms to the weighting curve, and reflects the perception of that sound emission by the normal human ear. (Gardner and Taylor, 1975:103).

Types of noise

Din

This is the most common type of noise experienced in everyday life e.g. sound of cars, typewriters, music etc. It consists of a wide variety of frequencies in the audible range between 20–20 000 Hz. We need to hear sound to give us information about our environment, but above a certain din, sound becomes noise.

Ultrasonic sound

This type of sound has frequencies higher than the audible range, and is experienced as vibrations. These can easily be shielded or absorbed and the control of this does not really present undue difficulty in industry.

Infrasonic sound

This is the noise below 20 Hz frequencies, and although it loses tonal qualities below 16 Hz, it is now believed that infrasonic noise is audible, and produces physiological effects such as changes in breathing, heart rhythms and disturbances in the functioning of the central nervous system.

Conventional ear protection is ineffective in attenuating infrasonic sound. Because of the physiological effects of this sound, whole body protection should be provided (Harris, 1984:249).

Impulse noise

Sudden impact noise, such as a gun shot or any type of industrial noise, may cause instantaneous hearing damage. These noises are characterized by discrete pulses of sound pressure, which have a sharp instantaneous rise in sound pressure.

Other unpleasant physiological reactions may also take place as a result of sudden unexpected noise e.g. a rise in blood pressure. increased pulse rate, and headaches.

Temporary threshold shift (TTS)

This condition in the hearing organ appears directly after exposure to excessive noise, and may last for a few minutes only or continue for a few days, depending on the kind of exposure. Physiologically this condition of temporary deafness can be explained as a metabolic disturbance in the cochlear cells of the inner ear caused by vasoconstriction of the local capillary vessels. This leads to a temporary shortage of oxygen to the organ of Corti and the auditory nerve cells.

When the noise exposure stops, the bloodflow of the inner ear returns to normal, and hearing with it. Recovery is highest when the exposure did not exceed many hours, and the ears are given a sufficient rest period before the next exposure takes place.

Permanent threshold shift (PTS)

Prolonged exposure to noise which causes a TTS, will lead to permanent damage. The physiology of this process is not quite clear, but according to Schröder and Schoeman, it appears as though prolonged exposure causes metabolic changes in the auditory receptor cells and nerves which eventually leads to degenerative damage to the cell structure.

This kind of damage leads to senso-neural deafness, which is non-reversible (1989:224–5).

Non-auditory effects

This includes a variety of symptoms such as:
— emotional effects e.g. irritability, stress and fatigue;
— physiological effects e.g. changes in sleeping pattern, increased excretion of adrenaline, lack of concentration, disturbances of the balance organ leading to dizziness, nausea, and sight disturbances.

Noise control

For the purposes of noise control in the workplace, the following methods are applied:
● modification of the noise radiation pattern;
● noise suppression;
● noise reduction;
● noise avoidance.
Although this is not the direct function of the occupational health nurse to introduce these measures, she should be familiar with them.

Modification of the noise radiation pattern

Noise is highly directional, and it is therefore possible to shield and reflect noise so that it can only be heard after it has struck some sound-absorbent surface.

Movable screens of absorbent material, and an absorbent ceiling covering can do much to reduce personal noise exposure.

Noise suppression

This may be achieved by introducing noise-absorbing physical barriers and/or enclosing machines which emit noise.

Noise reduction

Many mechanical processes used in industry produce noise e.g. cutting, hammering and vibration. For technical reasons these actions cannot be omitted, but with moderate additional costs, these processes can be made quieter. The fitting of dampers to machines may greatly reduce the noise emitted.

Noise avoidance

The changing of noise-emitting processes for equipment which emits low noise levels can reduce this hazard. Equipment must also be properly maintained if it is to remain quiet.

The Hearing Conservation Programme

Well organized, meaningful hearing conservation programmes, accepted and endorsed by management with the necessary supporting company policy, is an essential element in the control of this health hazard.

An effective programme should contain the following objectives:
- the prevention of noise-induced deafness;
- a decrease in noise interference with communication;
- legal compliance;
- a decrease in company expenditure for deafness compensation.

Steps in the organization of a programme

Schröder and Schoeman say that the primary responsibility for a hearing conservation programme rests with line management (1989: 232).

Organization of programme

A specific person should be responsible for the co-ordination of the total programme. This person may make use of the expertise of various specialists e.g. engineers, architects, health personnel and the administrative services.

Each worker should, however, also take responsibility for his or her own health and must be familiar with regulations and the dangers of noise exposure.

Effective policy and legislation

The Machinery and Occupational Safety Act, No 6 of 1983, makes provision for the safety of the worker. Regulations published under this Act, specify that workers may not be exposed to noise levels equal or above 85dB(A) in the workplace. Where these conditions do exist, specific conditions are prescribed for the control and/or protection of worker.

Hearing protection for workers must be provided free of cost.

Identification of noise areas

These areas must be accurately assessed and controlled. This can be achieved by monitoring through:
— Noise survey

Management and health personnel should take part in the assessment of noise in the workplace. The nature of the noise, its character e.g. frequency, type etc. must be established to design cost-effective measures for reducing the hazard.

— Pre-placement checks
During the pre-placement medical screening process, it is important that some form of hearing assessment be done. The person's hearing acuity should be assessed in view of job placement, and future hearing conservation.

— Pre-placement audiometry
Through the use of audiometry the effects of noise on a person's hearing can be measured. The person to be tested is placed in a quiet room, wearing headphones. Sound is produced in a pure tone, at measurable levels, to one ear at a time.

At the start of the test, the tone is played at a sound pressure level too quiet to hear. The level is slowly increased, until it is audible to the person tested, whereupon the level is again decreased to an inaudible level. The hearing threshold of the person is established at a particular level. The process is carried on for each ear at various frequencies and graphically recorded. This method provides for a course screening of a person's hearing.

— Serial audiometry
Where noise problems do exist, self-recording apparatus may be used for audiometry carried out at agreed intervals.

— Noise control
Control measures established for a dynamic conservation programme should be based upon the assessment of problem areas, and should include the following:

• principles of occupational standards;
• standards for the purchasing of equipment and design specifications;
• effective educational programmes.

Engineering departments contribute towards this programme by giving attention to the design of plants and machinery to be used; and the administration department can in turn control the exposure of workers through changes in production programmes, and the rotation of shifts of exposed workers.

The last and most important method used in noise control is the wearing of personal protective equipment. This will be discussed in a later chapter.

The role of the occupational health nurse in hearing conservation

The occupational nurse must be familiar with all aspects of noise and the hearing mechanism to enable her to play a meaningful role in the programme. Although hearing conservation is a team effort where many members and employees play an important part, the nurse is the person in the occupational setting who has a direct input when it comes to health matters.

Education and motivation of employers and employees forms an integral part of a successful hearing conservation programme and it is also in this area that the nurse intervenes.

The following are examples of areas where the occupational health nurse plays a role:

— noise measurement in the workplace; health surveillance of the worker; treatment of the affected worker;

— her role as educator enables her to take part in the health education of workers to educate them about the dangers of noise exposure and motivate them to take part in all activities instituted to protect hearing;

— as an administrator, she will maintain the necessary documentation so that an accurate record system of the worker's health is available.

The functions of the occupational health nurse in hearing conservation

Details of her job description may vary from one industry to another, but the following basic functions are usually required from the nurse in industry:

— observation of noisy areas, and comparing noise levels with the legislative requirements;

— liaison with management when reported levels are a health hazard;

— negotiation with management for a control programme if necessary;

— familiarization with actions taken to reduce risks, and actions for the application of ear protection; observation as to whether protection is worn;

— periodic visits to the workplace to consult with managers, and observation of the procedures applied to protect hearing;

— if she is involved in audiometry, she should ensure that tests are done regularly, and the line management notified on time; results should be discussed and used as an educational tool (Harris, 1984: 265), pre-employment and periodic screening of workers for hearing defects.

5.9.2.3 Lighting and **Lighting**
vision The complex technological developments of the last few decades set visual requirements which necessitate the assessment of the visual abilities of individual workers for specific jobs prior to job placement and also during the period of employment.

Light rays are emitted from various sources, and consist of rays of various lengths. Without light, vision is not possible. Proper lighting in the workplace will have numerous advantages, such as:

— saving of human energy, because poor lighting leads to fatigue;
— a decrease in the accident risk rate;
— the possibility of higher production;
— possible improvement in the work conditions;
— possible prevention of a decrease in production because of mistakes made in poor lighting;
— in general, the promotion of the efficient use of human and other resources.

Light for work purposes is mainly obtained from two sources:

● natural lighting e.g. sunlight rays;
● artificial lighting obtained from e.g. electrical sources.

The ways in which the above are utilized will determine effectivity.

The regulations published under the Machinery and Occupational Safety Act, No 6 of 1983 lay down specific requirements for lighting in emergency situations.

Sight Safety and visual protection programmes

Very many occupational accidents cause injury to the eyes, and it is important that these hazards be recognized and controlled.

Eye injuries are mainly caused by:

Burns

These can be chemical, thermal or radiation burns.

- Chemical acid burns cause rapid opacification of the corneal epithelium.
- Alkaline burns are deeply penetrating and the alkalinity may pass into the anterior chamber and cause deep-seated inflammatory conditions.
- Thermal burns may cause contracture of the lids, shrinkage of the conjunctiva, and corneal ulceration. These are slow to heal and often lead to permanent scarring of the cornea.
- Radiation injuries may be caused by any kind of radiation e.g. ultraviolet, infra-red or emissions from laser sources. Ultraviolet radiation may cause inflammation of the lids, conjunctiva and cornea; infra-red rays cause damage to the choroid, iris, ciliary body and retina. Prolonged exposure may cause cataracts. Laser radiation may cause retinal burns and choroidal damage.

Mechanical injuries

Small projectiles (foreign bodies) are the most common cause of mechanical injuries, and may lead to a variety of injuries depending upon the type of injury, nature of projectile and the tissue involved. Subconjunctival haemorrhages, corneal and conjunctival abrasions as well as extensive trauma may be caused by foreign bodies.

Penetrating injuries

Penetrating foreign bodies may cause rupture of and displacement of the inner structures of the eyes. If the foreign body is retained in the eye after penetration further complications such as inflammatory conditions may occur. All penetrating injuries must be referred to a doctor.

Visual protection

The use of goggles as eye protection cannot ensure total safety, but it should form part of a comprehensive protection programme.

Visual Welfare programme

Comprehensive programmes to ensure the visual welfare of employees is a fairly recent development in occupational health. Such a programme can bring about considerable advantages for both the employer and employee, e.g.

— improved quality and quantity of products manufactured;
— reduction in accident rates;
— collection of data on the visual level of the employee before and during employment, so that placement and problems can be detected and followed up.

Visual welfare programmes should be organized by a health team member who is a suitably trained person to carry out tasks such as screening, e.g. the occupational health nurse, with referral to an ophthalmic practitioner if necessary. This kind of programme should contain the following elements:

- Visual task analysis—e.g. lighting, distance of task, contrast, movement, colour recognition, duration of task and hazards involved.
- Lighting—e.g. minimum levels required for specific tasks.
- Distance of task—this is the working distance of all tasks, which may be: teloramic (more than 2 metres away) mesoramic (between 2 metres and 30 cm) ancoramic (less than 30 cm).
- Size of task—refers to the object, e.g. small, very small, medium, large.
- Contrast—determined by the degree of contrast between different light sensations, e.g. colour contrast, brightness and texture.
- Movement—movable objects make the perception of that object more difficult and require a high degree of visual acuity.
- Definition and legibility.
- Job detail—an analysis of each job is required to determine the visual requirements.
- Colour recognition—some tasks require a good colour perception, e.g. operators of machinery, marking of types of material.
- Duration of task should be noted, as prolonged performance may require some form of aid.

5.9.2.4 *Extreme temperatures* The human body has a very sensitive temperature control mechanism, which keeps the body temperature at a normal level, even though the skin temperature can vary considerably. Heat is generated in the body by the chemical processes of metabolism.

Temperature alone should not be considered in isolation, as there are many parameters concerned in the transfer of heat, e.g.

- *Radiation:* all materials absorb and emit radiant energy, some have low and others high emission rates. Matt surfaces will radiate less heat than highly polished metal surfaces.
- *Conduction:* this kind of heat transfers through material, and escapes into the environment. Poor conductors of heat are used to maintain acceptable thermal environments in extremely cold temperatures, for example.
- *Convection:* heat exchange from the human body is proportional to the square root of the wind speed.
- *Evaporation:* under normal environmental conditions, the evaporation of sweat from the body removes heat, and lowers the body temperature. This is influenced by the vapour pressure gradient between skin and ambient air, and the wet bulb temperature of ambient air. Evaporation can only take place if the temperature is below the body temperature. The air humidity describes the quantity of water vapour the air contains, and this must be linked to the air temperature to be of value in determining evaporation.

It is said that people can become acclimatized to heat. The body adapts to extreme conditions with the necessary accompanying physiological responses. This will, however, not be applicable in continuous exposure to extreme conditions for prolonged periods of time, as it may still lead to failure of the human body to make the required changes.

Heat illness

This term is used to describe the failure of the body to adjust to heat stress, and it may manifest in two ways:

- *Excessive salt loss* in sweat, with insufficient salt intake by mouth to replace it. This usually occurs when strenuous work is done in hot conditions. The term *heat exhaustion* is used for this condition. *Symptoms* are:
  — undue tiredness;
  — nausea;
  — muscle cramps;
  — collapse.
- *A rise in body temperature* due to failure of the normal cooling mechanisms of the body. This is common in extremely high temperatures. The term heat stroke is used for this condition. *Symptoms* are:
  — temperature of 40°C and higher;
  — convulsions;
  — coma and death.

Prevention of heat illness

- people exposed to such conditions at work should be physically fit and preferably acclimatized;
- an adequate intake of salt and water must be maintained (this may be as high as 15 litres of fluid and 30 gm of salt per day), one gram of salt can be added to a litre of fruit squash without affecting the taste;
- loose fitting and permeable clothing (cotton), but clothing should also be dense enough to protect from radiant heat where applicable;
- when exposure to radiant heat also takes place, resting periods in a cooled area at frequent intervals;
- physical exertion should be kept to a minimum, this is necessary to reduce internal heat production.

Cold environments

Outdoor occupations such as fishing and farming, and indoor conditions such as cold stores are often undertaken in extremely cold conditions.

The general effects of *extreme cold conditions* are:

- excessive heat loss from the body, with a fall in temperature;
- shivering (which is the body's normal reaction to try and increase heat production by muscular activity);
- local damage to fingers, toes and nose, known as frost-bite, which is the freezing of the tissues. The end result is similar to a burn.

Prevention of cold stress

- careful selection of work people (people with physical characteristics such as moderate fat and a muscular build seem to do better);
- protective clothing to insulate the body;
- wind and waterproof outerclothing which is also permeable to allow sweat to evaporate;
- special protection for extremities e.g. hands and feet;

- if the period of exposure is continuous, time for rest must be allowed in sufficiently heated rooms, with warm refreshments provided to stimulate metabolism (see NOSA requirements).

For the treatment of these conditions, refer to the chapter on emergency treatment.

5.9.2.5 Abnormal atmospheric pressure

High air pressures

This is a condition experienced by people working in areas of compressed air e.g. in tunnelling, diving and in caissons. The effect of abnormal atmospheric pressure is:

- an increase in the amount of air dissolved in the blood and body fluids;
- on rapid return to normal pressure levels, gas is released in the form of bubbles. These contain nitrogen. The bubbles can cause *decompression sickness*.

An ascent of 5 500 metres into the air is required to halve the atmospheric pressure, but a descent into only 10 metres of water doubles it. Every additional 10 metres adds another 1 kg of pressure per cm^2.

The change in the pressure of inspired air causes physiological disturbances because the effect of a gas is determined by its partial pressure. At a depth of 30 m the partial pressure of carbon monoxide is four times that at the surface. The major constituents of air, namely oxygen and nitrogen, also present problems in the form of nitrogen narcosis which can incapacitate divers. The increase in air density with depth means that more energy is required for respiration, and as the maximum breathing capacity is reduced, carbon dioxide retention occurs.

The amount of nitrogen dissolving in body tissues is proportional to its partial pressure, solubility coefficient and duration of exposure to pressure.

Four hours is considered to be the time it takes to saturate the tissues, and workers should be decompressed after a four to eight hour shift (Schilling, 1973: 284).

The reduction of pressure during decompression leads to:

- the expansion of the air in sinuses, ears and lungs;
- trapped excess air in the lung may expand and burst through:
  — the pleura to produce air pneumothorax;
  — into the lung to produce emphysema;
  — into the vascular system resulting in arterial air embolism.

Symptoms of decompression sickness

- pain in or near a joint;
- disturbances of the respiratory function e.g. shortness of breath, pain in the chest, coughing or collapse.

Prevention

- workers must be medically examined before work in compressed air areas starts. Regular surveillance is necessary.
- a person with a cold or respiratory infection should not be compressed or recompressed, as this may give rise to serious ear damage;

- the wearing of identification tags to indicate the area of work and the location of the nearest decompression chamber, for use in the case of decompression sickness.

Low air pressures

Aircraft pilots exposed to high altitudes without pressurized cabins may suffer from the effects of gas bubbles in the tissues.

Lack of oxygen can lead to black-outs, and if the cabin is not pressurized, oxygen masks should be worn.

At high altitudes mountaineers may suffer from hypoxia (above 4 580 m). Common symptoms are headache, lassitude, dyspnoea on exertion, nausea and vomiting. Adaptation to these conditions can take place, usually after 12–24 hours.

5.9.3 Mechanical hazards The invention of machinery in the eighteenth century brought new hazards to the worker. Many of these machines were dangerous and unguarded, and caused mutilation and deformities.

Today, the dangers of mechanical equipment are well understood, although not always treated with the necessary precautions. Legislation exists which prescribes the specific safety precautions required in the use of machinery (the Machinery and Occupational Safety Act, No 6 of 1983).

5.9.3.1 Vibration The increased use of machinery in the occupational environment represents another threat to the health of the worker, in the form of mechanical vibration. When handling or occupying these machines the whole body or certain parts of the body are exposed to the vibration.

Physical characteristics of vibration are:

- frequency and
- intensity.

Frequency is measured in Hz, and in human exposure the frequencies between 0 and 1 000 Hz is important. The intensity of vibration is the maximum displacement of energy from a central point, and is expressed in centimetres.

Sources of vibration are mainly machines and equipment e.g.

- turbines, compressors, electrical pumps, motors—these usually cause whole-body vibration;
- vibrating hand tools such as air pressure drills cause hand-arm vibration.

The extent of exposure to vibration is determined by factors such as:

- body size, posture and strain.

The effect of exposure is determined by the:

- frequency, intensity, time of exposure, direction of vibration and the isolation effect of clothing.

The physiological effect of vibration on the body

Vibrations do not affect all people in the same way—some people can absorb and/or tolerate more than others.

The human body is most sensitive to vibrations between 0,5 and 20 Hz.

The following symptoms may be experienced in the above range:
- general feeling of discomfort, muscle contraction, involuntary desire to urinate and defecate;
- chest pain, abdominal pain and difficulty in breathing;
- changes in heart rate and blood-pressure;
- vertigo and travel sickness;
- vibration may also influence achievement negatively—tasks requiring visual acuity and fine motor co-ordination may be affected.

Localized vibration (e.g. hand-arm system) may give rise to conditions such as:
— osteoarthritis of the bones in the hand;
— soft tissue injuries;
— vascular and sensory disturbances of the limb affected.

Control measures

These usually concentrate on the following methods:
— measures to control the mechanical environment, e.g. adaptation of equipment to lesson vibration exposure; proper maintenance of machinery and the replacement of outdated machines;
— administrative measures which may include the limiting of extended periods of exposure;
— the provision of personal protective equipment, e.g. gloves.

5.9.4   Biological hazards These constitute a particular hazard to people who work in laboratories and health institutions, as bacterial, viral or fungal contamination may occur in pursuance of the occupation. Workers who work with animals or animal products are also exposed to these hazards. Protective measures must be instituted in these work areas.

5.9.5   Psycho-logical hazards The mental health of individuals can be both positively and negatively influenced by their work.
Work situations which are very stressful may lead to mental illness, as well as all the negative influences it has on the human body. It is generally accepted that the following may lead to high levels of stress:
- certain occupations are of such a nature that they lead to stressful situations, e.g. high powered executive jobs; occupations such as the medical and nursing profession; occupations where the worker is exposed to highly dangerous activities like mining, flying, diving, etc.;
- relationships in the work situation may lead to tension and anxiety;
- job dissatisfaction and uncertainty.

5.10 THE ROLE AND FUNCTIONS OF THE OCCUPATIONAL HEALTH NURSE IN THE CONTROL OF THE ENVIRONMENT

Role

The concern of the occupational nurse for the prevention of ill health and the promotion of health in the worker, also means that she will be familiar with the workplace.

Knowledge of the workplace and its processes can only be obtained by investigating all aspects which affect or may be harmful to the employees.

The occupational health nurse must also be familiar with the work individuals are required to undertake.

This role, and the contribution the nurse is able to make in the promotion of productivity, may be a new concept to some employers. The contribution she makes also depends on the policy of the organization and their willingness to commit themselves to an environment which contributes to positive health.

The functions

The nurse in the occupational setting is one of a multidisciplinary team. Her functions therefore cover a wide spectrum of activities which may not be similar to those traditionally ascribed to her in the curative health services.

Brown says that expert occupational health nurses understand and utilize the concept of occupational ecology (1981: 43). The presence of the nurse in the production areas may initially be viewed with apprehension and suspicion, but if her approach is correctly handled through the necessary channels and with tact, she will eventually be accepted, and her functions understood.

Her functions can be described as follows:

- she makes herself aware of the potential hazards that appear in the workplace by doing an environmental survey;
- consciously observes the workers to establish the relationship between health problems and working environment;
- works within an interdisciplinary team—consults with the hygienist, safety professionals, engineers, medical team and management;
- assists in evaluating work procedures to establish their health risk, if any;
- maintains an efficient record system which will ensure complete and accurate data on all workers;
- plans clinic times in such a way that time will be put aside for visits to the plant; a notice giving details of where the nurse can be contacted must be displayed centrally so that she can be reached in times of emergency;
- identifies needs, equipment needed, deficits and problems noticed, and draw up written reports which can be presented to management.

Safety precautions and protective equipment will be discussed in the chapter on occupational safety.

5.11 BIBLIOGRAPHY

Brown, M. L. 1981. *Occupational Health Nursing*. New York: Springer Publishing Company.

Cralley, J. L. & Cralley, L. V. 1985. *Patty's Industrial Hygiene and Toxicology* Volume III. New York: John Wiley & Sons.

Gardner, W. and Taylor, P. 1975. *Health at Work*. London: Associated Business Programmes.

Girdano, D. A. 1986. *Occupational Health Promotion*. New York: Macmillan Publishing Company.

Harris, C. J. 1984. *Occupational Health Nursing Practice*. Bristol: John Wright & Sons Ltd.

Harrison, B. M. 1984. *Essentials of Occupational Health Nursing*. U.S.A.: Blackwell Scientific Publications.

Schilling, R. S. F. 1973. *Occupational Health Practice*. U.K. Butterworths & Co. Ltd.

Schröder, H. H. E. and Schoeman, J. J. 1989. *Inleiding tot Beroepshigiëne*. Goodwood: Nasionale Boekdrukkery.

Chapter 6: Occupational Medicine and Occupational Diseases

by J. T. Mets

6.1 LEARNING OBJECTIVES

At the end of this section the reader should be able to:
— define the concepts of occupational medicine and disease
— identify the main compensatable diseases
— describe the management of selected occupational diseases

6.2 OCCUPATIONAL MEDICINE

Occupational Medicine is concerned with the potential hazards for human health which workers face in their working environment. As part of the wider concept of Occupational Health, Occupational Medicine includes the prevention of and the early recognition of disease, the treatment and rehabilitation of workers and the promotion of health in the workplace. Because people 'bring their health status from home to work' in Occupational Medicine the doctor, nurse or assistant should consider health at work not only in relation to the physical and psychological work environment, but also to the home and community environment from which its clients come.

Occupational Hygiene is the other component of Occupational Health. Environmental and other ergonomic factors in the province of engineers, safety practitioners and health workers are important in Occupational Hygiene. Occupational Medicine is practised by doctors, nurses and their assistants after appropriate additional training and is concerned with man and groups of men defined by occupational characteristics. The objectives of those who practise Occupational Medicine are the prevention and management of medical problems associated with hazards in the workplace. As a medical speciality it is concerned with

'The appraisal, maintenance, restoration and promotion of the health of workers through the application of the principles of preventive and environmental medicine, emergency medical care, clinical medicine and rehabilitation.' (American College of Occupational Medicine)

Clinical medicine, which includes first contact primary health care, remains an integral part of the discipline, with regard to occupational diseases and injuries and to those diseases which prevail in developing countries like South Africa, and also to non-occupational diseases. The discipline rests, in its clinical aspects, on the basic medical sciences of which the most relevant are physiology and anatomy, pathology (in the sense of deviations which the human body and mind show from normal functions and structures) pharmacology, toxicology, biochemistry, immunology and the supporting discipline of epidemiology. Knowledge of clinical and industrial psychology and social science is of course of great value.

Table I shows the main elements of Occupational Medicine as practised in the field and as a component of Occupational Health. Although Occupational Medicine is essentially a clinical discipline, of necessity it incorporates a number of related 'non-clinical' elements.

Some of the elements listed fall under more than one of the 6 main categories reflected in the table.

TABLE I ELEMENTS OF OCCUPATIONAL MEDICINE

Preventive

1. Preplacement examinations
2. Screening, periodic health surveillance
3. Monitoring of special and vulnerable groups
4. Monitoring of personal protection methods, including immunization
5. Epidemiological surveillance
6. Health education and training (e.g. first aid)
7. Research (clinical, ergonomic, epidemiological)

Clinical

1. Emergency medical care (acute conditions)
2. Occupational diseases and injuries
3. Primary health care
4. Continuing health care (chronic conditions)
5. Health surveillance and biological monitoring, e.g. statutory, drivers, 'return to work' examinations etc.

Promotive

1. Health education (alcohol, smoking, lifestyle)
2. Health maintenance (general)
3. Rehabilitation and job placement
4. Counselling and referral (employee assistance programmes) and social aspects

Environmental

1. Hazard identification, recognition, evaluation and motivation for control
2. Legal requirements, monitoring
3. Extension to 'outside the factory wall' relations

Consultative

1. Placement and transfers on medical grounds
2. Professional to management, workers, unions, industrial relations and safety departments etc.
3. Co-ordination of activities of inside with outside health institutions and other agencies
4. Co-ordination of clinical management of worker patients
5. Community relations

Administrative

1. Medical, environmental, epidemiological and absenteeism records (not 'control')
2. Statutory records and reports, relevant legislation, e.g. Workmen's Compensation Act administration
3. Policies, procedures, hazard documentation, standing medical directives and protocols
4. Reference library and documentation
5. Applied appropriate research

One of the main aims of the occupational health nurse would be the prevention and early recognition of occupational disease. If prevention has failed the nurse would assist in establishing a diagnosis and in the management of the patient who is suffering a work-induced or work-related occupational disease. Nursing would include rehabilitation and follow-up. It deserves emphasis that in the South African context primary health care is also very much a component of Occupational Medicine practice.

As the main subject of this chapter is occupational disease no further discussion of elements of Occupational Medicine will follow here, except to state that the training of the occupational health nurse should at least incorporate the following subjects, to enable her or him adequately to deal with occupational health problems such as occupational diseases:

1. Toxicology of the substances and pathology of the medical conditions most likely to occur, e.g. dusts causing pneumoconiosis, substances causing asthma, some metals used in industry and mining, organic solvents, toxic gases and vapours, pesticides and also physical agents which may cause harm such as heat, cold, noise and radiation.

2. Relevant legislation pertaining to occupational diseases in the Workmen's Compensation Act, the Occupational Diseases in Mines and Works Act, the Machinery and Occupational Safety Act and its regulations. The last named provides for preventive measures backed by legal requirements and may also serve as a guide to select priorities, e.g. asbestos, lead, noise or any one of the 50 'high risk substances' listed in the General Administrative Regulations, wherever usage of the substance in question occurs. (Table V)

3. Clinical training in the nature and the scope of nursing practice which includes diagnosing and managing occupational disease.

4. Epidemiological aspects of occupational health with the emphasis on using these as a tool when dealing with groups of workers rather than with individuals only.

6.3 OCCUPATIONAL DISEASE

In general most so-called occupational diseases are indistinguishable from non-occupational diseases in terms of pathological manifestations. Many cases present with such non-specific symptoms as weakness, insomnia, sweating, malaise, nausea, vomiting, anorexia, dizziness and headache. A list of toxins which may cause headaches mentions 168 substances, the best known of which are perhaps carbon monoxide, (ethyl)alcohol and nitroglycerine, to which 'dynamite headache' is ascribed. Or, even more confusing, an occupational disease such as, for example, carbon disulfide poisoning presents with coronary artery disease.

Then there is usually an interval, when the disease is latent, between the onset of exposure and the first manifestation of the disease. This may make it difficult to link the two, especially in the case of carcinogens when the latent interval is long, e.g. mesothelioma developing 40 years after the first exposure.

Many occupational factors which have an adverse effect on health may act in the same way as those which are non-occupational. Some occupational hazards operate in concert with 'outside' factors. The effect of smoking and of certain dusts on respiratory function has the same end result.

Many substances used in the workplace which have an adverse effect on health if absorbed, are 'hidden' under a proprietary commercial name, without any indication of the generic, chemical name. Users are unaware of their potential hazardous nature, e.g. 'Genklean' is a chlorinated hydrocarbon solvent.

The effect of exposure to hazardous substances may be dependent on the dose taken—the degree of exposure and absorption determines if and when a noticeable effect occurs. The effect might become apparent at a time when the relationship between the two is not clear, unless the nurse is aware of such a possibility, of course. In the case of zinc fume fever the delayed effect may mimic an attack of 'flu' occurring many hours after work.

It is therefore very important for the occupational health nurse to know which potentially toxic substances and physically hazardous conditions occur in the working environment of the employees under her care. She must master the skills necessary to make a presumptive diagnosis or even just to suspect that a complaint or adverse effect may be linked to such a hazard. The most important of these skills is the taking of a detailed and thorough occupational history in addition to a general or specific medical history and then ascertaining the quality (type), quantity (degree and duration) of exposure and possible absorption by the patient. Through a structured inquiry into the occupational history it should be possible to detail all known or suspected exposures to potential hazards, in degree and duration. It is necessary to know where exposure occurred, in what type of job, and in which combinations, if any, with other stresses or hazards. Any effects, complaints, symptoms or signs which have been noticed earlier should also be noted; it is especially important to note whether these occurred during or after work, were worse on any particular days of the week, or during weekends, at the beginning or at the end of shifts, recurred after periods of holidays or other absences from work and whether other co-workers have had similar complaints or manifestations. All this must of course be complemented by a thorough knowledge of symptoms, signs and laboratory tests which would help the nurse to arrive at a presumptive or definitive diagnosis for the particular occupational diseases which may be expected to occur in a particular working environment. In addition the nurse should exhibit a high degree of clinical suspicion, based on such knowledge, and sensitivity to complaints presented by workers and alleged to 'arise out of and in the course of their occupation' to ensure early recognition of disease. Good relationships with and an understanding of other departments and their specific expertise, for example in the field of engineering controls and personal relations and close co-peration with other health workers are prerequisites for the nurse to fulfil her essential role. This role is *to prevent employees or groups of employees under her care to suffer significant adverse effects to their health*.

6.3.1   Definition In 1976 the World Health Organization, when reviewing its earlier
and recommendations on occupational health programmes, suggested
compensation that the concept of occupational disease should be broadened to
aspects incorporate medical conditions for which, although prevalent in the community and originating from many diverse factors, some contributory factor exists in the work situation of the patient.

Occupational diseases are defined as diseases which are solely or principally caused by factors which are peculiar to the working environment and are therefore 'arising out of and during work', with the qualification that the actual manifestation, i.e. the disease, may well arise 'after work'. Thus occupational diseases are only a sub-group of the so-called work-related diseases. The work related-ness of the multifactorial diseases which do not fall under this stricter definition of occupational disease comes from the fact that there are other hazards than occupational ones in Man's life at home and when away from work in the community. There cannot be an artificial separation of work hazards and those of the general environment. Hereditary factors and those deriving from a particular style of life influence human health in all spheres of life, at work and away from work. Lung tuberculosis is an example of a disease which may occur as a 'true' occupational disease in a healthy worker who has succumbed to an infection at work, or as a work-related disease in a susceptible worker elsewhere, resulting from excessive stresses at work, which are deemed to have 'caused' the illness. Impairment of health and breakdown of resistance to disease rather than an incident of direct infection would be the mechanism of pathogenesis in the latter case.

In the United States of America the National Institute of Safety and Health (NIOSH) published a list of 10 leading causes of work-related diseases and injuries in 1983. These are listed in **Table II**.

TABLE II   TEN WORK-RELATED DISEASES (NIOSH 1983)

1. Occupational lung diseases (incl. lung cancer)
2. Musculoskeletal injuries
3. Occupational cancers
4. Amputations, fractures, trauma, eye loss, death
5. Cardiovascular diseases
6. Reproductive disorders
7. Neurotoxic disorders
8. Noise induced hearing loss
9. Dermatological conditions
10. Psychological disorders (incl. alcohol abuse)

Frequency of occurrence, severity of outcome and also amenability to prevention were criteria used for listing and ranking. It is at once apparent that this is a list of broadly defined and mainly non-specific groups of conditions. It includes such multifactorial but work-related diseases as discussed earlier where the influence of factors at work may actually be minimal. On the other end of the spectrum are the 'true' occupational diseases such as noise induced hearing loss and the occupational cancers.

For compensation purposes the occupational diseases are more closely defined by adding restrictive clauses and scheduling as in South Africa, or prescribed in a similar way as in the United Kingdom.

For South Africa occupational diseases for which a workman can be compensated under the Workmen's Compensation Act of 1941, as amended, are those contracted under conditions which are scheduled in the second schedule of the Act. This second schedule contains a description of the disease together with a description of the occupation where these must have occurred to make them compensatable (**Table III**). The Act does however not exclude compensation for other occupational diseases, provided that the workman can prove that his claim falls within the scope of the Act. For example workmen who have contracted hepatitis B and lung tuberculosis have received financial compensation when it was proven and accepted that an 'accident', or rather an incident, of infection which had occurred at work had caused them to contract such a disease. A proposal to incorporate occupational asthma in the second schedule is under consideration.

TABLE III   SECOND SCHEDULE TO THE WORKMEN'S COMPENSATION ACT 1941

Industrial diseases (Section 89)

Ankylostomiasis (hookworm)
Anthrax
Arsenical poisoning
Poisoning by benzene or its homologues and their nitro and amino derivatives and its sequelae
Chrome ulceration
Cyanide rash
Dermatitis due to dust, liquids or other external agents present in the specific processes of the workman's occupation
Poisoning by the halogen derivatives of hydrocarbons
Lead poisoning or its sequelae
Manganese poisoning
Mercury poisoning or its sequelae
Pathological manifestations due to radium or other radioactive substances or X-rays
Phosphorus poisoning
Primary epitheliomatous cancer of the skin
Silicosis, asbestosis or other fibrosis of the lungs caused by mineral dust
TNT poisoning
Byssinosis
Mesothelioma

A description of the occupation associated with each disease is given in the Act.

The Occupational Diseases in Mines and Works Act of 1973, defines as 'compensatable disease' the conditions listed in **Table IV**. The common factor in these is that the worker must have performed so-called 'risk work', defined as work involving the risk of incurring a compensatable disease, as declared in a Government Gazette, or deemed to have been so declared under Section 13 of the Act, i.e. where exposure to potentially harmful dust, gases, vapours or chemical substances or factors may occur or where working conditions in the opinion of the Minister are (potentially) harmful.

TABLE IV   COMPENSATABLE DISEASES (OD in M and W ACT, 1973)

(a) PNEUMOCONIOSIS, a permanent lesion of the cardio-respiratory organs caused by the inhalation of dust in the course of performance of risk work, but excluding a calcified lesion.
(b) The joint condition of PNEUMOCONIOSIS AND TUBERCU-LOSIS.
(c) TUBERCULOSIS, which in the opinion of the certification committee was contracted while the person concerned was

performing risk work, or he became affected within 12 months immediately following the last exposure to such work.

(d) PERMANENT OBSTRUCTION of the AIRWAYS which, in the opinion of the certification committee is attributable to the performance of risk work.

(e) PROGRESSIVE SYSTEMIC SCLEROSIS which in the opinion of the certification committee is attributable to the performance of risk work.

(f) Any other permanent disease of the cardio-respiratory organs which in the opinion of the certification committee is attributable to the performance of risk work.

(g) Any other disease which in the opinion of the certification committee is attributable to the performance of risk work, and which the Minister by notice in the Gazette declared to be a compensatable disease.

Mesothelioma and certain cases of lung cancer have been attributed to risk work in certain mines and have therefore been regarded as compensatable.

It is clear that the certification committee has been given discretion as to what conditions should be compensatable subject to establishing that the condition is closely related to the work situation, i.e. that the patient has performed 'risk work'.

It is under consideration to consolidate all legislation for compensation of occupational diseases and injuries under one Act, covering these conditions irrespective of where they arose, in mines, works or any other workplace or work site.

It should also be noted that some of the occupational diseases are reportable to the Health Authorities under the Health Act of 1977. These are i.a. Anthrax, Lead poisoning, Poisoning from any agricultural or stock remedy registered in terms of the Fertilizers, Farm Feeds, Agricultural Remedies and Stock Remedies Act of 1947 as amended and also primary malignancies of the bronchus, lung and pleura. In the last category would fall such occupational cancers as mesothelioma and bronchial carcinoma resulting from occupational asbestos exposure, both compensatable under the OD in M and W Act mentioned earlier.

In the United Kingdom the list of 'Prescribed Diseases' which are compensatable under the Social Security Act of 1975 as amended covers many more conditions than the WC Act in South Africa does. In Finland the definition of compensatable occupational disease is much wider and more medically orientated than elsewhere, which probably accounts for the comparatively high rates of occupational diseases reported there.

6.3.2 Epidemiology of occupational diseases The major problem encountered when studying the epidemiology of occupational diseases, not only in this country but also elsewhere, is the lack of reliable data. Even where a legal duty to report occupational diseases exists there is under-diagnosis as a result of lack of recognition among health workers that many of the complaints about illness and diseases among the workforce may be work related. In South Africa the main sources of information about occupational diseases are the Medical Bureau of Occupational Diseases where diseases in mines and works are certified, the Workmen's Compensation Commissioners annual reports and the reports of occupational medicine clinics such as are run by the National Centre of Occupational Health and by a few other institutions and Trade Union medical services. Since 1985 the annual reports of the Workmen's Compensation Commissioner contain a table (no 12) which specifically lists the reported cases according to the second schedule (1985:632). This is over and above the listed cases due to poisonous and corrosive substances and agents for occupational disease reflected in Table 10 (5 310). The former table lists 414 cases of pneumoconiosis, 174 of dermatitis and a few cases of poisoning due to arsenic (7), phosphorus (5), manganese (4) and lead (1). It is confusing that Table 12 lists 139 cases due to arsenic preparations and 6 due to lead compounds. It is not possible to use these data to show priorities based on numbers. The Erasmus committee report of 1976 gives an estimate of the number of workers exposed to particular hazards but no reliable data on how many of those could be expected to suffer from particular occupational diseases in any one year.

The National Centre of Occupational Health report of 1985 shows that 75 cases of pneumoconiosis in non-mining workers were certified for compensation. It was also reported that of 442 workers examined at the clinic, 170 cases had been diagnosed as occupational disease. In 1988 a total of 460 cases were referred to the clinic, of which 48 were certified as having pneumoconiosis or mesothelioma, 94 had been suspected of suffering from asbestos and silica related disease and another 70 were classified as probable or definite occupational disease sufferers. It is not known how large the populations of exposed workers were among which these cases occurred, nor how representative the numbers could be. There are no reliable data to base expectations on to show how many cases of occupational diseases one would have to expect in South Africa or in particular industries. Finland probably has the most developed occupational diseases and injuries reporting system in the world. Their records show an annual average of about 5 cases of occupational disease per 1 000 workers. Skin diseases are reported as the most prevalent, as is the case in many countries, while occupational noise-induced hearing loss is also prevalent. If it is assumed that the workers in South Africa would not be better protected against occupational hazards than their counterparts in Finland, one could, basing one's assumptions on premises of dubious validity, expect that at least 22 000 cases of noise-induced hearing loss should be diagnosed in this country per annum. One would also have to expect about 10 cases of lead poisoning among the 15 000 exposed workers, about 200 cases of silicosis among 78 000 exposed workers, perhaps about 12 000 cases of dermatitis and in total 44 000 cases of all occupational diseases combined among a workforce of about 8 million in the formal sector alone. These figures are all rough estimates based on the expectation that it is likely that at least 5 out of every 1 000 workers would suffer an occupational disease of some sort in any one year. And that is a conservative estimate! It has been established that in the Western Cape a nurse working in industry may expect to find at least one case of lung tuberculosis, the most prevalent of the possibly work-related diseases, for every hundred workers under her care in any one year.

It is up to every nurse to determine for her/his particular work environment and worker population, based on knowledge of potential hazards and of the health status of those workers, what occupational diseases to expect and to look out for, with the emphasis on prevention. Keeping epidemiological records and scouting for epidemiological data in related industries and workplaces may help to establish priorities.

6.3.3 Management of occupational diseases

This chapter cannot take the place of textbooks which describe in detail, for each recognized occupational disease, the pathogenesis, pathology, toxicology of causal agents, clinical aspects (including prevention and early recognition), treatment and pharmacology of treatment modalities, emergency treatment protocols, follow-up and rehabilitation. Therefore the bibliography will contain references to information and recommendations for further reading about these and other aspects of occupational diseases.

In line with editorial policy the discussions to follow will be restricted to the occupational diseases listed in Table III, but additional space will be devoted to occupational dermatoses and lung disease, as these are most prevalent and not always recognized, and to occupational malignancies, which demand more and more attention.

These discussions will not be exhaustive but an attempt will be made to cover those aspects which are of particular importance to the occupational health nurse for her role as first line health worker in the workplace, with an emphasis on prevention and early recognition.

In 1986 the WHO published a guide for health professionals— 'Early detection of occupational diseases'. This is essential reading and reference material for any occupational health service. Part of what follows here is based on this work and on the NIOSH publication of 1977, 'Occupational Diseases, a guide to their recognition' and on the references listed in the bibliography. To assist readers in determining priorities for their own practice or service, this chapter will discuss the most prevalent or clinically important occupation-related diseases with the main responsible agents and the type of occupations or industry where these may occur.

There are a number of approaches possible when describing occupational diseases. One is to look at target organs and then discuss the deviations from the normal caused by known agents. Another way is to start with symptoms and signs and work back to describe which causal agents might be responsible for these and the toxicology and pathology related to these agents. This would reflect the actual situation in the field closely. A third way would be to start off with known hazardous factors, be they chemical, physical or biological and then to describe the adverse effects these may have on man, followed by a discussion on their management. The method to be followed here is similar to the one used in the WHO guide referred to above, i.e. to discuss particular adverse effects, defined and listed as a (compensatable) occupational disease, in relation to particular factors and occupations and then select aspects which are appropriate and relevant for the occupational health nurse for her/his particular role as a member of the occupational health workers team.

6.3.3.1 Ankylosto- *Occurrence:* Ankylostomiasis is scheduled for underground mining
miasis but other occupations exposed to risk are those where excreta are
encountered such as work on sewers, ditches, garbage, construction,
land excavation and farmyards, especially where a warm climate and
moist conditions favour the development of larvae of the hookworm.

Route of entry: Larvae invade the skin, usually interdigitally or via
the footsole.

Adverse effects: Localized erythema, oedema and itch. When the
larvae have migrated via the circulatory system and lungs to the
gastro-intestinal tract, non-specific gastro-intestinal symptoms follow, with chronic microscopic blood loss and subsequent iron-
deficiency anaemia.

Early recognition is based on a high suspicion and awareness of
possible infection, visual inspection of port of entry, stool tests for
eggs and blood test for anaemia in more advanced state. Diagnosis
and treatment with Pyrantel Pamoate for example, which is on the
WHO essential drug list, should follow. Monitoring of stools may be
considered in populations with a high infection rate.

Prevention: Education and sanitary disposal of excreta, personal
protection of exposed workers with boots and where indicated gloves
while at work.

6.3.3.2 Anthrax *Occurrence:* Handling of wool, hair, bristles and skins and work in
connection with animals and carcasses infected with anthrax.

Route of entry: The bacillus gains entry through damaged skin;
inhalation of spores may also occur.

Adverse effects: Local development of vesicles and a fiery haemor-
rhagic pustule ('malignant pustule') which may dry up and form a
black 'depressed' escar. Spread to regional lymph nodes and
bloodstream may result in high fever, septicaemia and, if untreated,
death. Inhalation of spores at first results in what may appear a
common upper respiratory tract infection which may be followed by
fever, respiratory distress, septicaemia, shock and death in a few
days.

Early recognition would require a high level of suspicion, early
presentation by the patient and visual inspection, the diagnosis is
made on clinical grounds and laboratory blood examination.
Treatment of restricted local inflammation is by antibiotics and rest,
hospitalization is needed for systemic symptoms and signs. Anthrax is
a notifiable condition under the Health Act of 1977.

Prevention: Zoonosis control by immunization of animals in enzootic
areas, certification as free from anthrax of wool, hides and hair,
abattoir animals and carcasses. Education and personal hygiene of
people at risk, immunization of high risk workers, personal
protection measures such as wearing gloves and masks when sorting
material (this used to be called the wool or rag sorters disease) and
dust suppression c.q. local exhaust ventilation where the risk of spore
laden dust aerosols arises.

6.3.3.3 Arsenical *Occurrence:* Arsenic compounds are used as insecticides, herbicides,
poisoning as a wood preservative, in the manufacture of some glass and enamel

products, in textile printing, tanning, metallurgy and for special paints. The principal form in which it is used is as arsenic trioxide (white arsenic). However, hydrogen arsenide, **arsine**, an extremely toxic colourless gas with a faint garlic smell, may be generated during certain processes in smelting, refining and in some chemical factories.

Arsenic occurs in nature and more specifically in seafood. Occupations at risk are found in agriculture, forestry, metallurgy, electronics, paper factories and many more industries. Arsenic is no 5 on the schedule of high risk substances which require registration with the Department of Manpower under the MOS Act of 1983.

Route of entry: Arsenic dust and fumes, as well as Arsine gas are inhaled; arsenic compounds may enter through skin abrasions but arsenic acids may permeate through contact skin. Some ingestion may occur by swallowing of contaminated saliva.

Adverse effects: The trivalent compounds are irritating to skin and mucosa; repeated or prolonged contact may cause vesicular and pustular eruptions, contact dermatitis (commonly of the wrists and with poor personal hygiene, the genitalia), skin sensitization (pentoxide), keratosis characteristically on hand palms and footsoles, hyperpigmentations and possibly skin cancers. Chemical conjunctivitis, rhinitis and pharyngolaryngitis occur, perforation of the nasal septum may follow. Chronic arsenic absorption results in widespread damage to skin, respiratory tract, liver, blood formation, kidney and the peripheral nervous system.

Inhalation of **arsine** may be fatal if in sufficient quantity. In acute poisoning vomiting of often bloodstained material follows within a few hours, with severe headache, abdominal pains, diarrhoea and pulmonary oedema. Massive intra-vascular haemolysis results in haemoglobinuria, with renal damage, uraemia and possibly death. Severe hepatic damage may occur, with haemolytic jaundice and cardio-vascular damage in surviving cases.

Sufficient ingestion of arsenic may result in a clinical picture of acute poisoning which resembles that which follows arsine inhalation, but with more delayed haemolysis, while muscle cramps may be a feature.

Arsenic compounds are regarded as co-carcinogens for man and are associated with skin and lung cancer as long delayed effects.

Early recognition: periodic visual examination of skin and mucosa of exposed workers, especially skin of wrists, hands, footsoles and inspection of the nose, combined with careful questioning about any perceived irritation effects would be helpful.

Hyperpigmentations, hair loss and white striations of nail beds may be present. Symptoms such as vague gastro-intestinal complaints and weight loss may be indicative of chronic absorption, in a later phase followed by sensory peripheral neuritis symptoms, 'glove and stocking' paraesthesia manifested as 'pins and needles' sensation.

Periodic examinations every 3 months, for instance, with biological monitoring tests on excretion of arsenic in the urine, are advocated. Full blood counts would only show deviations if absorption is already severe. Where long-term exposure over many years occurs routine chest X-rays have been prescribed to screen for lung cancer. However that is not a very sensitive test.

The ACGIH does not list a Biological Exposure Index for arsenic exposure, but according to Lauwerys excretion of arsenic should not exceed $220\,\mu g$ per g creatinine excreted in urine.

Prevention:

The ACGIH recommends as an acceptable exposure limit a value of $0{,}2\,mg/m^3$ of air for soluble arsenic compounds and of $0{,}05\,ppm$ for Arsine gas as a not to be exceeded time weighted TLV (threshold limit value). Arsenic trioxide is classified as a suspected human carcinogen (A2).

Personal protection methods should incorporate education and training with regard to the hazards of exposure. The use of personal protection such as face masks, gloves and proven impervious apparel where those are indicated as useful, should be worn. There should be education in personal hygiene. Daily showers and also clean working clothes daily should be made available where the extent of potential exposure warrants this. Medical surveillance following a protocol, at intervals determined by potential exposure, should lead to early recognition of problems and then lead to removal from exposure if necessary.

Treatment of chronic and acute arsenic poisoning with dimercaprol and other drugs should only be performed on hospitalized patients. Cases of acute poisoning especially after arsine inhalation should, after emergency supportive measures, be admitted at once.

6.3.3.4 Poisoning by benzene, its homologues and derivatives

The Second Schedule (Table III) lists benzene, its homologues and their nitro- and amino-derivatives and mentions involvement with production, use of or contact with these substances under occupation.

Benzene and homologues

Occurrence: **Benzene**, a typical aromatic hydrocarbon solvent has, because of its toxicity, mostly been replaced as a commercial solvent by its less toxic homologues, toluene and xylene. However these may, in commercial grade, contain appreciable concentrations of the substance benzene, as does petrol and aviation fuel. In parts of Europe the name benzine is used for petrol, and this term is also used to denote a mixture of aliphatic hydrocarbons, volatile components of petroleum also called 'white spirits'. These are much less harmful than the aromatic unsaturated compounds.

Benzene is used for the production of many other aromatic compounds, certain drugs and pesticides, dyes, paints and plastics. Those who are at risk are employed in the (petro) chemical industry, printing, leather, plastics, synthetic rubber and adhesive makers and paint sprayers. Also certain laboratory workers are at risk, while the presence in motor and aviation fuel should be kept in mind. Benzene is no 20 on the High Risk Substances (HRS) list of the General Administrative Regulations under the Machinery and Occupational Safety Act (MOS Act) of 1973. It may also evolve from no 9 (coal tar pitch volatiles) and from the distillation of coal and production of gas coke from coal. Its most important homologues are Toluene (methyl benzene), Xylene (dimethyl benzene) and Styrene (vinyl benzene).

Route of entry: inhalation of vapour may be supplemented by percutaneous absorption although these aromatic hydrocarbons are comparatively poorly absorbed by the intact skin.

Adverse effects: High concentrations of benzene cause narcotic effects with some local irritation on the eyes and the mucosa of the respiratory tract. Dizziness, nausea, confusion and staggering gait may be followed by coma and death due to respiratory arrest in fatal cases. Long term absorption due to exposure to lower concentrations may result in bone marrow depression and is associated with leukaemias. Liquid benzene has a degreasing effect on skin and may thus cause dermatitis. The main effect of benzene is its myelotoxic action. Counts of erythrocytes, leucocytes and thrombocytes may first increase, then aplastic anaemia may develop with leucopenia, thrombocytopenia, low haemoglobin and red cell counts. The bone marrow may be hypo- or hyper-active, which does not always correlate with peripheral blood findings.

Chromosomal aberrations have been noted for some time after exposure has halted. There may be a latent period of years before the onset of leukaemia, which is usually of the myeloblastic, non-lymphocytic type. However the prognosis of pancytopenia is relatively favourable in the majority of workers who are removed early from exposure, even though haematologic changes may be present for years.

Toluene has mainly acute narcotic effects and also some neurotoxic effects after chronic absorption but is not regarded as haematotoxic. **Xylene** has mainly narcotic effects but may also affect liver function, as does **Styrene**. The latter substance, at low concentrations of exposure, is less of an irritant to skin and mucosa than the other two but may be more neurotoxic and is reported as causing headaches at comparatively low rates of absorption. All three are solvents with a degreasing effect on skin and may therefore cause dermatitis.

Early recognition: Clinically there are no early symptoms or signs of haematotoxic effects. Acute effects such as dizziness, headache, nausea, confusion, uncoordinated movements are also symptoms of chronic absorption. Early neurotoxic effects are subjective and vague except perhaps headache, but may be indicative of excessive absorption. Skin manifestations may be useful pointers although skin absorption is less important than inhalation. Biological monitoring may help to diagnose incipient poisoning at an early stage.

For **benzene** which is metabolized to phenol and excreted in the urine as such at higher levels than by non-exposed people (normal value is less than 20 mg per g creatinine excreted) the determination of phenol in urine is useful. According to NIOSH the level should not exceed 75 mg phenol per litre of urine (at specific gravity standard of 1024). The ACGIH recommends that the level should not exceed 50 mg/ℓ when the sample is taken at the end of a shift. Benzene levels may also be determined in expired air as an indication of recent exposure and in blood. The urine test for phenol is more practical. In view of the haematotoxicity of benzene, periodic blood tests (full blood counts) are indicated for spotting myelotoxic effects as early as possible.

For **toluene**, which is metabolized into benzoic acid and then excreted as hippuric acid in the urine, Lauwerys advocates as tentative permissible maximum excretion 2,5 g of hippuric acid per g creatinine (or 1 mg ortho-cresol per g creatinine) excreted in the urine. The ACGIH recommends the same value as the Biological Exposure Index (BEI).

For **xylene**, a mixture of isomers, the determination of methyl hippuric acid in the urine is a useful test. The value should not exceed 1,5 g/g creatinine as recommended by the ACGIH and also Lauwerys.

For **styrene** the most practical test is to determine mandelic acid excretion in the urine. The value for this should not exceed 0,8 g/g creatinine (or 1 g/ℓ), the BEI advocated by the ACGIH, while Lauwerys regards 1 g/g creatinine as permissible.

In conclusion, early recognition of excessive absorption of these solvents is based more on biological monitoring than on clinical manifestations, combined with knowledge about potential exposure by workers and health staff.

Prevention: Apart from environmental control the need for adequate health education of the workers concerned is obvious. The use of personal protective devices, such as proven impervious clothing, gloves and boots and, where unavoidable, respiratory cartridge filters or air supply masks should be closely supervised.

Benzene should only be used in exceptional circumstances and then in closed systems or under special precautions, e.g. if used in laboratories. Wherever possible the least toxic substitute for a particular purpose should be used. The occupational exposure limit (TLV time weighted average) recommended by the ACGIH is 10 ppm for benzene, which is classified as a suspected human carcinogen (A2). For the homologues these limits are: Toluene 100 ppm, Xylene 100 ppm, Styrene 50 ppm according to the 1991–1992 table).

Treatment of over-exposure and acute poisoning is mainly symptomatic and supportive. There is no specific antidote for the haematotoxic effect of benzene. Long term monitoring is indicated once excessive, especially chronic, absorption of this substance has occurred.

Nitro and amino derivatives of benzene

Occurrence: Of the nitro derivatives **nitrobenzene** is used in the production of explosives, di-nitrobenzene, aniline dyes, paints, polishes and also for making celluloid. Nitrophenol and trinitrotoluene (TNT) are related compounds, the latter well known in the explosives industry. Among the **amino derivatives** of benzene **aniline**, used in the manufacture of dyes, the (synthetic) rubber industry, varnishes, pharmaceuticals and other chemicals is the most widely used compound. Used as intermediates in the synthesis of dyes are the related compounds listed under the 'High Risk Substances' as no 17 (4-nitro diphenyl) and 13 (4-amino diphenyl).

Route of entry: All these substances are readily absorbed by the intact skin when in liquid form, the main risk is however inhalation of vapour.

Adverse effects: The acute and subacute effects of these substances are the most important, although anaemia, liver damage and peripheral neuropathy has been reported after long-term absorption. The main direct adverse effect is the rapid development of met-haemoglobine resulting in anoxia.

There may be a delay of some hours after absorption has started before symptoms occur, commonly intense progressively severe headache without other symptoms of feeling unwell. Cyanosis of lips, nose and earlobes, usually recognized first by fellow workers, then follows (when the met-haemoglobine level has risen to 15 % or more). With increasing met-haemoglobinaemia symptoms such as dizziness, dyspnea or exertion, ataxia and tachycardia develop, followed by drowsiness, coma and death in severe cases, when the met-haemoglobine level rises to 70 % and more. The lethal level of met-haemoglobine is estimated to be around 85 g per 100 g Haemoglobine.

Most of the compounds are only mildly irritating to eyes and skin but dermatitis due to primary irritation as well as to sensitization may well occur.

Early recognition of symptoms of acute poisoning, of which headache is usually the first, is difficult and unreliable. This is compounded by the only mildly irritating effect of most of these substances. To expect other workers to notice incipient cyanosis in their colleagues is not of much use either. Therefore biological monitoring, over and above thorough and repeated briefing of potentially exposed workers by targeted health education, is probably the most helpful method for early recognition programmes.

Nitrobenzene is metabolized to nitro- and amino-phenol, which are excreted in the urine as p-nitrophenol in the case of nitrobenzene and as p-aminophenol for aniline. This is a non-specific but useful sign. Lauwerys recommends that no more than 10 mg of p-aminophenol should be found to be excreted per g of creatinine by people exposed to **aniline**, no more than 5 mg p-nitrophenol by those exposed to **nitrobenzene** (Maximum Permissible Value). This is much lower than allowed by the BEI as listed for aniline by the ACGIH which is 50 mg p-amino-phenol/g creatinine in a urine sample collected at the end of a shift, i.e. directly after exposure to aniline has occurred.

For **nitrobenzene** exposure the ACGIH recommends to determine p-nitrophenol, at the end of the shift or work week; the BEI value (similar to Lauwerys's recommendation) prescribes not to exceed 5 mg/g creatinine!

A confirmatory test which is of great value is to measure met-haemoglobine. The ACGIH recommends as BEI for all met-haemoglobine inducing substances that the value should not exceed 1,5 % in any exposed person at the end of a workshift. Lauwerys allows up to 2 % as normal value for non-exposed people and a maximum of 5 % for workers exposed to met-haemoglobine inducing agents. In practice it would be prudent to monitor workers suspected of absorbing any one of the substances discussed above at the end of a shift and regard 1,5 % of met-haemoglobine as the cut-off point for deciding that excessive absorption has taken place.

Prevention: Persons with known haemoglobinopathies or intractable anaemia should be kept away from potential exposure. Alcohol usage and cardiac conditions which cause poor oxygenation appear to increase susceptibility to adverse effects. Apart from environmental control avoiding skin contact and, where necessary, providing personal protective devices such as proven impervious gloves, boots and apparel is indicated. Workers should know the importance of and practise personal hygiene, daily showers after work for example, and be aware of the potential hazards and early symptoms. The frequency of planned biological monitoring should be based on assessment of the risk of contamination and exposure.

The occupational exposure limit for nitrobenzene is 1 ppm, for aniline and homologues 2 ppm, both annotated for skin absorption but not, as benzene is, as potential human carcinogen.

Emergency treatment of acute poisoning by inhalation (or massive skin contact) consists of administering oxygen, thorough washing of the whole body with soap and water when indicated, and hospitalization. Intravenous treatment with 1 g of ascorbic acid has been used as an emergency measure but its action is slow. Methylene blue in a dose of 1 to 2 mg/kg of bodymass intravenously, slowly injected, should be used with caution and preferably only in hospitalized patients. Met-haemoglobine levels should be monitored every few hours over a period of at least 24 hours.

Chlorinated benzenes are related compounds which do not fall under the terms of the second schedule in Table III. They are used as intermediates and as insecticides and are irritating to conjunctiva, skin and mucous membranes and may cause drowsiness, incoordination and even unconsciousness. Chronic absorption may affect the liver. Their toxicity generally decreases the more chlorine atoms they contain. Occupational exposure limits are listed by the ACGIH for ortho-chlorobenzene and the di-chlorobenzenes, the latter with skin absorption annotation.

6.3.3.5 *Chrome ulceration* There is more to adverse effects of chrome than ulceration resulting from 'any work involving the handling or use of chromic acid, chrome salts or other materials containing these substances as a constituent' as the second schedule of the Workmen's Compensation Act describes the disease, but the emphasis in this discussion will be on local rather than on systemic effects.

Occurrence: Apart from the metallic state chromium occurs mainly in a trivalent and hexavalent state e.g. as chromic acid and chromic salts. The hexavalent state is the more irritating and toxic one. Environmental exposure limits are set for chromic acid (mist), the trioxide (the most stable form) and for the particulate state as in metal fumes. Chromium is used in the electroplating and stainless steel industry, for pigments and photographic materials, in leather processing and it occurs in small proportions in portland cement. Consequently there are many occupations which expose workers to contact with irritating and sensitizing chrome compounds. Chromium is listed as no 4 in the High Risk Substances schedule in the G.A. Regulations of the MOS Act.

Route of entry: inhalation of chromic acid as droplets in mist, of chrome fumes and as fine dust may occur in certain workplaces. Absorption depends on solubility in water and on size of particle, also in the case of ingestion, while absorption through the skin may occur. Local contact results in irritation and potentially in sensitization.

Adverse effects: Chromic acid has a direct corrosive effect on mucosa and skin, irritation of the nasal mucosa may be followed by ulceration and perforation of the septum. Ulcers may develop in the upper respiratory tract and in the digestive tract with chronic ingestion. Lacrimation, chemical conjunctivitis, epistaxis, tracheo-bronchitis with cough and the development of oedema and asthmatic reactions due to chromium have been reported from the metallurgical industry. Contact dermatitis and chrome ulcers (deep, round 'punched out', with elevated margins (sometimes called 'Chrome holes')) have a tendency to develop on finger knuckles and hand palms. A faint itchy rash on forearms and on points of contact or friction on the legs may accompany this. Skin sensitization is relatively common and may pass unsuspected in construction workers who work with cement. Chrome dermatitis may manifest itself as seborrhoic or discoid eczema of hand and feet. Not only the hexavalent but also the trivalent compounds may cause an allergy to develop.

The hexavalent chromium compounds are considered to be causal agents for bronchogenic cancer and are classified by the ACGIH as A1 human carcinogens. They are suspected of leading to increased risk of cancer of the paranasal sinuses as well.

Early recognition: Awareness of the early symptoms of irritation, especially of the nasal mucosa, conjunctiva and skin is a prerequisite for early presentation by affected workers to the health services. This is especially important as chrome ulcers are difficult to treat. They are painful and do not heal well, nor does nasal perforation. Routine periodic medical examination should include rhinoscopy, over and above inspection of the skin and careful questioning as to the existence of early symptoms, including those heralding development of hypersensitivity. Screening for lung cancer by chest X-ray and sputum cytology has been advocated but is of dubious and limited value.

Biological monitoring by determining the excretion of soluble chrome compounds in the urine is recommended by Lauwerys. A tentative maximum permissible value is set at $30 \mu/g$ creatinine; the normal value in non-exposed people usually does not exceed $10 \mu/g$ creatinine. The ACGIH recommends that the excretion of hexavalent chromium compounds, measured as total Cr (Chromium) in urine should not exceed $30 \mu/g$ creatinine in a sample taken at the end of the shift at the end of the work week.

Obviously such monitoring is only valid for systemic absorption and does not take local effects in account. The diagnosis of chrome ulcer, nasal septum perforation and also chrome dermatitis is made on clinical grounds. A patch test may be necessary to establish whether sensitization has occurred.

First aid measures in cases where inadvertent ingestion has occurred include the administration of milk and a solution or tablets of ascorbic acid. Topical application of a 20 % solution of ascorbic acid repeated over a long period may assist healing. Alternatively treatment with 10 % Calcium di-Sodium EDTA ointment, repeatedly applied to mucosa or skin may be used. The earlier this is started the better! Both drugs tend to reduce hexavalent chromium to the trivalent state. Removal from exposure is indicated during treatment and in cases of chrome allergy forever.

Prevention: Technical control measures should ensure that the concentration of chromium in environmental air is as low as possible below the occupational exposure limit, whether it is in the form of vapour or droplets as chromic acid mist or particulate as in dusts and metal fumes generated by welding, for example. The recommended limits (TLV–TWA ACGIH), measured as metallic Cr are as follows:

As metal, bivalent and trivalent compounds: $0,5\,mg/m^3$. As hexavalent water soluble compounds: $0,05\,mg/m^3$. For chromates occurring in chromite ore processing the exposure limit is also set at $0,05\,mg/m^3$ while the A1 human carcinogen annotation is valid for these chromates and for certain insoluble compounds.

Skin contact must be prevented by i.a. the use of proven impervious long sleeved gloves, boots, aprons and the use of face shields where there is a risk of splashing. Specific barrier creams may be of additional value. Personal hygiene such as a shower after work and the daily provision of clean overalls are recommended. In Britain chrome ulceration is a notifiable disease.

6.3.3.6   *Cyanide rash*   For this compensatable disease the description of occupation reads: 'the handling of cyanide or any work involving the use of cyanide'. The most important risk of working with cyanide salts is of course that under certain conditions hydrogen cyanide (HCN) may develop, inhalation of which may cause sudden death.

Occurrence: Cyanide salts (sodium, potassium, calcium and complex salts containing iron as well) are used in the metallurgical industry, electroplating, extraction of gold and silver from ore and in photographic processes. Hydrogen cyanide (HCN) is released on contact of cyanide salts with any acid, it has a peculiar bitter almond smell. Derivatives of cyanide such as isocyanates are used in paints and in the production of resins and polyurethane foams, while acrylo nitrile (vinyl-cyanide) is used in the plastics industry. The latter substance is no 8 on the schedule of High Risk Substances of the GA Regulations under the MOS Act. It is an irritant and regarded as potentially carcinogenic. Combustion of cyanide containing chemicals, paints and foams may cause HCN poisoning if the smoke is inhaled.

Route of entry and adverse effects: Chronic exposure to skin contact with solutions of the alkaline and irritant cyanide salts causes itching and discolorations, resulting in a scarlet 'cyanide rash' which may be vesicular, papular or even weeping. Where the skin is mechanically scratched or irritated such a rash is more likely to develop. Whether sensitization occurs is still debated.

Irritation of nasal mucosa with bleeding, sloughing and perforation of the nasal septum may also occur where workers are exposed to mists or fine dusts containing these salts. Absorption through the skin is possible while inhalation of aerosols which contain cyanides may result in local irritation and resorption. The cyanide salts themselves are not considered as toxic but biotransformation leads to metabolites such as complex thiosulphates and HCN proper. The principal action of HCN is inhibition of cytochrome oxidase and of a host of other enzymes, leading to tissue anoxia, particularly of the brain. Chronic low level absorption may give rise to subjective symptoms such as nervousness, headache, changes in taste and smell, lassitude, dyspnoea on exertion and irritation of eyes, nose and throat. Chronic accumulation and high metabolic levels of thiocyanates may affect thyroid function.

Acute HCN poisoning is a dramatic event which may have a fatal outcome due to chemical asphyxia. Initial symptoms are weakness, confusion, headache, vomiting which may be followed by tachycardia, loss of consciousness, cessation of respiration and death. Emergency treatment consists of rapid removal from exposure (safeguarding the intervention team against inhalation), administration of oxygen and artificial respiration when indicated. Where skin contamination has occurred copious flushing may be necessary. Met-haemoglobine binds circulating HCN and inhalation of amylnitrite followed by intravenous sodium thiosulfate (50 ml of a 25 % solution over a period of 5 minutes) may therefore be used as first aid emergency treatment. Alternatively or in addition to this intravenous hydroxy-cobalamine may be given, followed when necessary by dicobalt-EDTA (Kelocyanor) in hospitalized patients.

Whenever a risk of acute HCN poisoning exists emergency kits and a first aid treatment protocol should be readily available on site.

Early recognition of skin effects rests on awareness of the workers themselves of the risk of developing dermatitis and on presenting early complaints to health services staff. The same applies to subjective complaints which may result from chronic low level absorption. For the management of acute poisoning the CN level in blood is of some significance. Determination of thiocyanate level in urine, which in non-exposed people normally does not exceed 2,5 mg/g creatinine excreted in the urine, may be used for monitoring. Smokers normally have higher levels than non-smokers. Lauwerys recommends that the ratio of the thiocyanate level in urine (measured as mg/g creatinine) and the carboxy-haemoglobine level in blood (measured as percentage) should not exceed a factor of 3.

Prevention of skin contact with cyanide solutions and of inhalation of mists and dusts should be ensured by technical control measures and the use of personal protective apparel where indicated, depending on the nature of the work process. Specific respirators may have to be prescribed, in principle only for emergency usage. Workers with chronic skin or respiratory problems may be more susceptible to adverse irritating effects than healthy men. Strict handling procedures should be adhered to while acids should be kept far removed from any cyanide salts.

The environmental exposure limit for cyanides recommended by the ACGIH is 5 mg/m^3 (measured as CN), for the salts (with skin annotation) and 21 mg/m^3 (or 10 ppm) for cyanogen itself. A ceiling value, the concentration not to be exceeded during any part of the work exposure, is set at 0,3 ppm for the highly irritating cyanogen chloride.

6.3.3.7   *Dermatitis* The second schedule (Table III) specifies that dermatitis, in order to be regarded as compensatable and thus occupational, must be 'due to external agents present in the specific process or processes of the workman's occupation'. There are textbooks and many chapters in textbooks available which deal with industrial or occupational dermatitis. The following discussion will be a brief summary of elements relevant to the practice of occupational health nursing.

Occurrence: Occupational dermatitis is widely regarded as the most prevalent occupational disease, even though perhaps under-diagnosed and under-reported to a great extent. Among occupational diseases it may well lead to the greatest amount of suffering, absenteeism and costs to all parties concerned. In Finland, which has perhaps the most reliable system of reporting in the world, it is reported as accounting for about one fourth of all occupational diseases cases. The Workmen's Compensation Commissioners report of 1986 lists in Table 12 under Industrial Disease cases a total of 49 cases of dermatitis, of which 26 were medical aid only, while 11 had been temporarily disabled and another 2 permanently disabled. Yet in Table 10, which shows the numbers of cases due to corrosive and poisonous substances and agents, among which it is likely that in many the skin was affected, a subtotal of 3 913 cases resulted from contact with acids and alkalis (1 293), cement and chromium (566), oils, greases, thinners, varnishes and paints (437) and 'other corrosive substances' (1 617). It is not unlikely therefore, that in fact many hundreds if not thousands of cases of 'industrial dermatitis' occur among the worker population in South Africa every year.

Occupational skin diseases are caused by hundreds of different chemicals which have irritant properties, while many may cause sensitization in susceptible individuals. Those substances which have a degreasing effect on the skin may cause a non-specific dermatitis. Physical agents such as ultraviolet rays may cause dermatitis, excessive cold chilblains, excessive heat burns. Skin cancers may arise from contact with pitches and tars and from ionizing radiation. Bacteria in cutting oils may cause infective dermatitis. The list is endless.

A more general descriptive term for occupational skin disease is occupational dermatosis, defined as an abnormality of the skin which is induced or aggravated by factors in the work environment. Inflammation is not always a feature as the term dermatitis would tend to suggest.

The diagnosis of an occupational dermatosis rests on a careful occupational history to elicit information about potential aetiological agents, on knowledge about such agents and their effects and on evaluation of the symptoms and signs presented with particular emphasis on chronology in relation to occupational aspects. The differential diagnosis with non-occupational skin disease may be very difficult at times. Where sensitization is suspected patch testing and laboratory tests may be indicated. The location of eruptions may indicate the site of greatest exposure, e.g. the backs of the hands, the volar surface of wrists, forearms and cubital areas, especially when dusts and liquids are the factors involved. Involvement of the eyelids, face, ears and the 'V' of the neck may indicate exposure to vapours and mists. Predilection to sites of friction may provide a further clue.

A rash which has not existed before and developed only after starting work in a particular job, with periods of worsening and remission related to periods of work and absence and disappearing during holidays or sick leave may well be occupational. Conversely a prolonged or recurrent eruption which develops uninfluenced by work periods may indicate an underlying disorder such as atopic dermatitis, psoriasis or nummular eczema.

The morphology of occupational dermatoses does not differ materially from that in other skin diseases. The major clinical manifestations are:

1. Acute contact eczematous dermatitis caused by an irritant, sensitizer or photosensitizer.
2. Chronic eczematous dermatitis with erythema, scaling, dryness, lichenification and fissuring, caused by degreasing and dehydrating agents such as solvents, detergents or weak alkaline solutions.
3. Folliculitis and acneiform dermatoses including chloracne which may be due to insoluble oils, waxes, greases, tars and certain chlorinated hydrocarbons and naphthalenes.
4. Pigmentary disturbances due to coal tar and petroleum products, hydroquinones, certain phenolics and fruits, vegetables and u.v. radiation, burns and chronic dermatitis.
5. Granulomatous dermatoses, chronic indolent focal inflammations with scar formation which may occur due to beryllium, silica, asbestos, viral and fungal infections.
6. Ulcerative lesions characterized by loss of tissue and necrosis of the skin or mucosa, such as caused by chemical burns, chromic acid, arsenic trioxide, calcium compounds, fluor and cement.
7. Neoplastic lesions, keratoses, papilloma, epithelioma, carcinoma on exposed areas such as caused by certain coal tar and petroleum products and derivatives, ionizing and non-ionizing radiation.
8. Miscellaneous other lesions, discolorations of skin, nails and hair, alopecia and sclerodermoid lesions.

Contact dermatitis appears in two forms, one caused by irritants, the other by sensitizers (allergens).

Primary irritant contact dermatitis is caused by agents which inflict direct damage to the skin when in contact at sufficient concentration and for sufficient time in most if not all people. There are differences in susceptibility. Most of the irritants in everyday life are not felt to irritate the skin at once but exert their influence gradually. Causation is often multiple with mechanical friction as an additional factor. The agent which started the irritant contact dermatitis may be different from the one which maintains it. People with a history of atopic eczema, dry skin and very fair complexion appear to be more susceptible. Predilection sites are the webs between fingers, backs of fingers and hands and the forearm. Occupational cumulative irritant contact dermatitis can take months to heal, even away from work and appears to result in an altered, often lower resistance to irritants. Even when the skin appears fully healed return to normal may take further time. Relapses may occur from activities which previously did not cause the patient skin problems.

Allergic contact dermatitis is caused by sensitizing agents (allergens) by inducing hypersensitivity to itself in the patient, usually by combining with a protein and leading to a so-called delayed, cell mediated (type IV) mechanism. The allergen protein combination is acted against by T lymphocytes as if it was a foreign protein. This is a different mechanism from that of developing hay fever or bronchial asthma. Contact sensitization occurs with chrome and platina salts, epoxy resins, chemical substances used in the rubber and leather industry, and some plants. Some substances are such powerful sensitizers that nearly every contact results in allergic reactions, e.g. dinitrofluorobenzene. Others evoke reaction in only a few susceptible people although many are exposed, as is the case with formaldehyde solutions. It is rare to see an epidemic of allergic contact dermatitis in a group of workers, but this may happen quite easily with irritant contact dermatitis, for example when a new irritant substance is newly introduced in a work process.

Sensitization may be triggered off by the very first contact, and not necessarily by a heavy dose, or it may develop over time, counted in months rather than years. It is a silent process and active dermatitis symptoms may suddenly and unexpectedly occur after a minimal exposure contact incident. It follows that, unless there has been past exposure, a case of contact dermatitis starting within a week or two after exposure to a particular agent will be irritant rather than allergic.

Contact sensitization is specific either to one particular substance or to a group of substances which are chemically closely related (cross- reaction) and is for practical purposes to be regarded as permanent. An allergic reaction may develop between 6 to about 48 hours after contact and may thus present as a series of attacks. An example is recurrent attacks of oedema of the eyelids, usually with itching, when a worker has been sensitized to epoxy resin in a pattern shop. More commonly a chronic dermatitis of hands and forearms follows sensitization to e.g. chromium in cement. The rapid and repeatable reaction to an allergen is made use of for the diagnosis of allergic contact dermatitis by diagnostic patch testing which is the single most useful investigation to be carried out in a patient suspected to suffer from occupational dermatitis due to a sensitizing substance.

The diagnosis of irritant contact dermatitis is usually based on the history, appearance of the dermatitis and knowledge about offending agents. A negative patch test may have supportive value. The risk of sensitizing a patient by performing patch testing is regarded as minimal and should not be used as an argument not to test when an indication to do so exists.

Mixed contact dermatitis also occurs, where irritant and allergic components of the dermatitis make diagnosis and treatment sometimes very difficult. A bricklayer who has been sensitized against chrome or cobalt, for instance, may develop an irritant dermatitis of the hands as a result of the alkalinity and grittiness of the mortar he uses concomitant with a chronic allergic dermatitis as cement may contain traces of both metals.

Cutting fluids are an important potential cause of both types of contact dermatitis. They are widely used in the process of machining metals and also of other hard substances such as glass. There are two main groups, one water-based as emulsions of mineral or vegetable oils, containing surfactants or wetting agents, the other based on mineral and other oils and not containing water. Formulations are often complex and many include bactericides to control growth of often anaerobe bacteria and also additives which may be sensitizers. The dermatitis caused by the water emulsion type of cutting fluids is often patchy and may mimic discoid eczema on the back of the hands and forearms. The oil-based cutting fluids tend to cause follicular dermatitis but both types may induce sensitization, resulting in mixed contact dermatitis, sometimes complicated by inflammation due to biological organisms in the cutting fluid.

Another form of occupational dermatitis, though rare, is photo-toxic contact dermatitis, which may occur in workers who handle coal tar products as in road building and roofing and are exposed to ultra-violet light from the sun. It usually occurs on the hands and face, its border being determined by shaded or covered skin areas.

Non-occupational irritant contact dermatitis does of course also exist where people are exposed to detergents, solvents and irritating substances away from work, or are sensitized by such metals as nickel and develop an allergic contact dermatitis as a result.

Prevention: Occupational dermatoses are not completely prevent-able but should be reduced to as low a level as possible. Targeted health education of the workforce and management is a difficult but essential means to that end.

Preplacement medical examinations should be used to establish whether there is a confirmed history of allergic contact dermatitis and if so what agent was responsible. Exposure to such an agent or group should then obviously be avoided to prevent recurrence. Whether a person has suffered from endogenous atopic dermatitis, hay fever or asthma is not very relevant for most occupations but should serve as a warning that it would be advisable to avoid heavy exposure to such agents as cutting fluids, degreasing solvents and detergents as this might facilitate recurrence.

Atopy is defined as the capacity, more readily than the general population, to produce immunoglobuline type E (Ig E) antibodies to the non-occupational common allergens in the general environment. Between 10 % to 30 % of workers may have such an inherent higher capacity. It may be anticipated that such individuals would also become sensitized more readily to those allergens in the occupational environments which cause Ig E mediated allergy. It has been established with reasonable certainty that this is the case for platinum salts with regard to allergic contact dermatitis and, in a different way, for animal allergens with regard to the development of allergic rhinitis (hay fever), asthma and also eczema. Atopic individuals do not necessarily develop such symptoms more often, but when they do it is likely that the effects are more severe, asthma in particular. This is not true, however, for the isocyanates and formaldehyde where no increased risk for atopic individuals has been established.

From a medical prevention point of view therefore, atopic individuals should only be considered as individuals who need closer medical supervision to protect them against the development of occupational disease, but not 'against work', unless there is adequate evidence that they would be at an unacceptably higher risk. Thus far this has only been established with reasonable certainty for contact with platinum salts and animal protein allergens. When workers who present for a preplacement examination already show clear symptoms of disease such as contact dermatitis or bronchial asthma it would be prudent not to allow them to work in contact with these groups of allergens, even if the history does not include these particular ones. Special precautions can always be taken by the informed worker to prevent problems but when sensitization has definitely occurred exposure to any offending agent should be prohibited.

Knowledge about potential irritant and sensitizing agents in the plant should be gained and be readily available. Where possible, alternative, less irritant or sensitizing agents should be used or advice to replace them be given. It is for instance well known that the major sensitizer in the group of epoxy resins is one with a low molecular weight. Using one with a higher molecular weight may prevent a lot of problems for workers. Restricting the use of potentially hazardous substances to confined areas and to a few well informed and trained people may also control a dermatitis problem.

Avoidance of contact by the use of proven appropriate protective apparel, such as impervious gloves and specific barrier cream may help. Imperviousness for particular agents should be established and ensured very carefully. Personal hygiene, frequent washing with soap and water, and using 'conditioning moisturisers and restoring skin creams' afterwards, would make prevention programmes more effective. Cleaning of skin by solvents or other degreasing or irritant solutions should be prohibited and controlled. The primary objective in rehabilitation would be to maintain worker patients who have suffered from occupational dermatitis in their own job by improving skin safety. The exception would of course be a properly diagnosed hypersensitivity to a particular agent present in that job if contact is absolutely not avoidable. For most occupational dermatosis patients it should be possible to return to their job if so desired after adequate treatment and training on prevention.

The first requirement for health services staff would be early recognition and early treatment as an urgent matter. Every week delay worsens the prognosis of treatment towards full rehabilitation. Change of occupation should be the last resort.

Primary epitheliomatous cancer of the skin is a dermatosis which is compensatable under the Workmen's Compensation Act and listed in the second schedule for 'any work involving the handling or use of tar, pitch, bitumen, mineral oil or paraffin'. Skin cancer may have a variety of causes amongst which the polycyclic aromatic compounds which occur in coal tar products, mineral and shale oils, anthracene, chrysene and creosote are well known. As a general rule those which are derived from mineral crude oils and bitumens are less carcinogenic than those which are found in coal tar derivatives. Ultraviolet rays as in sunlight may have a synergistic effect in people exposed to both factors, e.g. in road workers. Modern cutting oils are usually refined in such a way that the polycyclic aromatic hydrocarbons (PAH's) have been removed.

Occurrence: Occupations at risk are coal gas manufacturers, coal tar distillers, coke plant workers, certain refinery workers, roofers and roadworkers who use these products, carbon black makers, certain jobs in ammunition, paper and match factories and classically the chimney sweeps.

Route of entry or in this case of contact is adhesion to and resorption through the skin; inhalation of volatile PAH's has been reported as potentially causing lung cancer.

Adverse effect in this case relates to the development of primary epitheliomatous cancer of the skin. The substances in question first result in erythema with a burning sensation ('pitch smarts') after a few hours or days of exposure, intensified by sunlight. After repeated prolonged exposure folliculitis, thickening of the skin, hyperkeratosis, hyperpigmentation and comedones may occur. Wart-like papillomas may then develop, in particular on damaged skin, which may later develop into squamous cell cancers, keratoacanthoma and basal cell carcinoma. Skin cancers may take 5 to 50 years to develop. The scrotum is particularly prone to develop squamous cancers following exposure to tar and soot, more so when personal hygiene is lacking. An early sign of exposure to the volatile components is conjunctivitis with photophobia.

Early recognition rests on awareness of the possible results of exposure and contact with these substances and of the early symptoms, combined with routine medical examinations, usually at annual intervals, to elicit symptoms and signs. Biological monitoring by laboratory tests is not feasible.

Early diagnosis of skin abnormalities which may herald more serious effects, e.g. keratosis should lead to early medical intervention, when the prognosis is still good.

Prevention: Precancerous conditions such as keratosis or already developed skin cancers found on preplacement examination should preclude employment at risk of exposure to substances likely to cause skin epithelioma and cancer. Periodic examinations, combined with targeted health education and promotion of personal hygiene are useful elements in prevention of a condition which should not be allowed to occur in workers at risk. Technical control measures, including substitution with non-carcinogenic materials, the use of impervious protective clothing, gloves and boots, meticulous personal hygiene and provision of clean working clothes would all combine to adequately prevent adverse effects.

Occupational exposure limits such as have been listed by the ACGIH for asphalt petroleum fumes ($5\,mg/m^3$), for coal tar pitch volatiles ($0,2\,mg/m^3$ measured as benzene solubles), which value is also given for particulate Polycyclic Aromatic Hydrocarbons (PAH's), relate more to systemic effects than to skin effects. Notably however, coal tar pitch volatiles and also chrysene are categorized as A2 potential human carcinogens and considered as high risk substances (No 9 and 25 on the schedule of the GA Regulations under the MOS Act).

6.3.3.8   Poisoning The Workmen's Compensation Act's description of occupation under
byhalogen this heading reads: 'any work involving the manufacture of or use of
derivativesof or contact with halogen derivatives of hydrocarbons'.
hydrocarbons   The most important among these derivatives are those which are
used as solvents and degreasers, for dewaxing, dry cleaning, cleaning
of metals and in chemical extraction processes. They are mainly
chlorinated aliphatic hydrocarbons. The bromides and iodides are
more likely to be used as fumigants and in specialized chemical
processes, or for fire extinguishers, as is the case with fluorocarbons.

    The latter are also used as anaesthetics, refrigerants and propel-
lants, although in recent times the chloro-fluorocarbons (CFC's) are
increasingly displaced by more 'ozone-friendly' substances, because
of the reported adverse effect of the CFC's on the protective ozone
layer in the stratosphere.

    Aromatic halogenated hydrocarbons, some derived from benzene
and its homologues, are used as chemical intermediates for the
manufacture of dyes, pharmaceuticals and pesticides while the
chlorinated biphenyls (PCB's) are used in the electrical industry as
insulating material. In general the chlorinated derivatives are less
toxic than the bromide and iodide compounds, and the fluorocarbons
are the least toxic. Listed in the High Risk Substances list of the MOS
Act regulations are ethylene dibromides (no 30), methyl iodide
(no 38) and vinyl bromide (no 48). Moreover carbon tetrachloride
(no 23), which is extremely toxic to the liver and should not be used
as a general solvent, and vinyl chloride (no 11) are examples of
chlorinated hydrocarbons which carry potentially serious risks to
health.

    Chloromethyl ether (CMME no 15), and bis chloromethyl ether
(BCME no 12) as well as methylene chloride (no 50) are other
examples of chlorinated hydrocarbons listed in this schedule because
of their toxicity and potential carcinogenicity.

    The main adverse effects of the substances in this group are
depression of the central nervous system, defatting of the skin,
thereby facilitating the development of dermatitis, and liver damage,
while some, in higher concentrations, may cause primary irritation of
the respiratory tract and lungs, and damage to the haemopoietic
system.

    Both these groups, the aliphatic and the aromatic halogenated
hydrocarbons, are used widely and in great quantities, only a selected
number of these compounds can be discussed here.

Occurrence:

(a) Chlorinated hydrocarbons such as trichloroethylene and
1.1.1.trichloroethane are used as degreasers and solvents in the metal
and paint industry, for dry cleaning and in chemical processes
(1.1.2.trichloroethane, tetrachloroethane and the very toxic carbon
tetrachloride should not be used as general solvent or degreaser but
substituted by less toxic ones). Methylene chloride (dichloromethane) is used as a paint stripper and as a solvent for specialized
processes, as is chloroform, well known historically as an anaesthetic.
Vinyl chloride, notorious because of its having caused angiosarco-
mata of the liver in heavily exposed subjects, is mainly used as an
intermediate in the plastics industry. Chloro- and dichlorobenzene

compounds, in the aromatic group, are used in the chemical industry and for pesticide manufacture.

Categories of workers most likely to be exposed therefore are those in metal industries, paint and dry cleaning plants, some chemical industries and many other processes where the compounds are used as degreasing and cleaning agents or solvents.

Route of entry is mainly by inhalation of these volatile substances, most of which may penetrate the skin to some extent by virtue of their degreasing action.

Adverse effects vary; these can be due to acute massive absorption and poisoning which results in central nervous system depression signs such as dizziness, lack of co-ordination, confusion, narcotic effects, respiratory depression, arrhythmias, loss of consciousness, coma and death.

(Carbon tetrachloride poisoning also causes acute liver necrosis, abdominal pains, diarrhoea and renal failure, rapidly developing jaundice and secondary cardiac failure and may result in death). Chloroform, well known for its narcotic effects, is one of the more irritant substances of this group and may cause mucosal and skin burns, methyl chloride even frost-bite while methylene chloride (dichloromethane), apart from its irritant effect, also gives rise to the formation of carboxy-haemoglobine. All of these compounds, in varying degree, are irritant to the eyes, mucosal membranes and skin.

While chronic exposure to and contact with these substances may lead to chronic dermatitis, some give rise to chloracne (PCB's and chloro naphthalenes). Chronic absorption may lead to central nervous depression symptoms and liver function disturbances. Some have been implicated as being carcinogens, usually without indicating specific target organs except for vinyl chloride mentioned earlier.

Most also affect liver function in the long run, synergistic with damage caused by alcohol intake, and some induce arrhythmia. When heated or exposed to oxygen radicals (e.g. caused by ultraviolet rays in welding) decomposition to irritant gases occurs, one of which is phosgen, which may cause delayed and serious lung oedema after a few hours.

Generally speaking the least offensive and toxic substances in this group are 1.1.1.trichloroethane and trichloroethylene and tetrachloroethylene (perchlorethylene), although these still pose a potential risk to workers if not handled properly.

(b) Among the bromide and iodide derivatives ethylene bromide (1.2.dibromo ethane, no 30 on the HRS list), methyl iodide (no 38) and vinyl bromide (no 48) as well as methyl bromide are utilized as fumigants, pesticides, additives to petrol, fire extinguishers and in chemical processes. All except methyl bromide are regarded as potential carcinogens; they are irritating to skin and mucosa and have adverse effects on central and peripheral nervous systems, including a narcotic effect.

Methyl bromide, which is widely used as a fumigant for grain, warehouses and ships, may, after excessive absorption, cause delayed symptoms of neurological damage, tremors, convulsions, cardio-respiratory failure and death. In comparison, ethyl bromide is much less toxic and would therefore be recommended as a substitute.

(c) The fluorinated hydrocarbons are primarily used as refrigerants and as polymer intermediates but also as propellants, blowing agents and in fire extinguishers. They are also widely used in the electronic industry as solvents and degreasing agents. Their widespread use is largely due to their relatively low toxicity. For some purposes, as indicated earlier, their use has been restricted, particularly the CFC's, because of their adverse effect on the ozone layer around the globe. They are, however, mildly irritating to the respiratory tract and skin, especially their decomposition products. In very high concentrations a depressive effect on the central nervous system may occur.

(d) Aromatic halogenated hydrocarbons, as mentioned earlier, are used in the pharmaceutical industry, as chemical intermediates and for pesticides. There are chlorinated benzenes, naphthalenes and diphenyls in this group. Most are irritating to skin and mucosa and the respiratory tract on inhalation. Like the polychlorinated biphenyls, they may cause chloracne, affect the liver and are classified as potential carcinogens. In contrast to the halogenated *aliphatic* compounds, the higher the number of chlorine atoms in the compound, the less toxic it is likely to be.

Early recognition of effects is dependent on clinical awareness of the degreasing effect on the skin these substances have, and suspicion that early signs of dermatitis signify systemic absorption. With regard to chronic effects neurologic symptoms are usually vague and not very helpful, while the same applies to chronic effects on liver and kidneys.

Biological monitoring using specific laboratory tests for specific exposures is useful but not feasible for all these substances. Examples of guideline values for biochemical tests in blood and urine for the most important compounds, derived from Lauwerys (1983) and the ACGIH (1991/1992), the latter as BEI value (biological exposure index) are given below:

BLOOD and URINE
> Methylene chloride
> (dichloromethane) 0,08 mg/100 ml
> (carboxy-Hb 5 % (normal 1 %)) nonsmokers.

Methyl chloroform
> (1.1.1.trichloroethane) 50 mg/g creat.
> (sum of trichloroacetic acid
> + trichloro ethanol)

BEI end of week: 10 mg/ℓ trichloroacetic ac.
Trichloroethylene
> After 5 d exposure 0,06 mg/100 ml 125 mg/g creat.
> (trichloroethanol)
> 75 mg/g creat.
> (trichloroacetic ac.)
> BEI end of week: sum of both 300 mg/g creat.

Tetrachloroethylene

(perchloroethylene) 60 ppm (blood) 7 mg/g creat (urine).

(end of week)

The *diagnosis* of adverse effects rests, as usual, on a confirmed history of exposure and on establishing that effects are in accordance with those expected on absorption of the compound in question. Periodic health surveillance, using specific tests, combined with taking a detailed history and observing early signs when feasible, is much more useful than untargeted general medical examinations.

Prevention: Environmental control to keep exposure levels below acceptable limits, where necessary combined with personal protection devices such as gloves, aprons and even dedicated respirators where engineering control is not possible, are the basic measures to be taken to prevent excessive absorption and thus adverse effects. Health education to ensure appropriate and informed handling of the compounds (e.g. total prohibition of cleaning the skin with these substances!!) is essential, as is knowledge of adverse effects which may follow exposure and of the combined effect of alcohol intake as well as of the risk of decomposition products evolving on heating or exposure of chlorinated hydrocarbons to ultraviolet rays, ozone and oxygen radicals.

All information and education given should be geared to the substances used in the particular work setting. Occupational environmental exposure limits or guidelines for most if not all these compounds are published by the ACGIH and other sources annually.

Treatment of acute overexposure and absorption consists of, depending on the degree and manner in which exposure occurred, first aid measures such as administering oxygen, thorough washing of exposed skin, often of necessity followed by hospitalization for observation of delayed serious effects, such as lung oedema, liver damage or central nervous system effects.

6.3.3.9   Lead poisoning Lead poisoning is a reportable medical condition under the Health Act (no 63 of 1977). It is also a scheduled compensatable industrial disease on the 2nd schedule under the Workmen's Compensation Act, defined as 'lead poisoning or its "sequelae"', for workmen involved in 'handling of lead or its preparations or compounds'. Lead is incorporated as no 2 in the High Risk Substances list of the General Administrative Regulations under the MOS Act of 1983.

Occurrence: Pure metallic lead by itself is not dangerous but its oxide and salts, in the form of metal fumes or dust particles, present a hazard to health when absorbed on inhalation or ingestion. Inorganic lead poisoning is a potential risk where lead is smelted, burned or used in vitreous enamelling or glazing of pottery. Manufacture of lead batteries, lead pigments and additives and some specific processes in the metal industry and plastic industry where compounds in fine dust form or as fumes may contaminate the air are all potentially hazardous work situations.

Organic alkyl lead compounds such as tetra aethyl and tetra methyl lead, used as anti knock agents in motor fuel, cause a quite different clinical picture by virtue of their acute direct effect on the nervous system. Certain categories of refinery workers are at risk. The effects of organic lead compounds will be discussed separately.

Route of entry: Absorption of inorganic lead through the lungs is the most important route of entry although ingestion may play a role. Some lead salts, oily substances such as lead naphthenate and stearate, may be absorbed through the skin, as is the case, much more important, with the alkyl lead compounds. Risk of absorption of inorganic lead through the lungs depends to a great extent on particle size and solubility of the compound in body fluids. In lead mines where the poorly soluble galena (PbS) is mined, the risk of effects is much lower than where oxides and some more soluble salts are handled. It is estimated that about 30 % of inhaled lead will actually be absorbed, and only about 5–10 % of ingested lead. Once absorbed most of the lead will be bound to erythrocytes, some will be dispersed through soft tissues while accumulation in bone and teeth will form the bulk of the body burden. Elimination occurs through excretion via the urine for about 75–80 % and by the intestinal tract for about 15 %. When exposure and absorption are not at too high a level an equilibrium between absorption and excretion may be established without the worker suffering significant adverse effects on his health.

Adverse effects: Haematological effects of lead are inhibition of haemoglobin synthesis and shortened life span of erythrocytes, together leading to anaemia in exposed persons. Lead interferes with a number of enzymes and enzyme systems which gives rise to the accumulation of some of these as well as of precursors of haemoglobin in the blood. Increased excretion in the urine of some of these substances may result. Neurological effects are mainly on peripheral nerves, at first only recognizable by sensitive electro-physiological tests (nerve conduction velocity) but later resulting in disturbance of motor function, paresis and paralysis in severe cases. The central nervous system is also affected, encephalopathy with ataxia, convulsions and coma may occur, but these are more likely in children, who may also exhibit early behavioural and learning disturbances which are more difficult to spot in adults. Gastro-intestinal effects, diarrhoea, more often constipation, colic, loss of appetite and indigestion, occur after acute high level absorption as well as in chronic poisoning. Effects on spermatogenesis have been reported, but accounts of mutagenic and even carcinogenic effects need to be confirmed before these are accepted. Pregnant women should not be exposed to lead as the foetus is very susceptible to effects of lead, which passes the placenta.

Long-term effects on the kidney have also been reported, higher prevalence of hypertension in exposed worker populations, hyper-uricaemia and gout and other arthralgias have been linked with or ascribed to lead absorption. Susceptibility to adverse effects may vary. It is uncertain whether healthy women are more susceptible, but malnutrition, anaemia and haemoglobinopathies are factors which increase susceptibility.

Frank lead poisoning with clear clinical signs has become rare, as has the often described so-called 'Burton' line, a bluish line due to accumulation of lead sulphide in the gum adjacent to the molars.

Adverse effects of organic, alkyl lead compounds deserve special mention as these substances may cause acute intoxication of the central nervous system after absorption through the skin or by inhalation. Physical signs such as peripheral neuropathy or anaemia do not feature in this presentation while blood lead level, urinary excretion of ALA (amino-laevulinic acid) and coproporphyrines are likely to be normal and unhelpful for diagnostic purposes.

An acute encephalopathy with signs such as anxiety, delusions, hallucinations and convulsions may occur in the casualty.

A diagnosis of clinical lead poisoning rests on a substantiated history of exposure and potential absorption, clinical signs and symptoms corroborated by appropriate laboratory test results. The office of the Workmen's Compensation Commissioner would accept a claim supported by the well-known Lane's criteria, i.e. a blood lead level of more than 80 microg/100 ml would be regarded as 'excessive absorption', more than 120 microg/100 ml blood as 'dangerous' and as a sign of lead poisoning. Confirmatory test results would be a urine lead content exceeding 150 respectively 250 microg/ℓ and ALA excretion exceeding 20 respectively 40 mg/ℓ.

A distinction must be made between clinical lead poisoning, which is a reportable and compensatable medical condition and so-called 'metabolic lead poisoning' which is not accompanied by any clinical sign, not even anaemia, but is of great medical importance.

Early recognition of impending metabolic lead poisoning, also termed 'excessive absorption' as in Lane's parameters, is an essential function of health workers in occupational health services. Apart from knowledge about and evaluation of environmental lead exposure at work, this must be based on history taking and observation of working procedures, of adherence to personal protection and of personal hygiene preventive measures and on biological monitoring. When workers present themselves with symptoms and complaints resulting from excessive absorption of lead, it is already too late.

The acceptable exposure limit for lead in the working environment varies in different countries but is still 150 microg/m^3 of air in the United Kingdom standard as also recommended by the ACGIH as well as in the Lead regulations of 1989 under the MOS Act. In the USA however the Occupational Safety and Health Act adopted as standard a value of 50 microg/m^3. The Lead regulation stipulates as action level 75 microg/m^3 of air. Complementary biological monitoring tests are prescribed to safeguard the health of potentially exposed workers. These are blood lead level tests (not to exceed 80 microg/100 ml in adult men and 40 in 'women of reproductive capacity') and other biological tests such as Haemoglobin level. Also of use are tests for ALA and lead excretion in the urine, coproporphyrine excretion levels in the urine and zinc protoporphyrine levels in the blood.

The WHO proposes as health based biological limit for lead in blood the value of 40 microg/100 ml for adult males and 30 for females at reproductive age, as at these levels no significant adverse effect on haemopoiesis is expected to occur. The ACGIH regards a blood lead level of 50 microg/100 ml as an acceptable biological exposure index (BEI) with as alternative indices a maximum level of ZPP of 7,2 microg/g Hb and an excretion of lead in urine of not more than 150 microg/g creatinine excreted.

For screening purposes in an occupational health service concerned with workers who are potentially exposed to lead the following biological monitoring test results are recommended for a decision to withdraw the worker from exposure:

Blood lead 60 microg/100 ml

ZPP 7,2 microg/g Haemoglobin

ALA in urine 20 mg/ℓ

Coproporphyrine in urine 300 mg/ℓ

Lead in urine 150 microg/ℓ

Evaluation of excessive absorption, i.e. early recognition of persons who are at risk of suffering adverse effects on their health, would be served by a biological monitoring programme as set out above. Withdrawal from exposure should then be followed by monitoring of some of these tests, so that when values drop to acceptable levels return to work may be advised. The WHO supports this concept in its Technical Series report no 647, published in 1980.

Treatment when indicated may be preceded by a chelation provocation test in hospital to confirm the diagnosis, followed by chelation with Ca-EDTA and/or penicillamine.

Calcium gluconate intravenously has been used with success for lead colic.

6.3.3.10 Manganese poisoning The Workmen's Compensation Act lists manganese poisoning in the second schedule as industrial disease with the following as a description of occupation: 'any work involving the use or handling of or exposure to the fumes, dust or vapour of manganese or a compound or substance containing manganese'.

Occurrence: The main source of exposure to manganese oxide (MnO_2) is in mining of the ore (pyrolusite) which usually happens in open cast mines. As this is not soluble in water, absorption depends on fine respirable size of particles entering the body through the lungs. However, most of the manganese once mined is used in the iron and steel (ferromanganese) industry, for welding rods, dry cell electric batteries, for ceramics, in pottery and fertilizers. Manganese is an essential mineral for a number of enzymes in the human body and is mostly excreted in bile via the intestinal tract. Organic compounds which are more soluble give rise to higher concentrations of manganese in the urine than inorganic compounds.

Route of entry: mainly through inhalation of fine respirable dust particles, ingestion may occur; accumulation in liver and also the central nervous system follows absorption. Some of the organic compounds may enter through the intact skin.

Adverse effects are mainly of a chronic nature although very rarely substantial inhalation of manganese fumes may give rise to metal fume fever, high dust concentrations may lead to bronchitis and pneumonia. More important but also rare are the chronic effects on the central nervous system, 'manganism', resulting in a syndrome which resembles to some extent that of Parkinsonism. Individual susceptibility varies markedly.

Early recognition is based on awareness of exposure to and knowledge of the association of vague, aspecific symptoms with excessive absorption of manganese. Sleepiness, lassitude, perhaps some stiffness of leg muscles and twitching or cramps at night must give rise to concern. Tendon reflexes are increased, fine tremors and a disturbance of gait, 'high stepping' type may follow, with loss of expression of the face 'mask like', monotonous voice and psychomotor disturbances, all symptoms which resemble Parkinsonism. Estimation of manganese in blood and urine are not very helpful, that in faeces, though not very practical, may assist in making the diagnosis.

The acceptable environmental exposure limit recommended by the ACGIH is 5 mg per cubic metre of air for manganese dust and 1 mg for manganese fumes. No biological exposure index has been proposed. As indicated, the value of manganese in blood and urine is of limited value, analysis of faeces on a routine monitoring basis is not very practical. When an early stage suspicion on the grounds of symptoms exists removal from exposure may be indicated.

6.3.3.11   Mercury poisoning   Mercury and its compounds are listed as no 3 in the High Risk Substances list of the General Administrative Regulations under the MOS Act and mercury poisoning is a compensatable industrial disease scheduled in the 2nd schedule under the Workmen's Compensation Act. Under description of occupation this schedule reads: 'any work involving the use of mercury or its preparations or its compounds', a very wide description indeed.

Occurrence: Apart from mining and extraction of mercury which poses a hazard to mine workers, the use of mercury in laboratory, measuring and electrical instruments and in dentistry may expose workers to inhalation of mercury vapour or to skin absorption, the last especially but not exclusively by organic mercury compounds (alkyl and aryl compounds). Mercury is also used in electrolytic processes for the production of certain salts and for fungicides and pesticides, batteries and lamps, as well as for extraction of gold purposes. Methylmercury, regarded as the most toxic organic mercury compound, occurs naturally and may accumulate in fish and molluscs.

Route of entry is mainly by inhalation of vapour (mercury is volatile at room temperature and even below that) or of certain dusts through the lung. Metallic mercury but more so organic compounds may be absorbed through the intact skin while ingestion of contaminated material may also lead to poisoning. Organic compounds are mainly excreted with the faeces, inorganic ones with the urine. About 80 % of mercury vapour is actually absorbed, about 90 % of this will initially be bound by erythrocytes. Substances with a low solubility are usually less toxic.

Adverse effects vary from acute, irritational or systemic and chronic. Acute exposure may lead to skin rashes, bronchitis and pneumonia, in susceptible persons skin sensitization may occur. Chronic local and systemic effects are stomatitis, tremor and erethism (the classical triad) while gastro-intestinal disturbances, diarrhoea, nervous system effects and damage to the kidney such as tubular necrosis may follow. Erethism is characterized by increased irritability and excitability but sometimes unusual timidity, the originally developing fine tremor of fingers and facial muscles may develop into coarser tremors and inability to write legibly. Gingivitis with blackening of the teeth and loss of teeth is also a classic sign, extreme irritability and anxiety may occur. Clouding of the lens (mercurilentis) is a comparative early sign in some patients, restriction of visual field may also exist.

In poisoning with organic mercury compounds signs of sensory, ocular, auditory and cerebellar dysfunction are more prominent than in metallic mercury poisoning.

Pregnant women, the foetus (mercury passes the placenta), adolescents and persons already suffering from nervous system diseases are considered to be more susceptible to adverse effects than others.

Early recognition in the clinical sense rests on awareness of exposure to mercury, taking note of early relevant symptoms and signs such as minor behavioural changes, irritability, fine tremors (comparing a sample of handwriting with an earlier 'baseline' sample kept on file for that purpose), mild stomatitis and perhaps a skin rash. Increased salivation and swelling of salivary glands are further relevant signs.

However, biological monitoring tests are available and of value for complementing such clinical evaluations. Excretion of mercury should not exceed 50 microg/ℓ urine (or per g creatinine excreted) nor should a value of 3 microg/100 ml blood be exceeded. The ACGIH recommends as Biological Exposure Index (BEI) that total inorganic mercury in a urine sample taken before the workshift should not exceed 35 microg/g creatinine and that a blood sample collected at the end of the last shift of the work week should not contain more than 1,5 microg mercury/100 ml. The timing of sampling is dictated by the pharmacokinetics of mercury, which may be absorbed and excreted rapidly.

The WHO recommends, for long-term exposure situations, that the mercury in air concentration should not exceed 25 microg/m^3 of air. (The ACGIH accepts 50 microg/m^3 of air for all forms of mercury except organic alkyl vapour.)

For individuals the WHO recommends that the urinary excretion level should not exceed 50 microg/g creatinine excreted. This latter recommendation is a widely accepted and practical criterion.

In conclusion early recognition of adverse effects of mercury absorption should be based on biological monitoring complemented by routine periodical clinical evaluation whenever a suspicion that absorption takes place exists.

Environmental monitoring is of additional value for certain processes.

Treatment of mercury poisoning is to some extent controversial and should always be initiated in hospital. Dimercaprol (BAL British Anti Lewisite), d-penicillamine and less often Ca-EDTA have been used for treatment, but some authorities warn against the use of

Ca-EDTA and even dimercaprol in severe poisoning cases when the nervous system is involved.

6.3.3.12 Phosphorus poisoning The second schedule of the Workmen's Compensation Act lists phosphorus poisoning as a compensatable industrial disease for affected workmen if resulting from: 'any work involving the use of phosphorus or its preparations or compounds'.

Occurrence: Yellow (white) phosphorus is a waxy volatile solid substance which ignites spontaneously on coming into contact with air and may cause severe contact burns. It does not naturally occur in its free elemental form but as phosphates and acid. Red phosphor, its non-toxic allotrope, used to be used for matches. Yellow phosphor, usually handled submerged under water, is used for incendiary and smoke devices, explosives, ammunition, pyrotechnics and in certain metal alloy and electro technical products. Inorganic compounds are used for the manufacture of insecticides, fertilizers and pharmaceuticals. Other inorganic compounds such as chlorides and sulphides are used for agricultural chemicals, in the chemical industry and for insecticides. Phosphine, an extremely toxic gas, is used for fumigation but may be generated accidentally during certain processes in the chemical and metal industry. Relatively few workers would be exposed to elemental phosphor hazards, but potentially more to inorganic phosphor compounds. However, many more people who are engaged in agriculture and horticulture where the use of organic phosphorus pesticides (organophosphates) is widespread, would be at risk.

Route of entry: Elemental phosphorus causes severe burns on contact, also when ingested, but most of the phosphor compounds with which workers come into contact would be absorbed by inhalation of mists (liquids), vapours (from liquids and solids) and gas (phosphine). Skin absorption occurs readily with organic compounds, particularly the organophosphates, as well.

Adverse effects: Acute effects of contact with elemental phosphor and most toxic inorganic compounds such as phosphoric acid and chlorides are severe burns, irritation of eyes and mucosal surfaces, especially of the respiratory tract leading to acute bronchitis, and pulmonary oedema after a few hours. Absorption of phosphor in any form may lead to acute severe liver damage and cardiovascular collapse. Phosphorus pentasulphide, which is rapidly hydrolyzed to hydrogen sulphide, may lead to acute death as happens with inhalation of hydrogen sulphide gas which is as toxic as cyanide gas.

Acute effects of organophosphate compounds, perhaps only evident a few hours after exposure, are headache, vertigo, blurring of vision, lacrimation and salivation, tightness of the chest, heavy perspiration, dyspnoea and miosis. Fasciculation, ataxia, loss of reflexes, convulsions and coma may follow.

Most of these symptoms result from severe depression of cholinesterase activity due to organophosphate poisoning. Gastrointestinal symptoms are more common after ingestion.

Inhalation of phosphine gas causes irritation (it has a strong fishy odour) and acute central nervous depression, with similar symptoms as described above. It may lead to severe pulmonary oedema after a few or more hours, while acute cardiac arrest has also been reported.

Chronic effects of poisoning by inorganic phosphor compounds in small amounts over a long time manifests itself mainly by damage to the skeletal system and liver. Periostitis, ulceration of the gum and bone necrosis, loss of teeth especially in the mandible (phossy jaw) are classic signs, as are toxic hepatitis with jaundice. Chronic irritational 'contact' dermatitis, allergic dermatitis and non-specific chronic respiratory disease may follow on absorption of phosphorus in the body. Chronic poisoning by organic phosphor compounds gives rise to vague symptoms such as persistent headaches, loss of appetite, general malaise, sleeping disturbances, while chronic dermatitis, miosis and wheezing may also occur. Clinical symptoms as are described above usually only occur when cholinesterase activity is depressed by at least 50 to 60 %. Severe acute intoxication follows when inhibition of cholinesterase activity below 20 % of pre-exposure value occurs.

Early recognition: The irritant effects of phosphor and its inorganic compounds may serve as early warning that exposure is taking place. A certain degree of tolerance against the irritational effects of phosphoric acid (acceptable level in air is 1 mg per cubic metre of air, against 0,1 mg for elemental phosphor) appears to develop in exposed workers.

Phosphine gas is malodorous and smells of decaying fish; its acceptable exposure limit as recommended by the ACGIH is 0,3 ppm, for short-term exposure (STEL) 1 ppm.

No biological exposure index has been established for inorganic compounds as no appropriate assessment method is as yet available. Urinary excretion of phosphates, which happens normally, is not a useful sign.

However, for chronic absorption of organophosphates (and for the diagnosis of acute intoxication) determination of cholinesterase activity is a practical method for biological monitoring purposes. As individual variation around average values is wide, individual baseline, pre-exposure values for plasma, red blood cells or whole blood need to be established first. For the two last media an inhibition of up to 30 % may be regarded as permissible, for plasma up to 50 %.

For persons exposed to parathion urinary excretion of p-nitrophenol offers another measure for exposure and absorption as parathion is excreted in the urine for about 70 % in the form of p-nitrophenol. The maximum allowable value recommended is 2 mg per gramme creatinine excreted.

The ACGIH lists as biological exposure index (BEI) for organo-phosphorous cholinesterase inhibitors that 70 % of the baseline value of the individuals cholinesterase activity in Red Blood Cells should be maintained and for parathion that urinary excretion of p-nitrophenol in a sample taken at the end of the workshift should not exceed 0,5 mg/ℓ as confirmatory test for exposure to this substance.

Periodic screening examinations at relatively short intervals or after each exposure event are useful for early recognition of effects. Awareness of and skill in eliciting a history of early symptoms may serve as an early warning that absorption of phosphor has taken place. It should be noted that symptoms of organophosphates poisoning may be delayed for up to 12 hours or even longer. Acceptable exposure limits for various phosphor compounds are recommended by the ACGIH.

Prevention of adverse effects is possible through well-known procedures such as reducing the potential of contact, of reducing the escaping of vapour, mists or gas into the working environment (monitored by air sampling) and by the use of appropriate personal protective equipment.

Acute and chronic poisoning, when suspected or diagnosed, should be dealt with in hospitals where facilities for diagnostic radiographic and laboratory tests and treatment are available, particularly when organophosphates poisoning is suspected. High doses of atropine and artificial respiration as well as resuscitation may be necessary.

Poisoning by organophosphates which fall under the registered substances of the Fertilizers, Farm Feeds and Agricultural Remedies and Stock Remedies Act is reportable under the Health Act as a notifiable medical condition.

6.3.3.13 *Silicosis, asbestosis and other fibrosis of the lungs caused by mineral dusts* The second schedule of the Workmen's Compensation Act lists under description of occupation for these pneumoconioses: 'Any occupation (other than in a "dusty atmosphere" as defined in the Pneumoconiosis Act of 1956) in which workmen are exposed to the inhalation of silica dust, asbestos dust or any other mineral dust'.

The reference to the Pneumoconiosis Act or the present Occupational Diseases in Mines and Works Act serves the purpose to exclude cases in miners who perform 'risk work' (as defined) and whose compensation is covered by that Act. For practical purposes compensatability of these conditions as discussed here is applicable to workmen not working in mines or works.

Asbestos (no 1) and crystalline silica (no 7) are listed as high risk substances in the relevant schedule of the General Administrative Regulations of the MOS Act.

Occurrence: SILICA: Silicosis is a pneumoconiosis, a group of disorders of the lung which are characterized by being caused by inhalation of fibrogenic dust, fibrosis being the most important tissue reaction resulting from such inhalation. Crystalline mineral quartz respirable particles (free Silica oxide SiO_2) are the responsible agent, respirable referring to the fact that by virtue of size the particles can enter deep into the alveolar space. Apart from certain mining operations the following occupations involve a risk of exposure:

Stone dressing and polishing (monumental masonry and semi-precious stone work such as on tiger-eye etc.), sandblasting, casting and fettling in foundries, ceramic and other brick manufacture and manufacture of porcelain and earthenware for which silica containing substances are used.

Mixed dust pneumoconiosis, e.g. Coal miners anthra silicosis, is a form of silicosis which is codetermined by other dusts inhaled in addition to the free silica content of the total dust in question.

The characteristic pathological feature of silicosis is the silicotic nodule, a fibrous tissue reaction following inhalation and retention of free silica particles of a size between approximately 0,5 and 7 micron in diameter. Further fibrosis may then follow and also some calcification in lymph nodes. Workers who are exposed to silica are at increased risk to contract tuberculosis as well, the combination is known as silico tuberculosis.

ASBESTOS: This is the generic name for a variety of naturally occurring fibrous mineral silicates, the most important of which are chrysotile (white asbestos), crocidolite (blue asbestos) and amosite (brown asbestos). There are two subgroups, the serpentine group, to which chrysotile belongs, with curly longitudinal fibres and amphiboles, such as crocidolite which splits in shorter, straight fibres of variable length and diameter.

Apart from mining, milling, processing and transporting of mined asbestos, the manufacture and usage of asbestos containing materials such as roofing materials, tiles, coatings, insulation (lagging) and friction materials (brake linings), asbestos reinforced cement pipes and dusts and asbestos paper may put workers at risk. Most of these products would contain chrysotile, only a few and in declining degree also crocidolite. Substitution by other fibres, where technologically feasible, has reduced the utilization of asbestos fibres to a large degree. In some countries a virtual or real ban on the use of asbestos has reduced the risk to inhabitants of those countries to practically zero. The characteristic features of asbestosis are interstitial fibrosis and pleural plaque formation.

Route of entry for all dusts which may cause pneumoconiosis is by inhalation. Retention after inhalation is mainly determined by the size c.q. diameter of the particle. Long fibres of 200 micron but with a diameter of a few micron may penetrate the alveolae just as well as particles which measure not more than 5 micron in size. Asbestos fibres when ingested may possibly also cause harm, silica particles ingested are not thought to be significantly harmful for digestive tract tissues.

Adverse effects: SILICOSIS: Acute silicosis following massive inhalation of quartz particles in susceptible persons is a rare but rapidly progressive disease. Under extreme conditions breathlessness and cough develop over a period of a few weeks, accompanied by dyspnoea and incapacity to work within a few months and followed by respiratory failure and perhaps cor pulmonale in a few years. Especially if silicosis is combined with tuberculosis it may be a rapidly fatal disease.

Chronic low level exposure over many years (10 to 20 or more) will lead to silicosis of the lungs depending on level of exposure, type of dust (free silica content and size of particles) and biological factors in the host. Damage to the lymph nodes and lymphatics, lung tissue and small airways leads to fibrosis and scarring. This most frequently occurs more in the upper zones of the lung. Early stages are not accompanied by clinical symptoms such as cough, bronchitis and dyspnoea. Basic ventilatory lung function tests may remain normal for a long time. In later stages progressive dyspnoea on exertion and even at rest follows, based on a restrictive respiratory impairment. The disease process is progressive even after cessation of exposure. Intercurrent respiratory infections, cor pulmonale, hypertension and heart failure may be terminal events.

ASBESTOS: Acute asbestosis is not known to exist. A gradual, progressive, diffuse interstitial fibrotic process, with coalescing of lesions, pleural involvement and plaque formation takes place over years, eventually leading to incapacitating restrictive pulmonary disease. When chrysotile is the main fibre type inhaled, and especially in smokers, the risk of developing lung cancer, particularly adenocarcinoma, is increased manifold as compared with the normal non-exposed population. Amphiboles have also been associated with such an increase in lung cancer but crocidolite in particular is regarded as the main, if not the only, type of fibre which causes mesothelioma of the pleura, usually only after an interval of 20 to 40 years after first exposure. This tumour development does not appear to be influenced by smoking habits. Certain naturally occurring silicates, zeloites, used as building material, have also been implicated with mesothelioma in Turkey.

MESOTHELIOMA is specifically listed in the second schedule of the Workmen's Compensation Act for 'any work which involves the handling or use of asbestos or exposing the workman to asbestos dust, caused by the use of asbestos in connection with the employer's business'. The type of asbestos is not specified here but the type of tumour is. It is assumed that asbestos fibres other than crocidolite may also cause occupationally induced mesothelioma. Carcinoma of the lung, other than mesothelioma, is not scheduled as such as an industrial compensatable disease but claims for compensation could be awarded if it is proven to the satisfaction of the Commissioner that the lung cancer in question resulted from an exposure incident arising out of and during work.

In asbestosis abnormal radiographic signs tend to be more common in the lower zone of the lung than elsewhere, pleural involvement frequently shows up as obliteration of the costophrenic angles and pleural thickening and calcification (plaques).

OTHER MINERAL DUSTS which may cause fibrosis of the lungs but are less potent and less prevalent are silicates such as kaolin, bentonite and diatomite (possibly due to their free silica content), aluminium and beryllium.

So-called benign pneumoconioses, in which accumulation of dust in the lungs occurs without fibrosis as a significant tissue reaction, may be caused by iron oxide, tin, barium, calcium or chromate dusts. Deposits visible on radiography tend to disappear over time after cessation of exposure. These conditions are not compensatable diseases.

Early recognition: SILICOSIS, not giving rise to subjective symptoms, complaints or clinical signs in an early stage, can only be detected by periodic screening examinations which include chest radiography and preferably also lung function tests from the start, complemented by the taking of an occupational history and physical medical examination. The same applies, mutatis mutandis, to ASBESTOSIS.

Monitoring by chest radiography in accordance with the recommendations of the International Labour Office in their International Classification of Radiographic Changes in Pneumoconiosis, is essential for early recognition and indeed for arriving at a diagnosis, supported, when present, by clinical symptoms and signs, and by results of appropriate and carefully controlled lung function tests.

This requires special expertise and the availability of the standard set of radiographs published by the ILO for reference purposes.

Sputum tests may reveal the presence of so-called 'asbestos' or 'ferruginous' bodies but these only indicate that exposure to asbestos has taken place, not the existence of 'asbestosis' disease. When a suspicion that lung cancer is present exists, cytological examination of sputum may be helpful but this is not so for routine screening purposes. To diagnose silico tuberculosis sputum examination is a normal clinical procedure.

In conclusion, base line examinations of workers exposed to potential inhalation of mineral dusts should comprise of a properly taken chest X-ray and lung function test, in addition to the recording of a carefully compiled occupational history and a clinical examination. This should then be followed by routine periodic screening examination containing the same elements, at intervals determined by the type of dust workers are exposed to. This should be part of a well organized and maintained health surveillance programme aimed at early recognition of adverse effects, before significant damage to health occurs.

Prevention of adverse effects rests on sound industrial hygiene principles and may include, when unavoidable, the proper use of personal protective equipment, e.g. air supplied respiratory hoods for sandblasters.

The ACGIH recommends as acceptable exposure level for quartz and fused silica 0,1 mg per cubic metre of air, measured as 'respirable dust'. Lower values are given for crystoballite and tridymite. The WHO proposed tentatively that the concentration of 'respirable dust sampled in the breathing zone of workers' should not exceed 0,04 mg per cubic metre of air.

For asbestos the following limit values for fibres per millilitre of air are recommended by the ACGIH:

AMOSITE 0,5, CHRYSOTILE 2,0, CROCIDOLITE 0,2 AND OTHER FORMS OF ASBESTOS 2 FIBRES PER CC OF AIR.

The annotation A1 added to this signifies that asbestos is regarded as a confirmed human carcinogen.

The Asbestos Regulations promulgated under the MOS Act contain explicit standards, regulations and action levels aimed at the prevention of adverse effects to health of potentially exposed workers.

6.3.3.14 *TNT poisoning* The Workmen's Compensation Act gives as description of occupation under this heading: 'Any work involving the preparation, packing or handling of trinitrotoluol (TNT)'. Such kind of work would be expected only in the manufacture and processing of explosive devices. Trinitrotoluol (syn. methyltrinitobenzene) falls into the group of nitro-derivatives of benzene discussed earlier (no 4) but warrants a separate section.

Occurrence: exposure occurs in the manufacture of TNT in the chemical industry, and processing in the explosives industry, including the manufacture of bombs, shells, mines and other devices. TNT is a volatile solid substance.

Route of entry: Inhalation of vapour, which comes off at room temperature occurs to some degree (but less than in the case of liquid aniline) but skin absorption of the dust, especially in hot weather conditions when dissolved in perspiration may be the main mechanism.

Adverse effects: Acute intoxication is much less likely to happen than chronic poisoning as a result of absorption over time. TNT vapour and dust causes acute irritation of the eyes, nose and throat (with a bitter taste in the mouth) and skin (contact dermatitis) and may cause yellowish discoloration of hair, nails and skin. More important effects are toxic gastritis and hepatitis, sometimes severe with jaundice and potentially fatal in 30 % of cases. TNT also causes met-haemoglobinaemia and anaemia and in very rare cases even aplastic anaemia. This may manifest itself, late, even long after exposure to risk has ceased to exist.

Early symptoms are anorexia, nausea, constipation, headaches, lassitude, followed by anaemia, mild haemolytic jaundice, slight cyanosis and flushing of the face and the discoloration mentioned above.

Early recognition rests not only on knowledge of potential exposure and early clinical symptoms and signs but also on careful periodic medical examinations, including appropriate laboratory tests. Urinary excretion of TNT and its metabolites (dinitro-amino-toluene) may be measured routinely. The ACGIH recommends that the met-haemoglobine level should not exceed 1,5 % in a blood sample taken at the end of the shift. Lauwerys, who lists 2 % as the normal upper level for non-exposed people, suggests that up to 5 % is acceptable in workers exposed to agents which cause met-haemoglobinaemia. Full blood counts would indicate more advanced effects, while for the diagnosis of liver damage and hepatitis liver function tests and the determination of urocoproporphyrines and bile salts in the urine would be useful.

Prevention: The ACGIH lists as acceptable environmental level 0,5 mg per cubic metre of air, with the annotation that skin absorption occurs (usually the main route of entry). It follows that personal protection by protective and clean working clothes (changed daily), compulsory showers after work and strict personal hygiene are the most important measures to be taken. A special kind of indicator soap (akin to the Webster test with alcoholic sodium hydrochloride) which shows contamination with TNT up by an orange colour, would be useful to ensure complete removal of any TNT adhering to the skin.

When significant indications of adverse effects are noted and treatment is indicated the worker should be admitted to hospital.

6.3.3.15 Byssinosis Byssinosis is a chronic obstructive airways disease which is regarded as peculiar to the occupation of textile workers.

The Workmen's Compensation Act, second schedule, gives as description of occupation for byssinosis 'any occupation in which a workman is exposed to the inhalation of cotton or linen dust'.

The Greek word from which the name is derived refers to fine linen or flax. In general it is thought that not only cotton but also flax, hemp and sisal dust may cause byssinosis, a progressive condition which may eventually lead to total disablement if exposure persists long after first symptoms have appeared.

Occurrence: Industrial processing of the vegetable fibres rather than the growing of them appears to give rise to the risk of developing the disease in susceptible exposed workers. Thus the risk is greatest in textile mills, especially where spinning, winding and to a somewhat lesser extent where weaving is done, but also in the home industry.

Route of entry is by inhalation of the airborne dust at the workplace.

Adverse effects: Characteristic pathological changes in the upper and lower lobar bronchi are mucous gland hyperplasia and hypertrophy of smooth muscle, with varying degrees of lobar emphysema at a later stage. Symptoms are a feeling of tightness of the chest or difficulty in breathing which at first develops a few hours after renewed exposure to (cotton) dust, classically present on a Monday or other first day at work after a period off work. Initially symptoms will not be present on subsequent days but with increase of the severity of the condition will persist over other days of the week. Complaints of cough, dry or productive, may also be present. In later stages the disease resembles chronic bronchitis (with a spastic element) and emphysema, except that characteristically 'worst days' tend to be those first few days after return to work from non-exposure conditions. Corresponding to the symptoms a measurable but at first reversible decrease in pulmonary function test performance, notable FEV1 (Forced Expiratory Volume over one minute) develops. Smoking is a most important additional factor and may lead to similar, late and irreversible chronic lung disease and damage as byssinosis in its later stages. Workers may call their condition 'asthma' because their doctors and others may tell them that is what they are suffering from.

The principal mechanism leading to byssinosis is thought to be histamine release in response to contact with substances present in the vegetable fibre dusts. In established long-standing byssinosis the worker ends up with continually being dyspnoic, and has over distended lungs and emphysema. Chest radiographs do not show characteristic pathognomic changes.

People with pre-existing bronchial asthma, or perhaps even only with atopy, may react dramatically on inhaling these dusts. Such patients generally show reactions earlier in the day than byssinosis patients and on any one day of the week rather than with predisposition for the first day of re-exposure. Such patients usually do not persist with work in textile mills.

For clinical and epidemiological purposes a grading system has been in use for many years. At grade 1/2 the worker would suffer from chest tightness and cough only on the first day of re-exposure, at grade 1 on every first day of the work week, at grade 2 on more days of the week and at grade 3 symptoms would be complemented with evidence of permanent and irreversible lung function deficits. The WHO (Technical Report Series no 684, 1983) has proposed a simplified but extensive classification of symptoms, (B1 and B2), respiratory irritation signs (RTI 1 to 3) and lung function disturbances (acute or chronic, from nil through mild and moderate to severe effect).

Early recognition rests on awareness of exposure to and of the early symptoms, as well as of the confounding factors such as smoking habit, chronic bronchitis from other causes and pre-existing asthma or allergic constitution (atopy). Variation in susceptibility is a notable factor.

Periodic screening examinations are aimed at identifying those workers who are developing early symptoms. They should consist of at least the completion of a standardized specific questionnaire and a ventilatory lung function test before starting a shift (after a break of at least a period of 36 hours non-exposure) as well as a further test after 6 hours of normal work exposure on that first day of work after the break. Intervals between periodic examinations depend on exposure risk and individual factors but should not be longer than one year.

Pre-employment pre-exposure baseline data should be documented to enable evaluation of results at subsequent periodic examinations. A fall by 10 % or more of the pre-exposure test value of FEV 1 during one workshift, especially if occurring in groups of workers, should alert the health worker to take action.

Prevention: Environmental control of dust level by engineering methods is of course most important. Cleaning of machines, workrooms and equipment by compressed air should be prohibited. The United States (OSHA) Cotton Dust Standard sets as permissible exposure level of respirable cotton dust, measured in a standard manner, 0,2 mg per cubic metre of air for preparation and spinning operations, 0,75 for weaving. Other values are recommended for specific operations. The ACGIH recommends for raw cotton dust that the level in air, sampled with a cotton vertical elutriator, should not exceed 0,2 mg per cubic metre of air. High efficiency dust respirators may be used for certain maintenance operations but should not become a substitute for environmental control.

On pre-employment medical examination workers with pre-existing asthma, chronic bronchitis, abnormally reduced FEV 1 and heavy smokers, all at increased risk, should be evaluated by a physician before being allowed to start work in textile mills in places where they would be put at risk.

Treatment with standard bronchodilators and corticosteroids may relieve early symptoms of 'asthma'-like symptoms of byssinosis and with antibiotics those of chronic bronchitis. There is no effective treatment for byssinosis. Removal from exposure is therefore indicated. Symptomatic treatment may be prescribed but no therapy is available for the irreversible changes, which should not be allowed to develop, even though they are compensatable by law.

6.3.3.16 *Occupational noise induced hearing loss* Occupational hearing loss due to exposure to excessive noise in industry, i.e. impairment of hearing due to working conditions is only compensatable under the Workmen's Compensation Act in cases when audiometric readings show a decibel loss which is equal to a hearing impairment exceeding 25 % when the so-called 'three average formula' is applied. In South Africa this refers to loss at the frequencies, 500, 1000 and 2000 Hz.

The formula reads: 5 times $[1,5(a\text{-}26) + (b\text{-}26)]$, divided by a factor 6, $= n\%$ binaural impairment, where a is the average hearing loss expressed in decibels at the 500, 1000 and 2000 Hz frequency for the better ear and *b* that for the worse ear.

The maximum loss at each frequency is to be taken at 87 dB. Occupational hearing loss is not listed as a compensatable disease in the second schedule, but compensatability is based on schedule 1, which stipulates that total hearing loss in both ears is regarded as 50 % disability. Hearing impairment of up to 25 % is generally regarded as a mild hearing loss which is not disabling for employment. It should be noted that in this calculation of hearing impairment the decibel loss of the better ear (3-average value) is weighted with a factor 5 and that a factor of 1,5 is used to convert hearing loss values in decibels to percentage degree of impairment in each ear. In the United Kingdom substantial sensorineural hearing loss amounting to at least 50 dB in each ear, being due in at least one ear to occupational noise, and being the average of pure tone losses measured by audiometry over the 1, 2 and 3 kHz frequencies (Occupational Deafness) is compensatable.

Occurrence: Wherever at work the equivalent noise exposure level (N eq), measured in accordance with the SABS Standard 083- of 1983, (as amended in 1988 and 1989), exceeds 85 dB risk to sustain occupational hearing loss is deemed to exist. Then hearing conservation measures must be taken, which include audiography, since this standard has been incorporated into the Environmental Regulations of the MOS Act. Noise level meters and personal noise dose meters are available to determine whether the level of 85 dB (as integrated time weighted value corrected for impulse noise) is exceeded. This noise level is exceeded in many industrial working environments, e.g. the textile industry, stone crushers and mills, mines, foundries, metal industry and certain workplaces in the chemical industry, boiler rooms, power stations and engine rooms, as well as in many isolated operations. Excessive continuous noise, especially if exacerbated by intermittent impulse noise, will cause irreversible damage to hearing, the degree of which would depend on level of the noise, duration of exposure (per shift and over a working lifetime) and personal protective measures taken. Susceptibility to damage is variable but every worker must be regarded as susceptible if the exposure limit of 85 dB is exceeded.

Adverse effects are mainly auditory, viz. an insidiously developing hearing loss which usually manifests itself first at 4000 Hz in an audiogram, but then not only spreads to other frequencies but increases in severity over time. Only once that part of the spectrum which is necessary to hear conversational speech is affected significantly (by more than 25 dB) will subjective awareness of deafness occur. This is at the frequencies from 500 to 3000 Hz. Initially only those people who have an ear for high tones and music will be aware of earlier losses. The degree of hearing loss is proportional to the total amount of sound energy which has impinged on the ears. This dose can be estimated by calculating the Noise Emission Index, as defined in the SABS standard mentioned above. It is possible to predict, to some extent, what the expected hearing loss would be in individuals exposed to a certain noise level over a certain period of years. On epidemiological evidence it is also possible to calculate the risk of suffering a significant hearing loss for exposed populations. For practical purposes it is assumed that people exposed to noise levels not exceeding 80 dB are not at a higher risk than the general population.

Temporary threshold shift is the audiometric term for temporary reversible hearing loss which follows immediately excessive noise exposure occurs. This will wear off in about 16 hours after cessation of exposure, leaving only a slight, not measurable deficit in hearing. Over time the accumulative effect may lead to irreversible hearing loss, i.e. *permanent threshold shift*, eventually to severe and disabling occupational deafness.

The inner ear, in particular the organ of Corti, sensorineural cells which are the receivers of sound stimuli, bears the brunt of the noise assault. The resulting nerve deafness is similar to naturally diminishing hearing capacity associated with age (presbycusis) which is aggravated by occupational noise induced hearing loss.

Other causes of deafness affecting the inner ear, such as mumps and certain chemicals, and other forms of hearing loss such as conduction deafness resulting from middle ear infections may complicate and aggravate loss of hearing due to noise exposure.

Non-auditory effects are less well understood. Exposure to noise, especially intermittent impulsive noise, may lead to certain stress syndromes as a result of reactions of the autonomic nervous system and it is not impossible that these may act as an additional factor in the development of hypertension in exposed worker populations.

Early recognition is based on biological monitoring by audiography. In the early stages the audiogram of people exposed to excessive noise tends to show a threshold shift in the region of 4000 Hz frequency, i.e. a raised threshold for perceiving the pure tone stimulus used in audiometry which indicates a loss of hearing.

This is known as a 'dip' at 4 000 Hz and regarded as a valuable early warning sign of impending occupational hearing loss.

Under certain prescribed conditions it is also possible to predict to some extent what the potential permanent hearing loss would be for a certain individual if he were to be exposed to the same level of noise as presently for many years to come. Measuring the temporary threshold within about 5 minutes after the usual exposure for a workshift would give an indication of the expected permanent loss, but this test has not found general acceptance.

A pre-employment, pre-exposure examination of workers who are to work in a so-called noise zone, where the noise level exceeds 85 dB and hearing protection must be worn, must include a carefully taken history of previous exposure and previous ear disorders and an audiological examination which should include a baseline audiogram taken in accordance with the SABS standard (which is based on internationally accepted concepts). Audiography should then be repeated periodically, the first time within a year after which intervals of two years would be appropriate unless an appreciable hearing loss had already taken place or the noise exposure level defined as N eq exceeds 110 dB. In that case normal ear muffs might not adequately protect the worker against adverse effects and closer monitoring would be indicated. Prodromal symptoms of excessive noise exposure are complaints about 'ringing' in the ears, muffled hearing for a few hours after work and interference of speech communication while at work.

No treatment of permanent hearing loss is possible and in severe cases hearing aids may not be much help either. Prevention of occupational hearing loss is thus imperative. Engineering methods, reducing the noise at source and preventing noise impinging on the ear by isolation, shielding, noise absorption devices etc. may have to be complemented by personal protective devices such as approved earplugs or, at higher N eq levels, earmuffs. In that case, when the noise level cannot be reduced to below the acceptable limit, health education, supervision and even enforcement of the legal obligation to use hearing protectors, supported by audiography may become part of the duties of the health worker.

TABLE V MACHINERY AND OCCUPATIONAL SAFETY ACT
(General Administrative Regulations Annexure 4)

SCHEDULE

List of high-risk substances

1. All types of asbestos.
2. Lead and all its compounds.
3. Mercury and its compounds.
4. Chromium and its compounds.
5. Arsenic and its compounds.
6. Cadmium and its compounds.
7. All types of crystalline silica (dust).
8. Acrylonitrile (skin absorption).
9. Coal tar pitch volatiles.
10. Nickel sulphide (fume and dust).
11. Vinyl chloride.
12. Bis (chloromethyl) ether.
13. 4-Aminodiphenyl (p-xenylamine).
14. Benzidine.
15. Chloromethyl methylether.
16. Betanaphthylamine.
17. 4-Nitrodiphenyl.
18. Amitrol.
19. Antimony trioxide.
20. Benzene.
21. Benzo(a)pyrene.
22. Beryllium.
23. Carbon tetrachloride.
24. Chloroform.
25. Chrysene.
26. 3,3-Cichloro benzidine (skin absorption).
27. Dimethylcarbamyl chloride.
28. 1,1-Dimenthyl hydrazine (skin absorption).
29. Dimenthyl sulphate (skin absorption).
30. Ethylene dibromide (skin absorption).
31. Ethylene oxide.
32. Formaldehyde.
33. Hexachlorobutadine.

34. Hexamenthyl phosphoramide (skin absorption).
35. Hydrazine (skin absorption).
36. 4,4-Methylene bis (2-chloroaniline) (skin absorption).
37. Methyl hydrazine (skin absorption).
38. Methyl iodide (skin absorption).
39. 2-Nitropropane.
40. N-Nitrosodimenthylamine (skin absorption).
41. N-Phenyl-beta-naphthylamine.
42. Phenylhydrazine (skin absorption).
43. Propane sultone.
44. Beta-Propiolactone.
45. Propylene imine (skin absorption).
46. o-Tolidine.
47. o-Toluidine (skin absorption).
48. Vinyl bromide.
49. Vinyl cyclohexena dioxide.
50. Methylene chloride.

BIBLIOGRAPHY

TEXTBOOKS
1. Occupational Medicine, Principles and Practical Applications. Ed. Carl Zenz. Yearbook Medical Publishers, Chicago, 2nd edition 1988.
2. Environmental and Occupational Medicine. Ed. W N Rom. Little, Brown & Company, Boston 1983.
3. Occupational Health Practice. Ed. R Schilling. Butterworths, 2nd edition 1981.
4. Occupational Health, Recognising and Preventing Work-Related Disease. Eds. B S Levy and D H Wegman. Little Brown & Company, Boston 1983.
5. Aspects of Occupational Health. Eds. W M Dixon and Susan M G Price (SRN, OHNC). Faber and Faber, London 1984.
6. Handbook of Occupational Medicine. Ed. R J McCunney. Little, Brown & Company, Boston, 1988.
7. Clinical Occupational Medicine. L. Rosenstock and M R Cullen. W B Saunders Company, 1986.
8. Lecture Notes on Occupational Medicine. H A Waldron, 3rd and 4th ed. Blackwell Scientific Publications.

SPECIFIC TEXTS ON OCCUPATIONAL DISEASE RECOGNITION
1. Occupational Diseases, A guide to their recognition. NIOSH Publ. no 77–181. Ed. M M Key *et al* USA.
2. Early detection of occupational diseases. WHO publication. Geneva 1986.
3. Identification and control of work-related diseases. WHO Technical Report Series 714, Geneva 1985.
4. Early detection of Chronic Lung Diseases. WHO Euro reports and studies no 24, Copenhagen.
5. Health Promotion for working Populations. WHO Technical Report Series 765, Geneva 1988.
6. Notes on the Diagnosis of Occupational Diseases. Dept of Health and Social Security, London UK. Her Majesty's Stationery Office, Revised edition 1983.
7. Rapid revision in respiratory disease. F. Wiles, S Zwi and E Baskind. Medical News Tribune (SA) (Pty) Ltd, Rivonia.

8. Regulatory mechanisms for nursing training and practice: Meeting primary health care needs. WHO Technical report series 738, Geneva 1986.

EPIDEMIOLOGY

1. Epidemiology of occupational health. Eds. M Karvonen and M I Mikheev. WHO Regional Office for Europe. European Series no 20. Copenhagen 1986.
2. Epidemiology for the unitiated. G Rose and D J P Barker. B M A Tavistock Square, London 1979.

ENVIRONMENTAL ASPECTS

1. Rapid Guide to Hazardous Chemicals in the workplace. Eds. N I Sax and R J Lewis. Van Nostrand Reinhold Company, New York 1986.
2. The Hazards of Work: How to fight them. Patrick Kinnersly. PLUTO's Press Ltd, London (Workers Handbook no 1, 1973–1980).
3. International Labour Standards. A workers education manual, 2nd edition. ILO, Geneva 1982.
4. 1988 no 1657 HEALTH AND SAFETY COSH REGULATIONS. The control of substances hazardous to health. (HMSO) Her Majesty's Stationery Office, London, UK.
5. Guidance Note EH 40/88 annually revised, from the Health and Safety Executive UK (HMSO).
6. NIOSH Recommendations for Occupational Safety and Health Standards. Published annually as a supplement of the 'Morbidity and Mortality weekly report' by the US Department of Health and Human Services.
7. Threshold Limit Values for Chemical Substances and Physical Agents in the work environment and Biological Exposure Indices. Published annually by the ACGIH, 6500 Glenway Avenue, Cincinnati, OH 45211-4438 USA.
8. Recommended health-based limits in occupational exposure to heavy metals. WHO Technical report series 647. Geneva 1980.
9. Recommended health-based limits in occupational exposure to selected mineral dusts (silica, coal). WHO Technical reports series 734, Geneva 1986.

RECOMMENDED PAPERS PUBLISHED IN JOURNALS

1. Occupational Health Nursing in NURSING SA May 1987 vol 2, no 5, pp. 5–47.
2. Occupational Medicine in SA Journal of continuing medical education. April 1986 vol 4 pp. 5–128.
3. Proceedings of the International Symposium on research on work-related diseases, Espoo Finland 1984 in the Scandinavian Journal of Work, Environment and Health. December 1984, vol 10, no 6 (special issue).
4. Occupation and risk of cancer in Denmark. Scandinavian Journal of Work, Environment and Health, vol 13, special supplement 1, 1987.
5. Occupation and Cancer: Prevention and control, 2nd ed. Occupational Safety and Health series no 39, ILO, Geneva 1988.

Chapter 7: The Nurse in the Occupational Health Service

by J. Acutt and Y. Campbell

7.1 INTRODUCTION

Occupational health nursing has been defined by the American Association of Occupational Health Nurses as: 'The application of nursing principles in conserving the health of workers in all occupations. It involves prevention, recognition and treatment of illness and injury, and requires special skills and knowledge in the fields of health, education and counselling, environmental health, rehabilitation and human relations.' In order to achieve the major objective of health maintenance and disease prevention in an occupational setting the new occupational health nurse needs to adapt her basic nursing principles.

7.2 LEARNING OBJECTIVES

At the end of this section, the reader should have the knowledge to:
- Define occupational health nursing
- Describe the characteristics and responsibilities of the occupational health nurse
- Identify criteria for introducing the nurse into the organization
- Plan and establish an occupational health service
- Identify the functions of the occupational health nurse
- Apply the nursing process in occupational health nursing

7.3 THE OCCUPATIONAL HEALTH NURSE

The occupational health nurse must be a responsible and reliable person who can be trusted by management and employees alike. She must be professional and mature at all times, tactful, diplomatic and able to act with discretion in any situation. Professionally she must observe the provisions of the Nursing Act, 1978 (Act 50 of 1978) as amended (Searle, 1986: 114–28).

Good health is an attribute that is vital as she often works alone and cannot be replaced at short notice. It goes without saying that being well groomed, neat and clean, despite the dust and grease of industry, will gain the respect of management, the workers and professional colleagues and it is well to remember the regulations relating to nurses uniform in the Nursing Act, 1978 (Act 50 of 1978) as amended.

7.3.1   **Education and experience**   Occupational health nursing covers a very wide field and, the nurse may, for example, be faced with a gruesome accident or other emergency situation and may find herself counselling a young drug addict all in one day. On the same day, she may give a health talk to young mothers, motivate a health programme to management, and investigate a health hazard whilst attending to a steady stream of workers with day to day illnesses and injuries.

In order to cope she needs basic general nursing, midwifery, first-aid and specialized occupational health nursing training. She needs community health nursing training, communication skills, guidance to cope with administration, and specialized courses pertaining to specific hazards in her work situation, for instance, radiation, dust or chemicals such as organo-phosphates or hydro-fluoric acid. As in all fields of nursing, on-going education is vital, but the occupational health nurse has to keep up to date with the latest technology and new processes even before they are implemented in her type of industry—in order that she may warn management of possible health risks. She is expected to read nursing and technical journals, attend seminars and meetings of professional societies and above all maintain an interest and research new facts in order to keep up to date.

7.3.2 Responsibilities

7.3.2.1   *To the worker*   As in any form of nursing, the nurse's first responsibility is towards her patient, or in this case, the worker or even the work force, and her primary responsibility is to protect the well-being of the worker.

7.3.2.2   *To the employer*   The occupational health nurse owes a loyalty towards her employer and must protect the company from the adverse effects of work processes and hazardous substances on the worker. She can only do this if she knows the processes and chemicals, and should make it her business to find out what is being used and what possible health risks may result. She should also know how to prevent overexposure from the process or chemical.

7.3.2.3   *To professional colleagues*   The occupational health nurse has a responsibility towards the company physician, professional colleagues and also to the general practitioner of the worker. She should liaise closely with all three categories so as to benefit the worker.

7.4 THE DEPENDENT, INTERDEPENDENT AND INDEPENDENT FUNCTIONS OF THE OCCUPATIONAL HEALTH NURSE

7.4.1   **The dependent function**   The occupational health nurse is dependent upon the law that authorizes her to practise, as well as common and relevant statutory laws. She must ensure that she is, and remains, registered with the South African Nursing Council and a member of the South African Nursing Association.

As a professional nurse she is responsible for her own acts of omission and commission. She must utilize knowledge, skills and ability to the full to ensure quality health care and be accountable for any action she may take.

7.4.2 The interdependent function This function is a relationship between health professionals which functions for the benefit of the worker. The occupational health nurse must perform health care to the worker in cooperation with persons registered under:

- The Nursing Act 1978 (Act 50 of 1978)
- The Medical, Dental and Supplementary Health Professions Act 1974 (Act 56 of 1974)
- The Pharmacy Act, 1974 (Act 53 of 1974)

She must cooperate with other members of the occupational health team and accept responsibility for the manner in which she executes instructions or requests, and ensure that they are carried out accurately and on time. The keeping of an accurate record system is essential to ensure coordination of team effort.

7.4.3 The independent function The occupational health nurse, as a professional practitioner, is totally responsible and accountable for her own actions. She may make a nursing diagnosis, advise on treatment and give nursing care, but she must be aware of the extent of her knowledge, skills and abilities and also her limitations in performing her nursing duties. She may refuse to carry out instructions only in the case of an illegal act, over-prescription, inaccurate prescription or anything against the policy of the institution, the wishes of the worker or beyond her competence.

The company physician, her employer or the worker can expect the occupational health nurse to be competent and reliable and to carry out her function with accuracy and skill, but she has a duty to speak up if an instruction falls outside her scope of practice.

7.5 INTRODUCING THE NURSE INTO THE ORGANIZATION

The aim of all business organizations is to be productive, cost-effective and profit making. The task of the occupational health service will be to contribute to these aims by ensuring that:

- individuals are fit to do a specific job;
- their health is not adversely affected by their work and vice versa;
- employees who are incapacitated for any reason are returned to work as soon as possible.

This opens up broad new avenues of service and offers a grand challenge to the professional capabilities of the nurse. It is therefore important for the nurse to understand her own place within the organization. In the occupational setting, although the nurse will be concerned with the maintenance of health, this will not usually be the main aim of the employing organization. The aim of the organization will be to maximize output of goods and services, of which the occupational health service is a part.

The time to establish a correct professional understanding and working relationship with the employer is at the time of the interview and prior to acceptance of a contract of employment and the position charter (job description). The position charter is the most important document the occupational health nurse will have. Functions, duties and responsibilities should be clearly stated but be flexible enough to accommodate the nurse's changing and expanding role.

7.5.1 The position charter

- *Qualifications:* Education should be specified.
- *Reporting relationships:* It is essential for the nurse to know specifically to whom she reports, and from whom she will receive medical and administrative direction.
- *Ethics:* The charter should state that the occupational health nurse will comply with medical and nursing ethics.
- *Employment benefits:* As a professional, she should be accorded the same benefits as the other professional employees within the company.
- *Impartiality:* In accordance with nursing ethics, the nurse must maintain an attitude of impartiality in any controversy between employer and employee.
- *Remuneration:* The starting salary, increments, hours of work, shift differential, overtime pay, number of statutory holidays and length of leave should be confirmed in writing and understood before the position is accepted.
- *Benefits:* Sick leave, leave of absence, group health insurance, retirement plans and other benefits are usually established policies for all employees. These should be in writing if none exist.
- *Training:* In order to maintain her professional knowledge she should be given the opportunity to attend refresher courses, professional seminars and conferences.
- *Provision of reference material:* The employer should provide a library of current books and journals related to occupational health services.
- *Professional recognition:* She forms part of a team within the company to promote health and safety. Therefore it is imperative that she is recognized in this capacity and not isolated in her work situation.

7.5.2 The interview   To start off at a disadvantage is a handicap which may take a lifetime to overcome. For this reason, the interview provides the nurse with the opportunity to establish the scope and responsibilities of the post, the functions to be undertaken and the status, salary and conditions of work under which she will be expected to operate.

The interview may not always provide clarity about the proper role and function of an occupational health nursing service and if duties and responsibilities are suggested which have no bearing on this, the nurse should not accept the post unless changes can be negotiated which will allow the nurse to contribute her skills in an appropriate manner, for the maximum benefit of all employed in the organization.

The occupational health department, whether it is staffed by one nurse or a team of nurses and doctors, is a separate specialized functional department within the organization. The senior occupational health nurse should assume managerial control and responsibility for the smooth running of the department. Accountability should be to a senior member of the organization's management as well as to the company medical officer.

The success of an occupational health service depends on the establishment of effective relationships with members of the various departments within the organization. This relationship is sometimes hindered by the lack of understanding of each other's role and through a breakdown in communication. The occupational health nurse may feel threatened when instructions originate from non-medical or non-nursing personnel and contravene her equally ingrained codes of professional and ethical conduct. This situation arises because of the dual role that the occupational health nurse has to play. She is at the same time, an employee of the organization with duties and responsibilities to her employer and a nurse with professional responsibilities to the employees.

7.5.3   The role of   As a practitioner of first contact she must be able to exercise
the   professional skills in order to make an accurate diagnosis of the
occupational   condition presented and decide upon the action to be taken in the
health nurse   best interests of the person concerned.

She should continue to maintain a professional relationship with all employees whether they are fit and well or patients in need of specific nursing help. This relationship is a constant challenge based on the need for the occupational health nurse to adapt continually to changing circumstances, to refrain from taking sides in disputes, to remain a confidante and friend to all and to maintain a standard of excellence in all she does.

Any confrontation between employers and their employees should not concern her, as she needs to be very adept at playing a neutral role and must be careful to give the same advice to either side and not appear to be seen to support a management or union position. For this reason she should ensure that she participates as an impartial adviser in any health and safety committee established at the work place.

She should always respect confidences and protect the interests of the clients as well as the employer. It sometimes happens that these interests will conflict. Where this happens, the patient's interests must be protected so that no action should be taken by the nurse which may breach the code of confidentiality which must exist between the individual patient and her.

The exercise of tact and the development of good inter-personal relationships are the hallmarks of the occupational health nurse. The all-important ingredients of successful occupational health nursing are:

- The way nurses feel about the people they work with; the respect they have for the worker's dignity, and the worth and the value they place on the importance of gainful employment to good mental health. Nurses must work with all kinds of people, rich and poor, knowledgeable and ignorant, those who drink too much, those who belong to and support their unions, those who have family responsibilities which they handle easily and effectively and those who cannot cope.
- The way nurses feel about themselves and the importance they place on their contributions to the fulfilment of the health expectations.

- The professional image projected by the nurse is of vital importance, e.g. the correct uniform worn at all times with distinguishing devices, helps to portray the professional person the nurse is.

Occupational health nurses would do well to remember the statement made by a nurse: 'Occupational health nursing is the easiest job in the world to do badly—the most demanding to do well.'

7.6 SELECTED CRITERIA FOR THE PLANNING AND ESTABLISHMENT OF AN OCCUPATIONAL HEALTH SERVICE

7.6.1 Why have an occupational health service? A comprehensive occupational health programme pays dividends by:

- ensuring a safe work environment;
- controlling sick leave on a fair and realistic basis, to benefit both the worker and the employer;
- offering specialized health education services;
- good communication—acting as a link in the feedback chain;
- keeping the healthy employee healthy;
- facilitating pre-placement medical examinations, which would ensure that healthy employees are employed or that latent conditions can be treated;
- monitoring staff health on an ongoing basis—a healthy worker is a productive worker.
- The nurse has the first-hand knowledge of the end results of occupational accidents and exposures to occupational disease-causing substances and can go to great lengths to motivate the work force and management alike to promote the concepts of injury and disease prevention.

7.6.2 Establishment of an occupational health service Sometimes the occupational health service can be located in a new building or as part of a new facility housing other office functions. In many instances, however, it is necessary to accept and adapt an existing portion of the factory building. Whichever alternative is available, it is essential to realize that the successful planning of an occupational health service is only achieved through teamwork with other professional disciplines. The planning group should consist of the architect, building contractor, plant engineer, finance staff together with the senior medical and nursing representative.

Other factors will incorporate the company policy, its size and structure and the way it allocates its budget.

Factors which determine the health service requirements of an organization will also depend on the following:

- nature of employer business;
- number of employees;
- age and sex of employees;
- whether disabled persons are employed;
- hours of work including shifts and overtime;
- environment inside and outside the work place;
- raw materials;
- specific hazards;
- legislation;

- trade unions;
- location of new occupational health service;
- any existing occupational health service;
- company doctor—full or part-time;
- staffing of the occupational health service;
- access to local doctors;
- access to local hospitals;
- ambulance service;
- ancillary services;
- safety officer.

The relative importance of each of these factors will vary in differing situations. For example, the occupational health requirements of a mining group will differ greatly from the requirements of a supermarket.

As the functions of the occupational health service are planned, constant reference must be made to the factors both inside and outside the work place which will determine the individual requirements of the organization. The occupational health service must be planned in a systematic way if it is to be efficient. The first step is to define the aims of the service, the next step will be to plan how it can best meet the occupational health needs of the organization.

Once a service has been established and functioning, it is essential that a critical review should be made from time to time in order to identify any problems and to ensure that the service is fulfilling its purpose.

It is so easy to stay in a rut and use the excuse 'but we have always done it this way'. Practical changes are essential as the service grows and expands with the growth and expansion of the organization.

7.7 THE FUNCTIONS OF THE OCCUPATIONAL HEALTH NURSE

In 1959 the International Labour Organisation defined an occupational health service as being established . . . in or near a place of employment for the purpose of:

- protecting workers against any health hazard which may arise out of their work or the conditions in which it is carried on;
- contributing towards workers' physical and mental adjustment, in particular by adaptation of the work to the workers and their assignment to the jobs for which they are suited;
- contributing to the establishment and maintenance of the highest possible degree of physical and mental well-being of the workers.

There are several ways in which the occupational health nurse can achieve these aims.

7.7.1 Primary health care This means contact with medical personnel at the work place for the treatment of illness or injury i.e. care that can be given on site. This care includes care relating to day-to-day illness, the immediate treatment and follow-up of illness, and the treatment and follow-up of injuries on duty and workmen's compensation cases.

7.7.2 Environmental Various types of monitoring should be done on a regular basis in areas around employees to identify possible excessive exposure of employees to harmful concentrations of toxic fumes, vapours, dusts, aerosols, etc., in atmospheres where the possible presence of such concentrations cannot be excluded.

7.7.3   Biological Monitoring the biological functions of workers themselves are tested— blood, urine, tissue and exhaled breath tests are done, to ensure that they are not being poisoned by, inter alia, the substances with which they work or which might be present in the work environment.

7.7.4   Counselling Often a worker will come to the occupational health nurse first to discuss his problems. Every occupational health nurse must be aware of the limitations of her own capabilities and should not hesitate to refer the employee to the appropriate agency for further assistance. All discussions should be carried out in private and must be treated as confidential.

7.7.5 Rehabilitation One of the most important functions of the occupational health service is the rehabilitation of employees after serious illness or injury. Rehabilitation should begin as early as possible and the occupational health nurse will have to liaise with both the employee's doctor and the various departments in the organization where these workers are employed.

Both rehabilitated alcoholics and drug dependants need a lot of understanding and assistance, especially in the initial stages of the rehabilitation process. Her experience and sympathetic approach would make the nurse the ideal person to help these unfortunate people with their problems.

7.7.6   Services to the vulnerable groups

7.7.6.1 The women In most cases the women are trying to manage two jobs i.e. in the work situation and in the home environment. Working hours will be long as her day will start early and end late, especially if there are still small children at home. The occupational health nurse must be on the alert for these women who present with vague complaints and frequent visits to the occupational health centre. Careful questioning into the family situation is vital before diagnosis and treatment can be instituted.

7.7.6.2   The pregnant employee Should be carefully watched and where necessary be given advice on diets, health preparation for the baby, maternity benefits from the company, etc. In some cases the occupational health nurse may have to advise management that this employee should be moved out of the department to a more favourable type of employment.

7.7.6.3   The single parent In today's environment this is more evident and here many psychological problems will arise. The occupational health nurse should know who are the single parent employees and consider some counselling sessions with people who have the expertise to assist them.

7.7.6.4   The young employee Often the school leaver presents attitudinal problems by showing resentment to senior employees and by treating everything in a light-hearted manner. A great deal of tact will be required by the nurse who may have to counsel both the junior and senior staff. Here she must realize her limitations and not try to exceed them, thus causing further friction.

7.7.6.5 Late middle age group Often employees work beyond their retirement age and part of the problem is nature's way of the slowing down in one's capabilities. There is also the fear of retirement and the occupational health nurse, together with outside agencies, could arrange discussions regarding preparing for retirement, etc.

7.7.6.6 Chronically ill When new building alterations are planned, the nurse can play a vital part in advising management on various changes to accommodate the disabled employee, e.g. suitable toilet facilities, slopes instead of steps, doorways and desks to accommodate wheelchairs. At the pre-placement medical examination some disabilities will be found and again the occupational health nurse should liaise with the manager concerned to be aware of the situation and assist these employees to find job satisfaction.

7.7.6.7 The shift worker The occupational health nurse must be aware of the added stress on shift workers. Psychological problems associated with the adjustment to the changes in eating and sleeping patterns as well as fitting into the family life patterns.

7.7.7 Injuries on duty These must be treated as soon as possible and here on-going education to management and employees in the necessity of reporting all injuries is of vital importance. Failure to comply often results in unnecessary complications and excessive correspondence with the Workmen's Compensation Commissioner and private practitioners.

7.7.8 Placing people in suitable work To ensure that all new employees are both healthy and suitable for the work that they have been engaged to do requires a comprehensive knowledge of the work process, the various hazards that they will be exposed to, the effects, the legal requirements and the company policy.

7.7.9 The pre-placement medical examination The occupational health nurse can arrange for and assist with these examinations. Relevant documentation can be routed to all interested parties and records must be kept by the nurse. This service would include selecting the right applicant for the specific job. It is very important that these examinations be performed prior to employment, and also before the prospective employee gives notice of leaving for his current employment. No person should be employed before the results of a pre-placement medical examination is available. This examination should begin with a medical history form filled in and signed by the applicant to save time. The actual examination should be as simple as possible, but at the same time should convey the required basic information. All information supplied is treated with the strictest confidence.

7.7.10 Providing a treatment service The occupational health nurse should be able to assess any health situation and treat accordingly, e.g. emergency treatment, referral to employee's doctor or to the hospital, and then check the follow-up treatment and any further appointments. The use of outside agencies is sometimes essential and therefore the occupational health nurse must become an expert at choosing the correct system to use and in co-operating with the service that the agency provides and the individual specialists within each agency. When needing to co-operate with an outside agency occupational health nurses need to assess not only which system will be of most value to the client, but also which is the quickest, most flexible and most efficient, as well as the most acceptable to the individual concerned.

Observation of the work methods, substances in use and and factors affecting health is vital. The employee's family and social background is equally important. It is of course necessary to be fully aware of the housing, domestic and dietary situation of individuals.

It is imperative that the standard of treatment given by the occupational health service must be maintained at a consistently high level. The occupational health nurse must keep herself and her staff updated. There are times when the treatment is life saving. It is important that the occupational health team know the dosage, side-effects and contra-indications as well as the emergency treatment of the various medications that are used in the occupational health centre.

Adequate up-to-date stocks should be available and the emergency trolley be routinely checked for any outdated materials.

The occupational health nurse is always available to give advice and support but tends to involve outside agencies where there are special needs—help with alcohol or drug addiction for example, or crisis and stress counselling.

7.7.11 Controlling recognized hazards— secondary monitoring This term means the continuous supervision by either environmental or biological monitoring of a known occupational health hazard. Monitoring of the environment is, of course, the responsibility of the hygienist. Biological monitoring, however, requires the cooperation of medical and nursing practitioners.

7.7.12 Periodic health reviews The occupational health service's function is to control all known hazards causing injury and disease. Periodic health reviews are undertaken to screen fit, healthy workers to detect early signs of diseases or defects, through examination or tests. Employees must be told of the results of the examinations and of suspected or confirmed signs of disease. These cases must be referred for further medical investigation and/or treatment.

The periodic medical examinations of some employees are required by law, e.g. apprentices, radiation workers, public vehicle drivers, noise-exposed employees, food handlers etc.

7.7.13 Special examinations These would include the examination of employees exposed to potentially hazardous substances or processes and would vary from industry to industry. Note that it is therefore vital that the occupational health nurse should understand the production processes in her place of work and also know which hazards are generated by the processes in question. She should further know what risk exposures need to be examined in the employee e.g.

audiometry for noise exposure, blood for lead exposure, urinary tests for mercury exposure, etc.

Many other special examinations could be performed as and when required.

7.7.14 Identifying unrecognized hazards— primary monitoring

Conventionally, this term includes the discovery of new hazards by chemical analogy, evaluation of routine measurements or epidemiological survey. The nurse who provides primary medical care has a vital role to play in primary monitoring. She is in close contact with workers and therefore has the ideal opportunity to observe, record and interpret health changes in workers. Through her records she can quickly ascertain whether there is an undue prevalence of certain diseases in parts of the organization where she works.

It is also part of her normal routine to visit work areas regularly.This enables her to establish a correlation between the environment, the worker and his health. This facilitates the early detection of deviations from normal health. The occupational health nurse must be able to recognize new hazards by continuous surveillance of the work areas, as well as continuous contact with both employers and employees.

Abnormal trends seen in the occupational health centre must be investigated i.e. a survey of the area at fault may reveal the cause. When major building alterations are planned or new machinery and procedures are to be introduced, it is vital that the occupational health nurse be kept informed so that she is aware that new problems may be seen in the occupational health centre.

7.7.15 Avoiding potential risks

The occupational health team have first-hand knowledge of the state of health of employees and should be consulted when promotions or transfers are being considered. This would help to avoid potential risks, e.g. an employee with a cardiac condition or psychological problem being placed in a stressful work environment. It is not for the occupational health nurse to interfere with promotion or transfers but to advise management of potential risks that may arise.

7.7.16 Screening for evidence of non-occupational disease

Here is an opportunity for the occupational health nurse to carry out meaningful surveys on factors which are not solely occupational e.g. ischaemic heart disease, peptic ulcer, varicose veins, and so on.

When undertaking research, the occupational health nurse must remember that the ethical standards of general nursing practice are applicable. She should therefore ensure that:

- Freely given and informed consent is obtained from each employee involved. The procedure must be explained as fully as possible in terms which are readily understood.
- Each employee understands that he or she has the right to withdraw from the study. His or her wishes regarding this must be respected.
- Consent is obtained from any employee receiving treatment to consult the general practitioner concerning any implications of the proposed study.
- Bearing in mind that fully informing employees beforehand might invalidate results (e.g. when a control group is necessary), as

much information as possible must be given beforehand and additional appropriate information should be offered on completion of the study.

- Persons involved are protected against physical, emotional or social injury as far as the present state of knowledge allows.
- Employees are assured that the rules of confidentiality will be observed during the collection, processing, recording and presentation of data. This may be achieved by allocating a number to each employee involved, the names so indexed being accessible only to the occupational health nurse.
- If the organization has an ethics committee, the approval of this committee must be obtained.
- The person undertaking the study possesses the requisite knowledge and skills and is aware of personal limitations. This must be determined in the early planning stage.
- All findings are interpreted with integrity.
- Some responsibility for implementing recommendations is accepted by the investigator.
- Terms of reference are agreed at the outset and any departure taken only with the full agreement of all parties concerned.

7.7.17   Administration and management

Record keeping and statistics

Record: Each employee should have a medical record card. Accurate daily recordings of employees attending the occupational health centre must be kept. All records are confidential and only the medical staff should have access to them. Information can only be discussed with an employee's written consent, and then only the relevant information should be supplied.

Statistics: Meaningful statistics should be prepared and presented by the occupational health nurse on a regular basis to both the company doctor and management. To be meaningful, these statistics should be easy to understand and should not disclose any confidential matters. From these statistics management can judge the service offered by the medical centre.

Company policy

It is imperative to know and understand the company policies. The occupational health nurse should spend time with management or persons concerned to have these policies explained to her. She should have a copy of the policy manual in the occupational health centre for referral purposes as there are many areas that the nurse does not know but may be asked questions on when a worker comes in for treatment or advice.

This document is important if a proper service is to be given by the occupational health team because:

- Such a policy covers the objectives for the reason for health services and the various programmes that can be introduced to offer a good health service to all concerned.
- In specific areas, e.g. a hazardous working environment, the policy would list the types of investigations that are required, the types of on-going examinations of employees and specific emergency treatment and action in cases of accidents.

The nurse plays an important part in assisting management in keeping the company health policy updated.

Legislation

Copies of the following Acts should be on file, updated and at hand for easy reference:

- The Nursing Act 1978 (Act 50 of 1978)
- Medicines and Related Substances Control Act (Act 101 of 1965)
- Machinery and Occupational Safety Act (Act 6 of 1983)
- The Medical, Dental and Supplementary Health Professions Act 1974 (Act 56 of 1974)
- The Pharmacy Act (Act 53 of 1974)
- The Workmen's Compensation Act (Act 30 of 1941)

Any other Acts pertaining to the type of organization the nurse works in.

Medicine permit

She is responsible for completing the necessary documentation for application to have the occupational health centre registered with the Department of National Health and Population Development. This permit must be on display in the occupational health centre. As staff changes occur, the nurse must advise the authorities.

Recording of scheduled medicines

The issuing of scheduled medicines must be properly controlled and the occupational health nurse must realize the importance of correct recording in the drug books and the balancing of stocks.

Package inserts for medicines

For easy reference of all the medicines used in the occupational health centre, the nurse can make her own reference book by placing copies of the package inserts that come with the medicines in a suitable book. The occupational health team cannot remember all the side-effects and reactions of some medicines against others and so can refer to these package inserts if in doubt.

Stock-taking

Regular audits of all assets must be done accurately.

Reference library

Articles of interest and value should be clearly marked or photostatted, after permission has been obtained, and filed under headings for easy reference. To be effective this has to be continually updated.

Sickness absence control

All doctors' certificates and application forms for sickness leave should be routed to the occupational health centre where sickness absence can be controlled. Management is responsible for authorizing sick-pay but the occupational health nurse can keep an eye open for patterns that may arise, e.g. the same type of illness for employees working in the same area, frequent Monday absences, etc.

Referral letters

All referral letters, e.g. to doctors, hospitals, etc., should be photostatted so that there are always records to refer to in cases of dispute.

Budget

Some of the important items that should be included are:

- new and planned assets;
- medications and dressings;
- reference materials;
- seminars, conference fees;
- education materials;
- repairs and maintenance to the centre;
- overtime and shift work allowances for the medical staff;
- printing and stationery.

With experience and help from the financial management of the company, the occupational health nurse should be able to present a meaningful budget.

Workmen's compensation documentation

It is important that all the relevant forms are accurately completed and submitted to the Commissioner as soon as possible. A separate file should be kept for each employee who has suffered a major injury on duty. Photostat all correspondence. It is advisable to send this by registered post to Pretoria. The occupational health nurse should be advised by the personnel department when an employee is leaving the company so that she can record his forwarding address and send any compensation that might be due to him. Workmen's Compensation records should be kept indefinitely.

7.7.18   Education   For an educational programme to be effective it should be divided into two areas:

- education relating to the organization i.e. employee/employer;
- education relating to the occupational health nursing team.

People will change behaviour only when they understand what they must do and when they see the recommended action as a means to an end they themselves value.

The worker's right to know what the hazards of the job are and the employer's responsibility to provide a safe and healthful work environment are basic to an understanding of the MOS Act.

- *Education-for-health programmes:* These include teaching employees what they must do to prevent harm to themselves, to fellow-workers and to their families. Occupational health and safety education programmes should be attuned to the need of worker and industry. The aim should be to help employees learn how to take responsibility for the promotion, maintenance and protection of their own and their family's health.
- *In the work situation:* The nurse should assist in the education of management, supervisors and the work-force on the various

hazardous substances that they are required to handle; on other health hazards they are exposed to and also on what precautions to take to protect themselves.

- *Extended health education:* This category includes extended health education programmes to cover areas such as obesity, exercise classes, health menus offered in the canteen, stop-smoking campaigns, etc.
- *Educational methods:* Successful education can be achieved with the help of posters, pamphlets, films, videos and newsletters. Discussion of health-related topics can also be arranged, either on a one-to-one basis or in groups.
- *Safety committees:* Health topics can be discussed at safety committee meetings and safety representatives can be asked to spread the information in their daily contact with other employees. In this way, the usefulness of the safety representative, as an extra 'pair of eyes' can be extended.

Health and safety education activities are an integral part of every occupational health programme. If nurses are to help workers learn how to protect their health and how to make use of health care resources and safe work practices, the nurses must understand the concept of self-responsibility, that is, each person is responsible for determining and enhancing his or her own health potential.

Health is much more than the absence of illness—it is a dynamic state in which people do their best with the capacities they have and act the best they know how to maximize their strengths. Helping workers understand this concept is a challenge occupational health nurses must deal with as they assess the health status of employees in relation to their work. Helping workers to recognize hazards and to know when and how to see that the employer carries out his responsibility is an integral part of an occupational health nurse's responsibilities.

To maintain the well-being of the employee and to prevent ill health and offer a safe working environment the occupational health nurse plays an important part in the educational side, but she must keep up to date herself with new concepts, thus broadening her knowledge. To achieve this it is imperative that the nurse is involved on a regular basis in environmental visits throughout the plant, familiarizing herself and her staff with new projects, changes in the plant and any areas that could be the cause of a breakdown in the health of employees. With this knowledge the nurse can then explain to employees, where applicable, the necessary precautions to take and she would be speaking with that authority and proper knowledge which is essential for a successful health education programme.

The occupational health nurse can introduce an education programme either as group teaching sessions, and or on an individual basis from the occupational health centre but the nurse must always remember that in no way should she interfere with production, and she should always liaise with those in charge of departments to ensure a smooth running of her planned programme.

Quite often the occupational health nurse will find that the health education programme will not only be confined to the industrial/commerce situation but will also involve home and community health problems. Nurses experienced in this field know that many an employee is given inadequate basic instructions from hospitals or doctors when coping with illness in the family and they will often turn to the occupational health nurse for guidance. Thus the nurse's role is one of health promotion in its widest aspect, domestic, occupational and communal.

In considering the health programme, the occupational health nurse must first decide WHOM she is going to educate, WHAT health topics she should promote, WHEN she will do it and HOW it will be done.

The pre-placement medical examination is an ideal situation in which the nurse can start teaching health, either from observations made from the applicant's physical state or from the preventive health-safety aspect of the job for which the employee has applied.

Other types of educational programmes are through:

- the spoken word;
- the written word;
- visual education;
- practical teaching;
- personal example—this is an area often overlooked.

The nurse is constantly watched by the employees and she must be seen to do as she teaches. Her appearance should be spotless and her uniform complete. This gives the picture that she illustrates her teaching in hygiene and in the wearing of her uniform represents her profession. She should also be an example to the workers and wear the correct protective clothing and be seen to use safety equipment where applicable.

Much worker education can be accomplished through the use of a well-planned literature display and exhibit. Bulletin boards and health literature racks in the canteen, rest rooms, and throughout the plant can be used to make health information freely available to workers. Such display material should be chosen carefully and changed frequently. There should be a bulletin board in the occupational health centre for posters and for a display of health and safety information.

Carefully chosen pamphlets on health topics should be available in the waiting room for employees to read while they wait for the nurse or the doctor. Careful selection of literature is of utmost importance to get the message across, e.g. different cultures and different languages must be considered, as well as the employee's concept of the poster displayed.

The nurse will find it helpful to become familiar with the resources of these official agencies and learn how to use them. When the occupational health budget is developed each year, a line item for health publications should be included so that the necessary films etc., can be rented or purchased and pamphlets and posters purchased to support the health education programme.

Nurses will find it most helpful to have their names on the list of those to whom announcements of new publications and/or sample copies are mailed by commercial, voluntary and official agencies. In this way they can keep up to date on what is available and can share this with the members of the health and safety committee.

Periodic evaluation of the progress of a health education programme is necessary to find out whether one is accomplishing one's goals. There is no single way to measure the effectiveness of a health education programme. Each worker responds differently to the many and varied activities of a well-planned programme. How each person promotes, maintains, and protects his own and his family's health is an individual matter. Some need to develop different attitudes and learn new health habits, while others need only to modify their present attitudes and habits. The importance that members of the occupational health team attach to health education and the amount of attention they give to it are overriding factors in determining the success of the programme.

Although it is hard to measure, long-term results such as changed attitudes about health and certain other results can be measured. In so far as possible, specific objectives for the programme should be included in the master plan, so that progress can be checked against them. For example one objective may be to cut down on the number of eye accidents in a particular department. Progress towards meeting this objective is fairly easy to evaluate in that the number of injuries before the programme of eye safety was started can be compared with the number after it was put into operation. Lost time and medical costs are measurable.

When the objective is to help workers know the danger signals of cancer, the results are less easy to evaluate. One measure could be the number of pamphlets taken from the health literature rack over a certain period of time. A more revealing indication of success might be an increase in the rate of completed referrals, that is, the number of people who sought care from their physician or community clinic for one of the danger signals.

There are many sources of help available to the occupational health nurse in carrying out their role in health education. As the nurse identifies new needs for education she will find new sources of information by enquiring and by research. The most important aspect to bear in mind is to keep up to date and implement new ideas to keep the programme alive and functioning.

7.7.19   Research orientation It is imperative that occupational health nurses have a research orientation. It makes them ask why, it makes them look for relationships and it makes them use the problem-solving method.

Equally importantly, it helps them recognize the need for data generated by research as the basis for programme planning. When occupational health nurses understand research methods, they recognize the part their records can contribute to retrospective studies. When this fact is recognized nurses realize that what they record as current events and put into employee health records may many years later be used as data in a retrospective study. Well-designed records, which are promptly and accurately maintained, are essential to this function.

Occupational health nurses must be acutely aware of man-environment health problems. They must seek information about the environment of workers and must look for relationships between the signs and symptoms that are presented and the toxic substances and other hazards associated with the occupation. What they have learned from workers must be recorded so that others can use the data.

7.8 THE NURSING PROCESS IN OCCUPATIONAL HEALTH NURSING

The nursing process is a designated series of actions undertaken to ensure the client's well-being. The general rules of assessing, communication, planning, implementing, evaluation and research are applicable to both the employee and the organization.

Definition from Yura and Walsh 1973:23: 'The nursing process is an orderly, systematic manner of determining the clients' problems, making plans to solve them, initiating the plan or assigning others to implement it, and evaluating the extent to which the plan was effective in resolving the problems identified.'

7.8.1 Assessing The nurse begins the assessment of a potential problem when she first observes the client. Subconsciously she will note physical or mental features that may have bearing on the problem at hand. Her nursing diagnosis will be influenced by her observations as well as the history and signs and symptoms reported.

7.8.2 Communi- Communication contributes to all the aspects of the nursing process.
cation
Effective communication will elicit vital information without influencing the client subjectively, for instance 'What symptoms are you experiencing?' rather than 'Do you have a headache?'

In the implementation of the nursing plan, accurate instructions can influence the outcome of the intervention, and similarly effective communication will influence the extent of success in the evaluation of the intervention.

In the occupational health service, communication takes place at all levels and the nurse must use simple lay language to the uneducated layman, business terms when motivating for a new service to the organization, and technological terms when reporting on a medical condition to the medical officer.

7.8.3 Planning Once a nursing diagnosis is arrived at, planning commences with the priorities of the problem being arranged, appropriate nursing treatment applied, and an accurate record of the assessment, diagnosis, treatment, and even expected outcome, made.

7.8.4 Implemen- The implementation phase of the nursing process relies on the
tation intellectual, interpersonal and technical skills of the nurse for success. In a hospital this would mean the treatment phase where daily observations of temperature, pulse, blood-pressure and respirations are but a few of the observations made on a daily basis—and in the occupational health service the nurse would have to go to the client to see how he is responding. Not always feasible but follow-up of treatment is important and 'corridor consultations' must also be recorded.

7.8.5 Evaluation Effective intervention by the occupational health nurse can be reflected by sickness and absence from work, and the occupational health nurse keeps statistics of all consultations and types of problems reported and monitors the reasons given for sick leave and the number of days absent.

Biological monitoring and results of, for instance, dust samples or radiation exposure discs as well as injury on duty figures, are all forms of evaluation in a successful nursing process.

7.8.6   Research The nursing process is only complete when research has been undertaken to improve the assessment and communication phases but more important still are the planning and implementation phases.

7.8.7   Documen- Accurate record keeping, data collection, literature search, evalua-
tation tion and report writing is part of the daily routine in the occupational health service.

7.9 CONCLUSION

The ultimate aim or goal of a successful occupational health service should be to implement all the functions of occupational health nursing, but the establishment of a comprehensive occupational health service will take time. It will be only too easy for the enthusiastic nurse, working alone, to undertake more new projects than time properly permits. It is unwise to expect, or to try to implement, rapid changes. Familiarity with the aims and functions of the employing organization, and with the people employed within, is essential basic knowledge which every occupational health nurse requires. Therefore surveying the working environment and establishing effective lines of communication will figure high on her list of priorities, and time taken to acquire this knowledge and to establish relationships will be time well spent.

7.10 BIBLIOGRAPHY

Baker, M. and Coetzee, A. C. 1983. *An Introduction to Occupational Health Nursing in South Africa* Johannesburg: Witwatersrand University Press.

Brown, M. L. 1981. *Occupational Health Nursing* New York: Springer Publishing Company.

Harris, C. J. 1984. *Occupational Health Nursing Practice* Bristol: Stonebridge Press.

Harrison, B. M. 1984. *Essentials of Occupational Health Nursing* Oxford: Blackwell Scientific Publications.

The Journal of the Rhodesian Society of Occupational Health. Vol 3. No: 3 pages 13–17; Vol 3 No: 4 pages 21, 22 (October 1976).

Nursing R.S.A.: Vol 2 No: 5, page 5. May 1987.

Searle, C. 1986. *Professional Practice—A South African Perspective* Durban: Butterworths.

Slaney, B. 1979. *Occupational Health Nursing* Great Britain: Biddles Ltd.

Yura, H. and Walsh, M. B. 1973. *The Nursing Process* New York: Appleton-Century Crofts.

Chapter 8: Emergencies and Disaster Planning

by J Acutt

8.1 INTRODUCTION

Prompt and effective treatment of serious injury or illness at the place of work is usually the standard used by employers and employees alike to judge the efficiency of the occupational health nurse.

Preparation for this efficiency commences in the basic nursing training and continues throughout the occupational health nurse's career as she keeps her nursing, medical and technological knowledge up to date and uses her initiative to plan ahead for any eventuality.

The occupational health nurse receives her instructions for medical treatment in emergencies from her company physician. She requires written and signed 'protocol' that are updated regularly, for specific emergency situations. The medication and equipment required is checked daily and expiry dates noted so that new stocks may be ordered well ahead of time, and is kept at hand. Regular practice of first-aid procedures, cardio-pulmonary resuscitation, the insertion of intravenous injections etc., and updating of techniques and procedures is the responsibility of the occupational health nurse. Remember that the initial treatment and an accurate history of events including the time that it occurred may make all the difference to a complete and speedy recovery.

8.2 LEARNING OBJECTIVES

At the end of this section the reader should be able to:

- identify and, with the necessary medical protocols, treat injuries on duty and medical emergencies
- act effectively in case of occupational emergencies and disasters
- take part in the planning and implementation of an emergency plan
- identify her functions in case of death at work

8.3 INJURIES ON DUTY

Common injuries at the workplace include—

8.3.1 Lacerations and wounds By far the most common injury on duty that the occupational health nurse has to deal with are lacerations of the fingers and hands. Arresting the haemorrhage, assessing the extent of the damage whilst cleaning the wound, and obtaining a full history of the instrument that was being used, the force or weight involved, how the accident happened, the exact time that it happened and finally dressing the wound is part of the daily routine. Accurate history taking and completion of injury-on-duty forms is vital for good record keeping. Taking into account the wound and the history of the accident, the occupational health nurse may classify it as trivial and ask the patient to report back for dressings in order that she may monitor the healing but if there is any doubt as to involvement of nerves, tendons, bone, circulation or the amount of skin lost, the victim must be referred either to the company physician or an appropriate centre. Incorrect assessment and/or treatment may lead to a permanent disability.

The safety officer is normally responsible for investigating the cause of the accident, but the occupational health nurse can often get a clearer picture of circumstances surrounding the accident by visiting the scene and, by using the accident as a learning opportunity for fellow workers, she may prevent similar injuries in future.

8.3.2 Eye injuries Another common occurrence in industry is that of foreign bodies in the eye and burns caused by acids, alkalis or hot molten metal or glass in the eye. Superficial foreign bodies may be removed by the occupational health nurse (with a sterile cotton bud), but penetrating foreign bodies together with burns and any trauma of the eye should be referred directly to an ophthalmic surgeon or specific eye centre, as an extreme emergency. It is important to liaise with the specialist or unit beforehand, and for the company physician to issue clear instructions with regard to eye injuries in the event of him not being available at the time of the injury.

Arc eyes, as a result of intense ultraviolet irradiation during welding, will only give symptoms of irritation as if there is gravel in the eye, followed by pain, hours after the event, and the recommended treatment by the company physician should be available in the medical centre, as protocol. The occupational health nurse has an important role to play in the prevention of eye injuries through education of the workers and the enforcement of the correct eye protection during hazardous procedures in accordance with the company policy on health and safety. The strategic placement of eye fountains and their use for at least ten minutes following a chemical splash in the eye should also be taught to the workers.

Once the injury has occurred an accurate history of what the workman was using and how the accident occurred, including the direction from which the blow or foreign body entered the eye is important for the correct management of the injury by the specialist.

8.3.3 Multiple trauma Usually as a result of a major accident, whether it results in several injuries to one person or injuries to several people the principles of triage remain the same.

Triage means to categorize according to severity of injuries in order that lives may be saved. The occupational health nurse at the scene of multiple trauma would maintain an open airway, control severe haemorrhage with pressure and maintain in-line cervical spine support should the victim need to be moved. A well trained and co-ordinated first-aid team, usually made up of workers will provide invaluable support by carrying out first-aid procedures of cardio-pulmonary resuscitation, haemorrhage control, wound care, the splinting of fractures and basic shock treatment while the occupational health nurse co-ordinates the activities of the team, puts up intravenous infusions and gives emergency medical treatment according to the patient's condition.

8.3.4 Burns Localized burns on fingers, hands and forearms from touching hot objects and oven doors is another frequent case in an occupational health medical centre. Immediate cooling of the burn at the worksite arrests the damage done by the heat, appropriate dressings and not opening blisters promote rapid healing leaving little scarring and no permanent damage.

It is, however, the extensive burns from hot liquid and chemical splashes that need urgent medical treatment. Cooling the surface or rinsing away the chemical with copious amounts of cool running water can prevent further damage. Wrapping the patient in a sterile wet sheet, placing him in the shock position (recumbent with the feet raised about 25 cm), monitoring his vital signs, keeping an open intravenous line, whilst immediately transporting him to the local casualty department is recommended to prevent the complications of extensive burns from which the patient may succumb days later.

Significant burns may be caused by Beta radiation from electron accelerators and can develop two to four weeks later.

8.3.5 Heat exhaustion, heat stroke and hypothermia These conditions could be emergencies in areas where extremes of temperature occur such as near furnaces, in mines or cold storage rooms and workers work alone and do not realize what is happening when they start to feel tired.

Heat exhaustion can occur with physical exertion in a very hot, humid environment. It is the result of dehydration and electrolyte loss and presents with fatigue, headache, dizziness, thirst, muscle cramps, rapid and weak pulse, fast shallow respirations and a cool, clammy skin. Muscle incoordination, confusion, delirium and even coma could follow if the victim is not removed to a cool environment, given plenty of cool fluids to drink, if able to, and referred to hospital for intravenous fluid and electrolyte replacement if not. Heat exhaustion would occur more rapidly after a debilitating disease or a bout of diarrhoea and vomiting and therefore catch workers unaware after sick leave.

Heat stroke develops when the body can no longer regulate its temperature by perspiring. The first symptoms are similar to those of heat exhaustion, that is, the headache, fatigue, dizziness and thirst, but the patient soon becomes restless, the fast weak pulse becomes full and bouncing while the respiration becomes stertorous. The patient's skin becomes flushed and dry and the temperature will be over 40 °C and confusion, convulsions and unconsciousness will follow with possibly cardio-vascular collapse, cardiac arrest and death if treatment is not instituted without delay. The patient should be removed to a cool environment, clothing should be removed and the patient wrapped in a wet sheet and fanned. Cardio-pulmonary resuscitation may be necessary, oxygen must be administered and the vital functions monitored, whilst an intravenous infusion of Ringers lactate is given. Medication needs to be administered according to standing orders and the patient referred to the nearest casualty department.

Hypothermia could occur when the body temperature falls below 35 °C in an environment of below freezing point, or with prolonged exposure to low temperatures especially with the use of alcohol and drugs, or even some medical conditions such as diabetes mellitus. The victim feels very cold and exhausted, becomes pale and shivers uncontrollably, until incoordination with slurred speech sets in. The pulse and respiration rate become very low and the patient becomes confused before lapsing into unconsciousness.

The patient must be removed to a warm area, wet clothes need to be removed and dry insulating covering applied to the whole body, except the face. Cardio-pulmonary resuscitation may be necessary, but check carefully for a slow pulse first. Vital signs must be monitored and warm sweet drinks may be given. Transfer to hospital.

8.4 MEDICAL EMERGENCIES

Emergencies as a result of medical conditions are less frequent if there is an efficient health service at the work place. Pre-placement and periodic medical examinations highlight medical conditions, ensure early advice and treatment and the condition can be controlled by regular follow-up by the occupational health nurse.

A register could be kept of all known epileptics, diabetics, hypertensives, asthmatics and even those with tuberculosis and other health problems. Treatment in an emergency would be discussed with the company doctor and protocol drawn up for specific emergencies including medication to be given in the case of cardiac arrest and anaphylactic shock.

8.4.1 Cardiac arrest Perhaps the most common cause of cardiac arrest is a myocardial infarct or coronary thrombosis.

The victim or his co-workers usually inform the occupational health nurse that he is not feeling well, has indigestion and/or a severe chest pain. The pain could be described as a vice-like or crushing pain in the centre of the chest possibly spreading to the left arm or throat. The victim will feel weak or dizzy, perspire profusely, be cold to touch and anxious. His face will become ashen-grey with the lips, tip of nose and ear lobes becoming cyanotic. It is imperative that the victim does not exert himself, is reassured and placed in the semifowlers position. Oxygen and medication must be administered according to the doctor's orders. Immediate transfer to the nearest casualty centre in an appropriately equipped ambulance with constant monitoring is required. An intravenous line should be kept open with a very slow infusion.

Should cardiac arrest occur and defibrillation not be available the occupational health nurse should commence cardio-pulmonary resuscitation.

Cardio-pulmonary resuscitation

Take time to ascertain that the pulse has in fact stopped by feeling carefully for the carotid pulse. If absent place the victim on a hard surface (usually the floor) and open the airway by extending the head or lifting the jaw forward and upwards (the jaw lift is recommended if there could be a neck injury). Clear the mouth of fluid, vomitus or loose dentures.

If spontaneous respiration did not occur when the airway was opened, take a deep breath and closing the victim's nostrils with two fingers, and placing your mouth over the open mouth of the victim, sealing the lips, blow the air from your lungs into the victim's mouth. The victim's chest should rise and then fall when you take your mouth away. This is an indication that the airway is open. If the air is rushing past your mouth and you cannot feel it entering the victim's airway and the chest did not rise, clear the airway again and extend the head or lift the jaw more firmly. If the airway remains blocked try closing the mouth and blowing into the nostrils.

After two quick but full breaths, check again for a carotid pulse. If absent measure the sternum to find the midpoint and place the heel of one hand on the centre of the lower half. Place the heel of your other hand on top of the first, lock your fingers and lift them from the chest wall. Keeping your elbows straight and your shoulders directly over your hands press down on your hands in order to push the breast bone 4 to 5 cm down thereby squeezing the heart between the breast bone and the spinal column and emptying the blood in the chambers into the circulation. Release the pressure and blood will flow into the chambers again. These compressions are kept up rhythmically for 15 counts before the airway is opened again and two full breaths are given to be followed by another 15 even compressions.

Check for a pulse again after four cycles or the first minute and thereafter after every 12 cycles.

If a first aider comes to help the rhythm can be changed to five compressions to one breath after initially giving two full breaths.

It is imperative that this procedure is practised regularly with the medical staff and first aiders at the place of work, to perfect the rhythm which is crucial to successful resuscitation. The procedure should be continued until the victim's heart starts beating and breathing is restored. Improvement in his colour and a pulse in the carotid artery may merely indicate that the resuscitation is effective.

8.4.2 Anaphylactic shock Anaphylactic shock is a condition that may be fatal within minutes and one in which a gram of prevention is worth many kilograms of cure.

Prevention starts with good history taking at the pre-placement medical examination and health education of the worker to emphasize the importance of reporting allergies and good record keeping of possible signs and symptoms of previous reactions. Before administering any medication the patient should be informed as to what he is getting and asked if he is aware of any allergy towards the drug, or any other for that matter. Skin tests before administration may prevent, but have been known to cause, a major reaction. Anaphylaxis is commonly caused by parenteral administration of a drug, serum, vaccine or venom (e.g. bee sting) to which the patient has been previously sensitized.

The first signs and symptoms include the patient's statement that he feels strange, perhaps with a tingling scalp or a thick tongue. He is apprehensive and may look flushed or have an itchy rash or paresthesia. A tight feeling in the chest, wheezing respiration, fast thready pulse, a fall in blood pressure is soon followed by laryngeal oedema, bronchospasms, unconsciousness, vascular collapse and death.

The prescribed course of drugs could include an anti-histamine, adrenaline, hydrocortisone and aminophyllin to be given under specific circumstances, in specific doses either intramuscular or intravenously and these should be readily available together with syringes, swabs and files, butterfly needles, intravenous infusions and administration sets and oxygen in a pack that could be grabbed and taken to the patient should an emergency call come through. The patient is put into the shock position, is reassured, kept warm and given oxygen whilst being closely monitored for bronchospasm, fall in blood pressure and significant changes in the pulse rate. Keeping an open airway and an open intravenous line while the company doctor is sent for if he is on the premises or nearby as well as an ambulance to transport the patient to the nearest casualty department. It is vitally important that the occupational health nurse clarifies the desired treatment with her medical officer on the first day that they work together and that she keeps her 'anaphylactic kit' instantly available.

8.5 OCCUPATIONAL EMERGENCIES AND DISASTERS

An emergency due to occupational hazards could just as easily involve only one person as it could the whole work force and they are therefore dealt with under one heading.

A disaster is any sudden occurrence that results in loss of life, injury and property damage. It can range from a minor to a major disaster depending on the number of fatalities and injured and the costs of the destruction. If incorrectly handled a minor disaster could become a moderate or even a major one due to increased loss of life or destruction of property by for instance a fire following an explosion.

Classification of disasters

Disasters are classified according to their cause. *Natural disasters* refer to storms, floods, mud slides, tornadoes, earthquakes, etc. and even epidemics. *Man-made disasters* include fire, bomb threats or explosions, riots and panic. Also included here would be transport disasters such as aeroplane or train crashes and of course industrial disasters.

The following industrial accidents specifically need mention—

8.5.1   Mining accidents Rock slides, explosions caused by coal dust or methane gas leaks, and even flooding of mine shafts. In recent years improved safety measures, mining techniques and rescue methods appear to have reduced the frequency of major mining disasters. (Garb and Eng 1969: 212–24.) Mines usually have well-defined emergency procedures and the occupational health nurse will be involved in the treatment of the injured in a hospital situation.

8.5.2   Radiation emergencies or nuclear reactor accidents Although uncommon, the disasters at Three Mile Island in the United States of America and Chernobyl in the Union of Soviet Socialist Republics rocked the world by the immensity of the implications.

There are three levels of radiation where the victim can be contaminated by the radioactive material or have ingested or inhaled it or become irradiated as a result of exposure to gamma rays or X-rays.

8.5.2.1 Management of radioactive contamination Radioactive material such as dust, solid particles or in a liquid form adheres to the victim's skin and clothes. The victim needs to be decontaminated in a special decontamination zone. Evaluation of the level of contamination should take place throughout the decontamination process with a suitable radiation detector. Urine and faeces samples should be saved and measured for the amount of radioactivity.

8.5.2.2 *The decontamination zone* This should be a room or area away from the contamination area that should be prepared by removing all surplus furniture and other items, and placing a disposable waterproof covering on the floor. A free water supply and a large container for all contaminated water must be arranged. Protective clothing with waterproof shoe covering and respirators for the decontamination personnel if there is a risk of airborne radioactive particles as well as suitable containers for contaminated clothes and for urine, faeces or nasal swab samples must be arranged beforehand.

The treatment of life-threatening conditions and open wounds which should be irrigated with copious amounts of sterile saline, take precedence over the general decontamination process, the victim is completely undressed and his clothing sealed in a plastic bag. Initial monitoring for the level of contamination is done and monitoring is repeated throughout the process. The nostrils, mouth and external auditory canals are swabbed with cottonwool applicators and these are sealed in glass test tubes and placed in a lead lined container for monitoring at a later stage.

The ears, eyes and nostrils should be irrigated with a normal saline solution. The skin is then gently scrubbed with soap and water at body temperature. Vigorous scrubbing should be avoided as it stimulates the circulation and can cause breaks in the skin, which will assist absorption of radioactive elements into the body. Only if monitoring reveals persistent contamination of the skin should more abrasive scrubbing be used to remove dead skin and contaminants that adhere to the skin proteins.

Hair should be shampooed as well and if there is evidence of resistant contamination it should be cut off. (Shaving is risky as there is a chance of nicking the scalp.)

Should contamination persist chelating agents can be used to bind the radioactive contaminant into a complex agent as it is removed from the skin. These patients are always followed up regularly and thereafter yearly for possible module formation in wounds.

8.5.2.3 *Internal contamination* When radioactive material has entered the body by inhalation or ingestion, therapy must be directed at elimination and excretion of the radio-nuclides and decreasing the gastro-intestinal absorption. This is a medical emergency! The use of emetics, gastric lavage, purgatives and enemas and even lung lavage may be recommended by the medical officer-in-charge. Reduction of gastro-intestinal absorption will be aided by agents such as aluminium containing antacids, alginate or Barium sulphate.

Once the agent has been absorbed blocking agents such as Potassium iodide which reduces the uptake of radio iodide by the thyroid gland can be used. Mobilizing agents increase the natural turnover process of some radio-nuclides and chelating agents bind the radioactive ion into a non-ionizing ring complex that can be excreted by the kidney.

The time involved in carrying out the above procedures is crucial in minimizing the effects of the radiation accident and careful planning and preparation for such an event is part of the occupational health nurse's duty in an industry where radioactivity is used.

8.5.3 Exposure to toxic substances One of the most important duties of the occupational health nurse is to identify all the chemicals and gases that are brought into the work place, how they are used and what by-products are formed during the process. In larger industries she will liaise with the safety officer, industrial hygienist, buyer, production manager, horticulturist or head gardener as well as the worker himself. By doing 'factory rounds' and asking workers about their work she will discover interesting and sometimes horrifying facts as uninformed or careless people go about making their daily tasks a little easier, albeit unsafe. Toxic substances enter the body by inhalation, skin absorption or ingestion. The most common acute poisoning in industry is through inhalation.

8.5.3.1 Respiratory emergencies The commonest respiratory emergency that the occupational health nurse has to deal with is that of occupational asthma.

Occupational asthma

Careful history taking, lung auscultation and physical examination as well as an accurate lung function test would preclude an asthmatic from work areas that have respiratory irritants. Allergies to natural substances such as skins, hair, fur, feathers, mites, flour, grain dust, fungi, moulds or even wheat weavils amongst others and chemicals including chromium, cobalt dust, epoxy resins, formaldehyde, gum arabic, isocyanates, nickle, organo-phosphates, phenol, phenylene-diamine platinum salts, pyrethrin, tannic acid, toluene, tetrachloropthalic anhydride, tragacanth and vanadium to name but a few, could result in bronchospasm.

Standard asthma treatment applies in occupational asthma; remember to remove all traces of the causative agent from the patient.

8.5.3.2 Respiratory irritants All irritants produce an inflammatory reaction of the mucous membranes of the entire respiratory tract causing mild symptoms such as rhinorrhea and watery eyes with low dose exposure through to oedema of the larynx and lungs followed by death in high dose exposure or exposure to highly-toxic gases.

Examples of respiratory irritants include:
- *Ammonia* whose particularly pungent smell does prevent more serious accidents from happening. Used mainly in the fertilizer industry, the symptoms of exposure vary from upper respiratory tract irritation to pulmonary oedema and death. Bronchiectasis may follow as a permanent lesion after exposure.
- *Bromine* is a reddish brown gas used in the chemical and petroleum industries with similar symptoms and treatment as chlorine inhalation.

- *Chlorine* is a yellowish green gas with a sharp odour used mainly in paper, chemical and mining industries as well as in water purification and sewage treatment plants. High concentration exposure can cause panic due to choking, coughing, dyspnea, chest pain and haemoptysis. Emergency treatment for shock with oxygen and bronchodilators is followed by urgent referral to hospital where they will be admitted for observation for possible pulmonary oedema.
- *Fluorine* is a yellowish green gas with a pungent odour, used in the chemical, petroleum, uranium, aluminium and glass industry. High dose exposure gives similar symptoms to that of chlorine exposure and requires similar treatment.
- *Nitrogen oxides* are usually colourless and odourless and are found mainly in farm silos where fodder ferments, fertilizer manufacture and in metal cleaning processes and welding. High exposure gives similar symptoms as chlorine exposure and requires similar treatment.
- *Phosgene* is a toxic gas used widely in the manufacture of dyes, isocyanates, pharmaceuticals, polyurethane resins and is present in welding fumes and burning polyurethane fumes. Whilst initially causing only slight upper respiratory tract irritation, exposure is often followed by a latent period of a few hours up to three days, when pulmonary oedema arises, leading to respiratory failure if medical intervention is delayed. Admission to hospital for three days for observation is vital following exposure to phosgene gas.
- *Sulphur dioxide* is a colourless gas with an unpleasant pungent odour. It is used in bleaching and paper manufacturing but is a by-product of many industrial processes as well as fuel and oil combustion. Active high dose exposure may prove fatal due to obstruction of airways. Treatment: Oxygen, bronchodilators and even cortisone may need to be administered prior to urgent hospitalization.

8.5.3.3 Asphyxiants Asphyxiants deprive the vital organs of the body of oxygen in one of two ways:

Simple asphyxiants

These are physiologically inert gases that displace atmospheric oxygen and thereby deprive the victim of oxygen. These gases include carbon dioxide, ethane, methane, nitrogen and then smoke which is a chemical irritant as well as an asphyxiant.

Treatment can only be given once the victim has been rescued which is a hazardous procedure. Rescuers must wear self contained breathing apparatus. Cardio-pulmonary resuscitation, oxygen and urgent hospital treatment is required.

Chemical asphyxiants

Chemical asphyxiants are gases that disrupt cellular respiration by preventing oxygen from reaching the cells. The effect of chemical asphyxiants depends on many factors including the duration of exposure; the concentration of the gas in the area; the victim's health status and lung function; the use of personal protective equipment;

the presence of other toxic gases in the area; and most important of all—the emergency medical management. The three most common chemical asphyxiants are carbon monoxide, hydrogen cyanide and hydrogen sulfide.

Carbon monoxide

This gas is present in any enclosed area where incomplete combustion of organic materials takes place, especially in tanks, garages and mines where ventilation may be poor. Victims will at first complain of headaches, dizziness, a tight feeling of the chest and nausea. As the carboxyhaemoglobin level rises symptoms become more severe with a shortness of breath, racing pulse rate, vomiting and eventually collapse and coma. With high carboxyhaemoglobin levels the mucous membranes become a cherry red colour.

Treatment: Remove the victim from the area and oxygenate him and if necessary do cardio-pulmonary resuscitation. Paramedic treatment of intubation and establishing an intravenous line with a Ringers lactate solution for drug administration may be required. Monitor for cardiac dysrhythmia and transfer to hospital.

Cyanide

Hydrogen cyanide is used to make monomers for plastics and also in electroplating, fumigation and ore extraction. In a fire or an explosion cyanide is often released and inhaled by the victims together with the smoke. It has a characteristic bitter-almond smell. Liquid hydrogen cyanide is easily absorbed through the skin.

Treatment: Remove the victim from the area. Immediate use of the cyanide antidote kit, whilst simultaneously doing cardio-pulmonary resuscitation and decontamination of the skin with water requires a team of first aiders.

The cyanide antidote kit consists of Amyl nitrate capsules, an ampule of sodium nitrate 3% and an ampule of sodium thiosulfate 25% and is used in this sequence. The Amyl nitrate is crushed in gauze and held by the victim's nostrils for 30 seconds. Then the sodium nitrate is administered intravenously slowly, taking three to five minutes, followed by 50 ml sodium thiosulphate intravenously over a period of ten minutes. These injections may be repeated after two hours and must be verified in protocol from the medical officer in charge. The patient should be placed in the Trendelenburg position and the intravenous line should be kept open. Constant cardiac monitoring is essential for early detection of dysrhythmia and atriventricular blocks.

Hydrofluoric acid

Hydrofluoric acid is often used to remove potting, cement and lacquer from glass, ceramics and fine wires as used in the electronic industry.

After exposure the skin may at first only appear wrinkled and feel strange—severe pain follows hours later as the fluorine combines with the calcium in the system to form calcium fluoride and only subsides when the fluoride ions are saturated which may be days later.

Immediate removal of contaminated clothing and rinsing of the affected area under running water for at least ten minutes to remove as much of the acid as possible, before giving the patient a jar of calcium gluconate gel to massage into the area continuously in an effort to saturate the fluoride. Continue the application en route to hospital where he will be given a calcium infusion. Liaison with hospital personnel beforehand is imperative to ensure correct treatment as permanent scarring of the affected areas and nailbeds occur.

8.6 MANAGEMENT OF HAZARDOUS MATERIAL ACCIDENTS AND TOXIC EXPOSURES

The management of accidents involving hazardous substances begins with good planning. The occupational health nurse must know exactly which hazardous substances, whether in their original form or as a result of combination with other substances during a process, are on the premises.

Planning would include the following:
- *A chart* should be drawn up to include each substance, its trade name, its ingredients, description of colour, odour, consistency etc., the area and the process in which it is used, the clinical signs and symptoms of exposure and the first-aid treatment.
- *Education* of all the workers in the area, from the manager to the floor sweeper, as well as the staff from the receiving depot and store in the identification of hazardous substances in the area, their effects on the body and emergency procedures, including who to inform, decontamination, evacuation, first-aid procedures and personal protective equipment.
- *Liaison* with local emergency services to ensure good relations and correct treatment for specific toxic substances.
- *Safety and health committee* would include the company physician, the general manager, safety officer, industrial hygienist, production manager and the occupational health nurse. New procedures and substances to be used should be discussed as well as fresh information regarding the toxic substance, its substitution or treatment of exposure. A company policy on safety and health aspects is another duty of this committee.
- *Protective equipment:* Policy and procedures for the supply and the correct use and enforcement thereof is drawn up by the safety and health committee. Continual updating of information and new appliances as they become available is the duty of the occupational health nurse in the absence of a safety officer.
- *Decontamination zones:* Eye fountains and showers should be provided with correct drainage so as to prevent contaminated water from entering the general drainage system and spreading the contamination. Education in the correct use of these showers for at least ten minutes while the occupational health nurse is sent for is vital rather than a quick rinse and the victim then making his way to the medical centre.
- *Rescue and first-aid teams:* Basic training in rescue and first-aid should be supplemented with information on specific hazards and

regular practising. Team members should be issued with the correct personal protective equipment. Depending on the extent of the accident they may need to set up a command post and secure the area.

- *Follow-up:* A special meeting of the safety and health committee should be called following any spill or exposure in order to learn from the experience by ironing out any misunderstandings about procedure in an effort to reach optimal health and safety standards.

8.7 A DISASTER PLAN AND EMERGENCY EVACUATION

Although the most senior official of an organization is responsible for the planning and execution of an emergency plan, he often delegates the task to an appropriately qualified official, whilst giving active support to the programme. The occupational health nurse has a specific role to play in the provision of first-aid in an emergency but all too often in smaller industries she needs to initiate the disaster programme by drawing management's attention to existing hazards on the premises and possible consequences of accidents, as well as the ever present threat of fire, rioting, explosions or even natural disasters.

8.7.1 The disaster plan An industrial disaster is any sudden occurrence that results in loss of life, injuries to workers and property damage. It will disrupt production and may even hold further threats to the well being of the workers by way of escaping gas or radiation for instance. A well executed disaster plan could prevent a disaster from happening and would certainly minimize the effects of one.

8.7.2 Prevention of a disaster Any disaster plan should commence with the prevention of a possible disaster by way of planning the building or the utilization of space in a work area with safe storage, good ventilation, good housekeeping, strategically placed fire extinguishers and first-aid boxes etc. Education and training of the workers in the hazards of the procedures that they carry out daily, safety precautions and protective equipment as well as first-aid and emergency procedures and orderly evacuation. Minimizing the effect of a disaster could be achieved by thorough planning, identification and training of the emergency controller and coordinator, as well as key personnel in each area, including fire fighters and first aiders and training the workers in emergency procedures and evacuation.

8.7.3 The emergency controller Appointed by the general manager, this person has the responsibility of designing the emergency plan, organizing drills and streamlining his plan to iron out problems. He will require:

- a plan of the whole site together with the floor plan of the buildings indicating all entrances and the different areas;
- the floor plan must indicate main electricity boards, hazardous substances, inflammable materials, gas cylinders etc.;
- all fire extinguishers, first-aid boxes and emergency equipment including rescue equipment must be indicated on this chart;

- updated lists of names, addresses and telephone numbers of all emergency personnel, senior management and local emergency services;
- an effective communication system;
- an identification system for emergency personnel;
- an emergency transport system; and
- an efficient evacuation system.

8.7.4 Scene security The company security department will isolate the scene, evacuate it and control onlookers, news reporters and volunteers as well as incoming emergency personnel and equipment and outgoing evacuees and victims. They will report to the emergency controller in the command centre.

8.7.5 Command centre A central command post, headed by the emergency controller and staffed according to the extent of the disaster will:
- assess the extent of the disaster;
- establish a communication system with radios and runners;
- liaise with internal security, fire fighting, security and first-aid team leaders;
- liaise with external emergency teams;
- implement a pre-arranged identification system;
- control the transport of victims;
- control information to outsiders and the press.

8.7.6 The communication system This operates between the command centre and coordinators at the scene, as well as at evacuation points and rescue teams, the first-aid transport and security posts. The alarm system must be checked regularly as well as the radios and their effectiveness in all areas of the buildings. Runners may have to be used if the radios cannot be heard in certain areas.

8.7.7 The first-aid post An area must be identified that is large enough to accommodate many injured, is easily accessible, has running water, toilets and storage space. The dining hall is often used for this purpose. Stocks of emergency supplies, blankets and even refreshments are stored at the site and checked regularly.

8.7.8 Evacuation points Gathering points at a safe distance from the building are identified for each exit of the building in order that workers may evacuate via the quickest safest route. The evacuation procedure must be made known to each employee and practised at least twice a year.

8.7.9 The rescue and fire fighting teams In smaller industries these teams consist of specially trained workers who practise their procedures regularly and are au fait with procedures followed by local emergency teams with whom they liaise closely. Appropriate easily identifiable personal protective clothing should be worn by team members.

8.7.10 First-aid teams These are specially trained workers who control first-aid boxes and equipment in their areas, and practise regularly as a team with a team leader, at least once or twice a month. The occupational health nurse is often involved with the training and certainly takes an active interest in their practise sessions and gets to know the capabilities of each team member. When local emergency teams are called in they take command of the first-aid post and the first aiders should be able to work with them, and must be identifiable by their armbands and white coats or similar dress.

8.7.11 Transport Appropriate vehicles should be identified to transport casualties should the need arise and also to transport workers home in the event of major disruption of production.

A disaster plan must be known to everyone on the work site, it must be adaptable according to circumstances and carefully evaluated after every practise session and certainly after a disaster of whatever magnitude. Experience has shown that reaction time decreases, co-ordination improves and the disaster controlled to have the least effect on the workers, production and the company as a whole when emergency procedures are known and practised regularly.

8.8 DEATH AT WORK

It is a devastating experience to have a death at the place of work and the occupational health nurse has specific legal and ethical responsibilities, whether the death is caused by an accident or as the result of an illness. By law the occupational health nurse may not certify death and should attempt life saving procedures, unless it is obvious that resuscitation is impossible as with gross mutilation. The company physician or in his absence a local practitioner may be called in this case and once death has been certified the coroner must be informed. All cases of death due to unnatural, sudden or instant causes should be reported to the coroner and the scene must be left as it was found until all investigations are completed.

Accurate record keeping of all relevant facts, including the names of witnesses is as always important. Ethically the nurse must do all in her power to preserve life, but when death is certified she must preserve dignity in death, remembering also that to fellow workers and onlookers the body is still the person that they knew. She should carefully cover and screen the body and arrange for removal as soon as possible.

The nurse will be aware of the effect of the stressful event on the fellow workers and will reassure them and arrange for them to get back to work. It is the nurse's duty to inform management of the event in a concise report. The personnel department also need to know and they should inform any relatives who may also be employed at the same firm.

If possible the occupational health nurse and a senior member of management will inform close relatives at home. If not, the police will do it. It is at times like these that the professional status of the occupational health nurse stands her in good stead.

8.9 BIBLIOGRAPHY

Baker, M. and Coetzee, A. C. (eds.) 1983. *Introduction to Occupational Health Nursing in South Africa*. Johannesburg: Witwatersrand University Press.

Garb, S. and Eng, E. 1969. *Disaster Handbook*. New York: Springer Publishing Company.

Harrison, B. M. 1984. *Essentials of Occupational Health Nursing*. Oxford: Blackwell Scientific Publications.

MacMahon, A. G. and Jooste, M. (eds.) 1980. *Disaster Medicine*. Cape Town: A. A. Balkema.

Nelson, R. N., Rund, D. A. and Kellar, M. D. 1985. *Environmental Emergencies*. Philadelphia: W. B. Saunders.

Rosenstock, L. and Cullen, M. R. 1986. *Clinical Occupational Medicine*. Philadelphia: W. B. Saunders.

Waldron, H. A. 1979. *Lecture Notes on Occupational Medicine*. Oxford: Blackwell Scientific Publications.

Chapter 9: Psychological Adjustment of the Worker in the Work Environment

by Z. C. Bergh

9.1 INTRODUCTION

Psychological adjustment or mental health as a comprehensive concept refers to certain behaviours and conditions in individuals, which in the context of their environment or situation and related norms, characterize their psychic or psychological welfare. The degree of psychological adjustment refers pre-eminently to the behaviours or methods whereby the individual acts in his environment, solves his problems and copes with life and work stress. Mental health can include behaviours such as the degree of satisfaction with life and job, emotional control, kinds of interpersonal relationships, social behaviour, actualization of potential and skills, stress experiences as well as the presence or absence of psychopathological (abnormal) conditions and even physical handicaps.

Because work has an integral place and meaning in most people's lives, personal success and psychological adjustment is often linked to some or other criterion of job success or attainment of goals in a career. The study of work adjustment or occupational mental health deals with the adjustment or maladjustment of an individual in the context of the work organization's functioning. Therefore individual work adjustment can be separated neither from the 'organization's health' nor from the environment in which both the individual and the organization exist and function. It is thus also necessary to understand the interaction between the worker and the organization because the degree of adjustment or maladjustment is not caused only by the situation or the individual's traits, but is rather the result of the type of congruence or fit between the individual and his work situation. Understanding of both the individual and the organization and their interaction will not only aid our diagnosis of symptoms and causes but also in managing work adjustment, for instance, counselling the problem employee or intervening with aspects of organizational malfunctioning.

In the broad field of human resources management the interaction between worker (individual) and his environment, such as the work situation, is represented by, inter alia, the organizational psychology, career psychology, ergonomics and the so-called interactional psychology or person-environment fit theories. As a matter of fact one of the main objectives of the theoretical and practical personnel psychology, as well as disciplines such as career counselling and the different therapeutic practices, is to facilitate the best fit between the individual and his environment, not only in terms of productivity but also with respect to psychological adjustment. In our modern times surely psychological work adjustment must be equal in importance compared to aspects such as quantity and quality of products and services, the physical health of the worker and the hygiene of the work place.

The statistics in 9.3 on the incidence, as well as cost and personnel implications of mental health in general and in the work place might serve to highlight the importance of effective mental health management.

9.2 LEARNING OBJECTIVES

When you have studied this chapter you should:
- understand the scope and complexity of mental health problems;
- understand the interaction between the individual (worker) and his work environment;
- grasp the importance of work in personal and work adjustment;
- be able to define and describe personal and work adjustment;
- be able to mention criteria for personal and work adjustment;
- recognize causes for personal and work adjustment problems;

- be able to interpret certain psychopathological conditions with reference to their implications for work behaviour;
- be familiar with specific work-related adjustment problems;
- be familiar with personal or self-management strategies for better work adjustment;
- be familiar with organizational and therapeutic approaches to improve work adjustment.

9.3 THE INCIDENCE, COST AND PERSONNEL IMPLICATIONS OF MENTAL HEALTH PROBLEMS

It is obvious that the *effects of maladjustment* spread further than the immediate place of incidence because of the interactive nature of human behaviour, and the fact that the individual daily finds himself in different systems where he as a self-system forms part of other systems. There can be a *circular relationship* between an individual problem, a social problem, a work problem and their symptoms. Thus the policy on such a problem and the responsibility for it could become a community, an organizational, an economic and even a political problem. Health, especially mental health remains one of the world's greatest and most expensive problems. The discussions that follow form merely the tip of the proverbial iceberg.

In 1978 approximately 120 000 000 cases of maladjustment were reported in the U.S.A. This involves between twenty-five and thirty million people, which amounts to virtually ten per cent of the U.S. population.

Recent research indicates that between fifteen and twenty-five per cent of the world's population in different parts of the world suffer from at least one type of psychological disorder. If less serious emotional problems are also counted in this figure, it may even be higher than fifty per cent (Louw et al., 1989).

Furthermore, Syme (1974) and Kasl (in Cooper and Payne, 1978) estimate that more than half of the American population are affected by a stress problem.

In the U.S.A. more than forty per cent of the beds in State hospitals are occupied by people with psychological problems; in 1976 approximately 200 000 of the beds in private institutions were occupied by psychiatric patients. It is estimated that three million Americans annually receive constant psychiatric or psychological treatment.

It has been estimated that, depending on the type of condition, between six and fifty per cent of the people who consult medical doctors on physical illnesses are actually experiencing psychological problems, especially psychosomatic, neurotic and stress conditions. Blythe (in Greenwood and Greenwood, 1979) maintains that seventy per cent of the medical patients in the U.S.A. and Britain display symptoms that can be attributed to stress. These symptoms occur more often among the general American population than more serious conditions like alcoholism, organic problems, psychoses and personality disorders. On the other hand, although the last-mentioned group of conditions occur more rarely, they have more serious direct and indirect costs in terms of the restrictions of the person's functioning, his hospitalization and treatment (Follman, 1978).

Psychological maladjustment costs the U.S.A. at least twenty to thirty million dollars annually for treatment, services and hospital administration. This amounts to fifteen per cent of the annual health budget of 140 million dollars, and to eight per cent of the total American budget. The loss of productivity annually amounts to another fifty million dollars.

The mortality figure in the U.S.A. because of psychological problems is much higher than is commonly believed. Cardiac diseases, which are normally associated with stress and psychosomatic conditions, are responsible for more than half of all the deaths; lost working days because of this amount to 132 million per annum. It is estimated that for every death because of an industrial accident, fifty people die because of cardiac disease. It seems ironical that organizations (in South Africa as well) spend millions more on security and on the prevention of accidents than on the prevention of cardiac disease.

In South Africa the total cost of public health services (including the provinces and the homelands) administered by the Department of Health amounts to more than R230 358 000 for 1981/82. This represents a rise of approximately ten million rand on the figure for 1980/81. If general administration, welfare and pensions, and ancillary services are also included, the amount comes to R935 339 000. Out of this total figure, an amount of R78 993 000 has been voted for mental health services, which amounts to 34,2 per cent of the total health budget. The greater portion of the amount for mental health, R65 554 700, has been spent on hospital treatment, and more than six million has been spent on out-patient services. Expenditure on training for this period has amounted to a mere R3 424 200, despite staff shortages that make proper services difficult. The number of resident psychiatric patients for 1981 came to 14 616, and most of the cases occurred in the age groups 19 to 39 (4 707), 40 to 59 (3 276) and 60 years and older (2 267). The total number of admissions for 1981 amounted to 26 471; 17 014 of the cases occurred in the age group 19 to 39, 5 601 in the age group 40 to 59, 2 291 in the age group of 60 years and older, and 1 565 in the group 0 to 18 years. We must also include 3 975 resident mentally retarded persons and 2 772 'dangerous' patients, as well as another 8 149 patients in private and licensed institutions.

In terms of broad diagnostic groups the numbers of resident and discharged patients are as follows: mental retardation: 5 924; nonpsychotic aberrations: 5 679, of which anxiety-based disorders (neurosis) (1 108), personality disorders (1 153), addiction to alcohol (1 339), organic and nonpsychotic conditions (241) and depression (316) occurred most frequently. The number of psychotic disorders amounted to 27 698, of which schizophrenia (15 439), affective psychoses (2 597), transient organic psychoses (2 289), alcohol psychosis (1 096), senile and presenile organic psychoses (1 397), other organic psychoses (1 630), paranoia (250) and other nonorganic psychoses (1 385) occurred most frequently. As far as alcoholism alone is concerned, almost 10 000 people were treated at rehabilitation and registered centres for alcoholism and drug addiction in 1981, and the State subsidy amounted to more than two-and-a-half million rand. In 1981 the social responsibility for this problem and concern about it were underlined by a congress on 'Alcohol in perspective' in Johannesburg. The necessity for a more system-oriented approach to the prevention and treatment of alcoholism in South Africa received special attention.

These data show some increases and warning signals if compared to the information from the 1987/88 Annual Reports.

Trends in industry

Warshaw (1979, p. 5) says the following about the incidence of work stress: 'In the business world, stress seems to be the number one by-product of success. There is no escaping it.'

Forbes (1979) asserts that about eighty per cent of all the emotional problems experienced by workers derive from stress. Warshaw (1979) and Greenwood and Greenwood (1979), however, refer to the necessity and positive value of work stress for a productive work life. Nevertheless, everywhere in life and in the work situation there are people for whom work stress and other psychological symptoms have no advantages. Their behaviour has a dysfunctional effect on their personal lives and on those of others, and it is counter-productive to, say, the work organization and the community. Underachievement, absence, dissatisfaction, accidents, personnel turnover, poor work relations, unhealthy attitudes to work, strikes, lower production, bankruptcy in business, the closure of businesses, and certain psychopathological and emotional maladjustments can be signs of poor individual or organizational and community mental health.

It is estimated that more than twenty-five per cent of the labour force in the U.S.A. consisting of approximately 100 million people, have an emotional, personality or another more serious psychiatric problem. Du Plessis (1973) already puts the figure for South Africa at twenty per cent. In studies undertaken by Vlok (1971, 1981) he found that alcoholism is the main problem in the South African industry and that emotional problems are also increasing. These phenomena are manifested at all levels in every type of occupation, although there are differences in the frequency and type of maladjustment at different levels of an occupation and in occupational groups (Follman, 1978).

The total losses in the U.S.A. because of occupational maladjustment amount to at least fifty to seventy billion dollars per annum. Forbes (1979) puts the losses in the U.S.A. because of lost working days, hospitalization and untimely deaths at the level of management at between ten and twenty billion dollars.

Between twenty and thirty per cent of the absences from work in the U.S.A. are attributed to severe psychopathology, personality disorders, neuroses and emotional problems. Truancy occurs more frequently among women than among men, while age and the type of occupation also affect the frequency of absence. In 1976 the total costs of absenteeism amounted to twelve billion dollars. A considerable portion of this can be attributed to neuroses and psychoses (Follman, 1978).

It has been estimated that emotional and stress problems may be the cause of between eighty and ninety per cent of the industrial accidents in the U.S.A. (Forbes, 1979). The 1973 report of the Workmen's Compensation Commissioner in South Africa shows that insurers for all racial groups have reported almost 355 000 disability claims. Thirty-four per cent of these cases merely needed medical treatment, fifty-four per cent were temporarily disabled, nine per cent were permanently disabled, and about one per cent had died. The number of lost working days amounted to more than four million; together with the unreported cases the number of lost working days have been put at five million. If we include the fatal and permanently disabled cases, the total number of lost working days amounts to more than 32,5 million. Disability claims and medical costs have cost the Workmen's Compensation Commissioner over R361 million.

Reports of alcoholism and drug addiction as work-related and major problems in industrial mental health are received from all over the world, but specific diagnoses and statistics are not readily available. It seems as though the frequency and intensity of these problems will continue to increase. Kane (1975) estimates that eight per cent of the American labour force are full-scale alcoholics, found at all levels of work, in any type of occupation, among both sexes and organizations of any size. Forbes (1979) asserts that about twelve million Americans experience alcoholic problems which, according to Warshaw (1979) costs the State forty-three billion dollars; twenty billion dollars of this amount represent loss of production, and thirteen billion dollars medical costs. As early as 1974 Louw reported that untreated alcohol problems in the RSA cost the industry more than R136 million. Vlok (1971, 1981) has found that alcoholism is an ever-increasing problem in the work situation and that management is becoming more conscious of this problem. Kane (1975) and Forbes (1979) point out that apart from the direct costs and consequences of alcohol abuse, it also has indirect consequences for the individual and the organization.

Warshaw (1979) reports that about thirty-three million people in the U.S.A. were using some form of drug at the beginning of 1970.

Psychosomatic diseases caused by stress—headaches, peptic ulcers and cardiac diseases, for example—affect between ten and twenty per cent of Americans. At least half the deaths are attributed to cardiac diseases, which causes a loss of 132 million working days. Forbes (1979) estimates that the Americans annually spend more than 200 million dollars on sedatives, and that the effect of these remedies may be the direct or indirect cause of work-related problems, for instance accidents and absences.

As far as insurance claims are concerned, the percentages are as follows: 55,4 per cent for neuroses, 12,3 per cent for psychoses, 18,5 per cent for personality disorders, 7,5 per cent for psychophysiological problems and 6,2 per cent for organic conditions. Between ten and twelve per cent of all the claims can be attributed to the aforementioned conditions (Follman, 1978).

Managerial stress with its cost implications is a sphere that is receiving considerable attention in our time. In a systems model to calculate the cost of stress Greenwood and Greenwood (1979) found the following cost implications of managerial stress in the U.S.A. as set out below. The statistics are based on three cost factors, namely loss of work, hospital costs and death costs.

In 1970 about 21 545 000 executive officers (15 681 000 men and 5 864 000 women) received a total remuneration of approximately $198 170 811, which implies an average of about $9 198 per annum. In terms of loss of work because of stress problems it cost these managerial people about four billion dollars while the State had to pay another four billion. If we accept Blythe's estimate that seventy per cent of the problems were caused by stress, the direct personal costs still amount to $2 861 billion. Hospital fees amount to $248 million and the cost of out-patient services to $131 million. The mortality figures for these managerial people come to 288 526 for both sexes (244 000 men and 44 000 women) between the ages of twenty-five and sixty-four. The figures also include early deaths because of cardiac diseases, cancer, accidents, suicide and smoking problems—all associated with stress. In projections the life incomes of these people have been estimated to amount to more than 23,5 billion dollars; at a stress aetiology of seventy per cent it amounts to about sixteen billion dollars.

Greenwood and Greenwood (1979) also refer to the tremendous increases in the cost of disability premiums because of the effects of stress. Furthermore, in 1970, 10 748 of the 284 000 new industries in the U.S.A. failed, which cost the U.S.A. more than $96 million; in 1973 this figure came to approximately $134 million.

Carone et al. (1978) discuss the implications of the 'misfits' in the industry on the unemployment figures for the U.S.A. They include 'underemployed', 'overeducated' and 'mistrained' people. Carone et al. point out that, despite economic prosperity, unemployment is increasing at an average rate of approximately 7,6 per cent (in 1976): in some groups it is as high as fifty per cent. According to Carone (1978) there were about 1,2 million unemployed people in the U.S.A. in 1976. He maintains that they should be regarded as 'discouraged' rather than 'unemployed' persons; they are no longer interested in looking for work because of lack of job opportunities, rapid urbanization (sometimes forced) or other reasons. The problems of these 'qualified unemployed' persons in the U.S.A. (2,8 %) are also attributed to the high birth rate directly after World War II, which caused an oversupply of well-qualified workers between 1970 and 1980. The oversupply is diminishing, however, because of a dramatic decline in births in the U.S.A. after 1960; experts envisage that the U.S.A. may finally face a shortage of manpower. Carone (1978) believes that one of the main problem areas in industrial mental health has been the tremendous increase in female workers since 1945 (122 % compared to 30 % among the men). This has given rise to a change in role behaviour and to problems with children in households where both parents work (in the U.S.A. more than 6 500 000 young children out of a total of about 27 600 000 children under the age of eighteen).

In this regard Carson et al. (1988) report that in the U.S.A. about twelve per cent of all school children are clinically or psychologically maladjusted.

These cost statistics refer particularly to what is often described as the direct burdens of industrial mental health. They may include the following: lower or total loss of production; reduced or loss of income for the individual and the organization; the loss of financial investment in selection and training; the loss and misuse of equipment and other materials; the loss of working time; fees for medical and other treatment; hospital fees; advance pension payments; disability claims; legal fees; unemployment insurance premiums; bankruptcies in industry; and death claims and fees.

Indirect burdens can have an even more severe effect on the individual, the organization and the community. They include the following: personal pain, discomfort and inconvenience experienced by the individual and his family, relatives and friends because of physical or psychological problems; and quality of life and of working life which is affected by these factors; negative attitudes to work and difficult interpersonal relationships; a lack of initiative and risk-taking that are needed in the work situation; lack of motivation that leads to inertia; inefficiency and inadequacy; incorrect and poor decision-making; rigid behavioural and communication styles; the loss of clients; and mistrust among clients and in the community. These factors usually relate to particular problems and direct costs. It has been estimated that in 1974 $19,8 billion of the $36,8 billion spent on occupational maladjustment in the U.S.A. can be regarded as indirect costs.

The above-mentioned statistics, like many others, are probably inaccurate and may be an overestimation. In most cases, however, they underestimate the cumulative negative effects of mental disorder on the individual, the work situation and the community.

Mental disorder and the concomitant occupational maladjustment create a personnel problem. The industrial psychologist and organizational management must take note of this problem; in point of fact, they are confronted with it. We shall merely refer to a few of the consequences.

The potential of the organization's manpower lies in the quality of the human potential within the organization, and especially in the environment. The quality of the 'organizational life', which includes its effectiveness, efficiency and health, is also a function of the feedback between the organization and the systems surrounding it. In this context mental health or maladjustment can become part of the organization and its functioning, irrespective of whom management wishes to hold responsible for it or of its policy on mental health. In its policy and functions management must consistently tackle the prevention, diagnosis and treatment of occupational maladjustment. This means that the quality of not only the working life will be improved, but also that of the problem worker. In this way the risk of and financial investment in, say, research into occupational maladjustment and in its management will become a profitable rather than an unprofitable venture.

Every organization has its own problems with regard to the interaction that takes place inside it and with its surrounding systems. Because of its heterogeneity and rapid development, South Africa now has to face new challenges generally, and in particular in relation to individual adjustment and interpersonal relationships. Think of the implications of the new developments in labour relations and the political-economic prospects. A projection of the future human-work interaction seems complex. Organizations become bigger, more differentiated, technologically more refined, perhaps more impersonal for the worker. Since posts become more demanding and intellectual demands are higher, the worker becomes more sophisticated and sensitive, and he wants to know more, to participate more and take more decisions. He wants to become more deeply involved and he wants to communicate more. In the midst of these more intense stressors the worker has to satisfy his need for achievement and his social needs. It is the task of management to make use of creative job design to prevent the alienation of the worker from his place of work, and to teach him how to adjust, especially in the event of change.

9.4 A MODEL FOR UNDERSTANDING WORK ADJUSTMENT IN CONTEXT OF ORGANIZATIONAL FUNCTIONING

9.4.1 **Premise** An *organization*, functioning as a whole or as a unity, is formed to achieve objectives that cannot be achieved by individuals on their own.

Individuals join an organization to achieve objectives and to satisfy needs in a work context that would be impossible or difficult to accomplish on their own.

The type of *interaction between individual and organization* finally contributes to the meta-objectives for organizational and individual success, namely efficiency, effectiveness and 'health'—the last-mentioned quality includes individual physical and mental health and also organizational health.

The chief *premise* is that the individual as a self-system in all his modes of behaviour (biological, social and psychological) can be best understood by first examining his functioning in the context of the wider and hierarchical systems that surround him.

The study of individual behaviour maladjustment, and its diagnosis, understanding and treatment, are never possible if one has a purely simplistic point of view. For the purposes of your study and practice you will have to think in terms of systems which means that you may have to review former views and attitudes, or that you may have to conceptualize and apply them differently.

9.4.2   A systems interactional model Figure 9.1 is a diagram representing an adapted model by Beer (in Cummings, 1980), and the integration of ideas from various approaches to stress, therapy and behaviour.

In your study in the different nursing disciplines you should be fully conversant with systemic paradigms and with various applications of systemic premises to hygiene management, for instance, in occupational health or medical diagnosis. This knowledge could be an important source of reference for this chapter.

This approach does not endeavour to deal exhaustively with all aspects of organizations. However, because of the interaction it is impossible to omit certain aspects of organizations from the model. You must bear in mind that the emphasis in this chapter is always on the individual in a specific context.

9.4.3   An operational description of the model The individual as a *self-system* brings certain individual qualities and characteristics to the work organization because of his unique frames of reference. The personality of the individual consists of behaviour patterns or relationship styles formed by learning and experiential processes in all his hierarchical systems, and in turn determines his behaviour in his relationship with the organization. The *organization* also has specific and characteristic inputs because of its culture and its influential hierarchic systems (environment). Its characteristics—for example, certain structures—will determine the type of contact with the individual and also the type of behaviour and process that can be expected. Through a process of reciprocal, continuous and circular *interaction* determined by specific behaviour and communication styles, structures, rules, transactions, and so on, the individual and the organization define certain types of relationships and a particular climate. This leads to certain *outputs* (attitudes, behaviour, feelings, etc.) by the individual and the organization, which in turn finally result in certain *consequences* for the individual and the organization. The consequences reveal the extent to which individual and organizational objectives, needs and expectations have been satisfied. The interaction between individuals and between individual and organization is constantly monitored by means of *feedback* which also determines the extent to which the individual accepts or rejects the outputs and consequences. It is important to remember that there are certain *dominant influential factors* in both the individual and the organization. These dominant 'coalitions' can determine the extent to which individuals and organizations are selective in their interactions, observation and acceptance so as to gain the maximum benefit from events and situations.

Following is a very brief description of model 9.1. Aspects of it which will become more evident in other discussions of this chapter.

FIGURE 9.1

A systems interactional model for the study of work adjustment

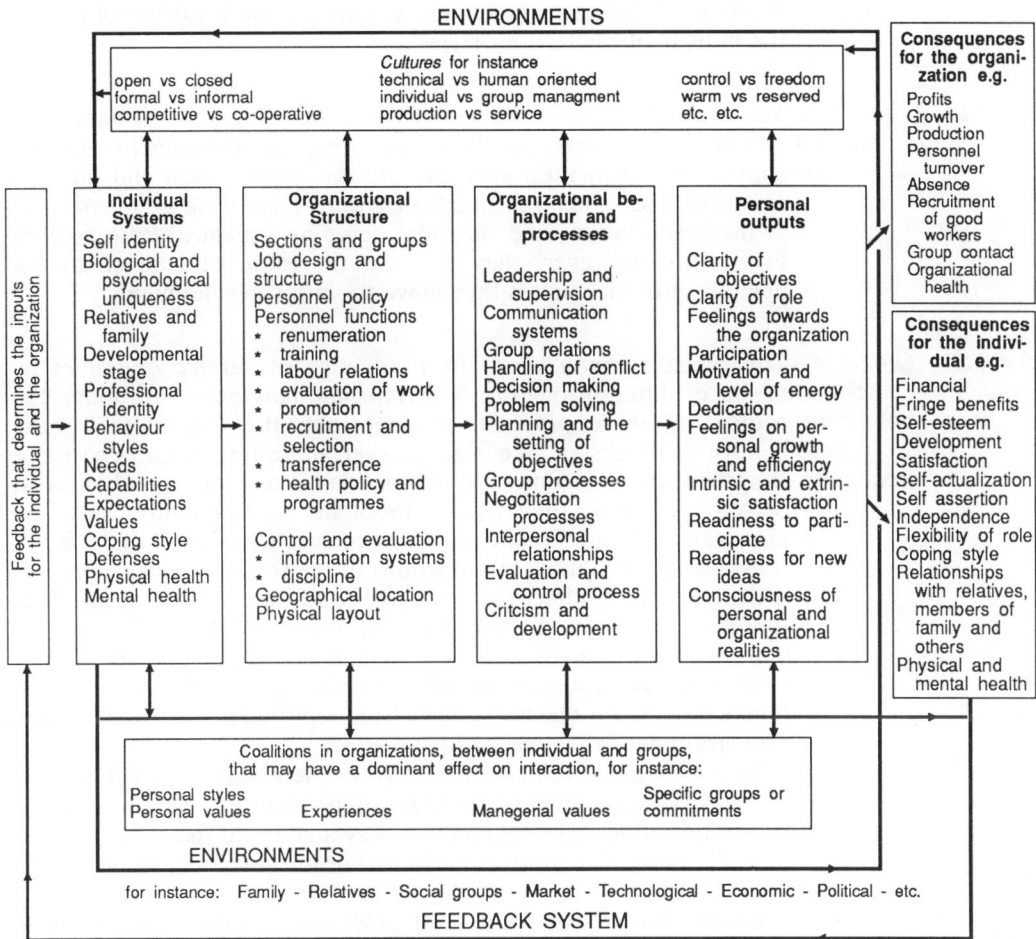

ENVIRONMENTS

	Consequences for the organization e.g.
Cultures for instance open vs closed — technical vs human oriented — control vs freedom formal vs informal — individual vs group managment — warm vs reserved competitive vs co-operative — production vs service — etc. etc.	Profits Growth Production Personnel turnover Absence Recruitment of good workers Group contact Organizational health

Feedback that determines the inputs for the individual and the organization

Individual Systems	Organizational Structure	Organizational behaviour and processes	Personal outputs
Self identity Biological and psychological uniqueness Relatives and family Developmental stage Professional identity Behaviour styles Needs Capabilities Expectations Values Coping style Defenses Physical health Mental health	Sections and groups Job design and structure personnel policy Personnel functions * renumeration * training * labour relations * evaluation of work * promotion * recruitment and selection * transference * health policy and programmes Control and evaluation * information systems * discipline Geographical location Physical layout	Leadership and supervision Communication systems Group relations Handling of conflict Decision making Problem solving Planning and the setting of objectives Group processes Negotitation processes Interpersonal relationships Evaluation and control process Critcism and development	Clarity of objectives Clarity of role Feelings towards the organization Participation Motivation and level of energy Dedication Feelings on personal growth and efficiency Intrinsic and extrinsic satisfaction Readiness to participate Readiness for new ideas Consciousness of personal and organizational realities

Consequences for the individual e.g.

Financial
Fringe benefits
Self-esteem
Development
Satisfaction
Self-actualization
Self assertion
Independence
Flexibility of role
Coping style
Relationships with relatives, members of family and others
Physical and mental health

Coalitions in organizations, between individual and groups, that may have a dominant effect on interaction, for instance:

Personal styles
Personal values   Experiences   Manegerial values   Specific groups or commitments

ENVIRONMENTS

for instance: Family - Relatives - Social groups - Market - Technological - Economic - Political - etc.

FEEDBACK SYSTEM

9.4.4 The components of the model

9.4.4.1

The individual (people)

The individual can be *described in terms of various systems*, for instance biological, social, marriage, family, relatives, culture, and so on. The individual's potential for the organization lies in the qualities (capabilities, knowledge, skills, etc.) he brings to his work. We have to remember that the individual—his self-image and occupational concepts, his interpersonal and other adjustment skills, his behaviour and communication styles, even his problems—has been formed and is being formed by a process of continuous *interaction* with his environment and with culture. The success of the individual's productive role and his intra- and interpersonal relationships—in other words, his mental health—can be largely a function of the interaction with the organizational systems.

We have to acknowledge that every individual has *idiosyncratic* (unique) qualities that can be important for mental health. The way in which these idiosyncratic qualities affect behaviour and relationships is crucial for a psychological study of mental health. As soon as the individual joins the organization, the organization should, by means of its personnel functions, be conscious of possible problems in the individual's behaviour styles.

9.4.4.2   The organizational structures These are the *formal aspects* of the organization, for instance the various departments, job design and structure, personnel functions, control and evaluation systems, and the geographical and physical situation. The structures largely *determine the individual's behaviour* in the organization, and they may serve as a means of motivation. Frequently, however, they are also the cause of conflict and of negative attitudes unless they leave room for development.

9.4.4.3   Organizational behaviour and processes The organization *achieves* its productive or service *objectives* by means of different types of *behaviour and interaction*. Although the content of these processes is important, the *way in which* the behaviour processes take place is even more important. The more congruent the behaviour and interactions in terms of the objectives, the more effective their results. Problems are frequently caused by management being so concerned with technical processes that it is not sensitive to the complex transactions of the social behaviour process which constantly affect the objectives and, hence, the results. It is therefore necessary to be aware of the role played by existing behaviour and processes in the problems or symptoms of maladjustment that are reported. In other words, one has to establish the function of the problems that have been reported in the context of the organizational behaviour and processes.

In *intervention techniques* it may be necessary to facilitate the change or development of processes in the sociotechnical structure of the organization. The intervention may amount to the actual change of behaviour in the group or individual or the development of specific social skills.

Organizational behaviour and processes include things such as leadership and supervision, communication, group relations, the handling of conflict, decision-making processes, problem-solving, planning and the setting of objectives, group and meeting processes, interpersonal relationships, evaluation and control processes and criticism and renewal processes.

9.4.4.4. Individual or human outputs The attitudes or psychological conditions shown in figure 9.1 basically represent the *individual behaviour* that results from interactions between individual and organizational systems. The quality of this behaviour should initiate important feedback and should be an indication of the individual's adjustment to the work situation and of its 'cost' for the organization. The analysis of the behaviour outputs can indicate the effect of, among other things, the work situation, the organization structures and the management processes. This is where serious individual or group problems should be spotted. These human attitudes, feelings and behaviour obviously relate directly to the type of consequences for both individual and organization.

9.4.4.5 *Culture* All the elements in figure 9.1 can determine organizational (and individual) cultures. Organizational culture implies the type of 'climate' (especially a *psychological climate*) that exists, which can be defined and maintained within certain sectors (and perhaps the entire organization). The characteristics of the climate determine the type of behaviour, attitudes, values and customs in the organization. The psychological climate in the organization can contain elements—for example, personal versus impersonal, trust versus mistrust, warmth versus reservedness, acceptance versus prejudice, understanding versus insensitivity, rigidity versus openness—that are important for an individual's self-esteem and through which he will display behaviour important (or unimportant) for himself and for the organization.

In the same way the individual (or self-esteem) influenced by all his systems, also has a particular psychological climate. This is manifested in the way in which he forms relationships and his communication with the organization. Individual and organizational cultures can probably be defined as symmetrical, complimentary or parallel; the type of contract that is finally formed will be based on the definition of the relationship.

It is important to remember that *intervention techniques* for the individual and for the organization can amount to an intervention in one or several aspects of the culture, including values and attitudes. This is why someone who wishes to 'diagnose' or treat an individual or an organization has to proceed from their internal frame of reference. Therefore it serves no purpose to apply the identical 'package' technique to all organizations. The same principle applies to individual methods of treatment.

9.4.4.6 *Environ-* Individuals and organizations exist and function in *particular* *ments environments*. This fact implies that there must be interaction. The boundaries between individual, organization and environment are not clearly defined, since an individual may be a 'member' of various systems. It may be a problem if the *boundaries* and other characteristics of individual organizational or environmental systems are so rigid that development inside them becomes restricted, so that growth within and outside the system is either impossible or uncertain. Fortunately absolute closedness is impossible, since the organization consists of people. Wherever there are people there can never be 'no communication' or 'non-behaviour'.

In figure 9.1 we mention specific types of environmental systems for the individual and for the organization, which are probably the most relevant. The environment that affects different organizations or individuals may vary, depending on the context in which they act or on which aspect you wish to study. In *diagnosis and interventions*, one of the things that management also has to do in its staff and management functions, is to be aware of what is happening in the environment and of how a *problem* that has been reported *can be functional in a specific environment*. In this regard you *know* (or will later learn) how technical systems, for instance automatization, have been associated with job alienation among other things. We must also remember that, as in the case of culture, the adjustment or maladjustment of the individual and the organization—in other words, the way in which problems are handled—can largely be determined by the support from the environment.

9.4.4.7 Dominant influences (coalitions) Certain elements or combinations of elements in individual or organizational systems can have a *strong influence* on the functioning of systems or subsystems, or on elements of them. For instance, in an organization the technical divisions may be the most important, and for an individual religion may be the dominant influence from the environment. In the system of the family the mother may be the dominant figure for an individual, or the coalition between mother and son may be a strong and controlling influence in the family and, hence, in the work situation.

In the *analysis and treatment* of individual and organizational problems it is important to note the existence and functioning of dominant influences and coalitions that may have a destructive influence on the functioning of the whole system. If individuals or organizations lack strong qualities such as authority, structure, care or support—the purpose of intervention may need to be to establish and to reinforce these dominant influences.

9.4.4.8 Consequences for the individual and the organization Particular consequences for the individual and the organization are a function of, but also an input for, all the system components mentioned so far. What has been achieved through the behaviour of and the interaction between the individual and the organization can lead either to either the achievement of the objectives or to failure, to need-satisfaction or to frustration, to survival or dismissal. The type of result is again an important input in the cyclic process of *feedback* which will cause the interaction between individual and organization to continue, to change or even to stop. In other words, the *evaluation of the consequences* for both individual and organization is an important diagnostic technique, not only to establish what has happened in the interaction between the individual system and the organization, but also to find out how it happened. Once again the use of *intervention* techniques based on the evaluation of consequences will depend on what they mean in the setting of all the individual and organizational systems.

Now that you understand the model you should realize the importance of assessing an individual's problematic behaviour in the context of his other environments. It is, for instance, necessary to assess the individual as a total entity, realizing that deviant behaviour may often be a function of not only his behaviour but rather his interactions and the rules and boundaries which control his actions, furthermore that it is often of no avail and counter-productive only to treat the individual when he is merely a symptom-bearer of a broader problem. Maybe the most important application of this model is the realization that we as behaviour scientists and practitioners always form part of our diagnosing or treatment systems. This, for one, means that we definitely always influence, either positively or negatively. The healing or helping factors advocated in the different therapeutic or other helping methods are really embedded in the characteristics of the relationship between us as the helper and the helpee. The person with problems learns other more acceptable forms of behaviour because he sees and experiences examples of such behaviour within the intervention or counselling relationship.

9.5 WORK AND HUMAN BEHAVIOUR

The relationship between work and mental health must be seen in the context of the importance of work in man's life and the meaning it has (psychological, social, ethic-moral, religious, economical, political) for each individual and community. The importance of work as a field of study is reflected in the vast volume of publications, some of them best-sellers, on the influence of work in man's life, career development and guidance in respect of work stress, career choice, and so forth. The entire issue of the development of work values and work attitudes, which should, for instance, lead to further studies and career choices has become an integral part of the educational and value systems of man. The theory and practice of vocational guidance, the enhancement of the quality of the working life and stress management have become independent 'industries' in their own right. The issues of job creation, unemployment, automatization and related matters have also become emotional matters over which power groups, such as employers and unions, are continually negotiating.

It is after all clear that, from the Protestant work ethic which regards work as noble, virtuous and necessary, right through to the changing attitudes which consider work to be unpleasant, detrimental and in decline, that work in some form or another is here to stay and that it will always have a large influence on the individual and the community. As Ruskin (in Levitan and Johnson, 1982, p. 141) puts it: 'Distribute the earth as you will, the principle (sic) question remains inexorable—who is to dig it? Which of us, in brief word, is to do the hard and dirty work for the rest.' Camus (in Levitan and Johnson, 1982, p. 63) expresses this unavoidable interaction between man and work as follows: 'Without work all life goes rotten. But when work is soulless, life stifles and dies.' Implicit in this point of view is the challenge to the individual and the psychologist or health worker to optimalize work and work adjustment—particularly in view of continual changes in the work place and changing work values and attitudes. In addition, the unemployed—for various reasons—and the maladjusted worker will always be around. It is clear that man, his work and career, the work place, the surrounding environment and the interaction between these variables have characteristics that affect human health in general and mental health in particular. O'Toole (in Healy, 1982, p. 115) says: 'Effective performance of challenging, socially meaningful work enhances self-esteem and overall mental health, while labouring in an unchallenging, undesirable job, reduces self-esteem and correlates with many physical and mental disorders.'

Views on work differ (Levitan and Johnson, 1982; Furnham, 1984):

- The Protestant work ethic and morality postulates that work is good and noble and that man has a duty and a mission to develop his potential, while laziness and idleness are condemned. Proponents of this point of view consequently accept that the development of a 'sound working personality' and a productive role is the norm and that the future of work is ensured. Levitan and Johnson, for instance, indicate a number of trends in the U.S.A. which, in spite of everything, reflect a positive attitude to work.

- On the other hand there are those who argue that man had greater freedom before the Fall; and that work only became a burden and a constraint afterwards. Proponents of this view may hold that man works purely for economic reasons (to live) and that work is gradually disappearing in view of the modern worker's greater demands for freedom, as well as the role of modern technology where man has in some cases become a mere extension of the machine.

- Those who see the matter from a more practical point of view stress the change in the nature of work, from a physical and production orientation to a more intellectual and service orientation.

- Another view, which fits in with the concept of work alienation, points out that work will disappear as a result of factors such as technology, which will lead to greater unemployment and increased job dissatisfaction since the worker is no longer involved with his work activities and with the end-product of his labour.

In view of these considerations it is interesting to note that contemporary work values differ greatly from the traditional attitudes towards work.

Traditional

- strong loyalty towards the work organization
- great need for money, status and promotion
- stronger identification with work roles than with personal roles

Contemporary

- lesser loyalty and obligations towards the organization
- less emphasis on work security and stability
- greater emphasis on personal roles, more free time, need for stimulating work, participation in decision-making, creative work, non-routine tasks, better communication with management, greater opportunity for personal growth and development.

Virtually all findings about workers' job requirements and complaints about work confirm that on almost all occupational levels the complaints deal with matters that influence self-esteem and self-image, and are therefore concerned with mental health rather than with physical well-being, money, et cetera. When one looks at the above findings, one finds also the implication that management objectives, which are mainly economic, and the more personal aims of the worker are always likely to show a certain degree of conflict.

In times of crisis in particular, it seems as if man's needs are repeatedly sacrificed to, among other things, economic considerations. This is reflected in increased unemployment, dismissals, and so forth.

Perhaps the meaning of work can best be understood by considering the serious consequences for the individual when a possibly long and meaningful interaction and involvement with the work situation is severed. Gechman (1974) defines *unemployment* as a process of exclusion, through which the individual is defined 'as a non-member of the society with severe consequences for the person, his family and society' (p. 749). According to the A.P.A., on the other hand, retirement is often a process of dying as a result of boredom. 'The sudden cessation of productive work and earning power of an individual, caused by compulsory retirement at the chronological age of 65, often leads to physical and emotional deterioration and premature death' (in O'Meara, 1977, p. 7). Gillet (in Isaacson, 1985) also gives a striking description of the consequences of unemployment: 'The personal loss of these changes is deep and tragic. A rise in alcoholism, mental illness, heart disease, suicide, child abuse or wife beating follow a rise in unemployment rate. When a plant closed in Chicago, eight out of 2 000 workers committed suicide. In Wayne County, Michigan, where unemployment approaches 20 %, a community hotline recently reported that calls about spouse abuse jumped over 300 % in a year's time. Mental health clinics report huge rises in case loads within the past two years.' If the situation in South Africa during the past three to five years is considered, and one takes note of news reports on unemployment, tragic family murders, crime figures, alcohol abuse, political unrest, bankruptcies and liquidation of businesses, et cetera, the above-mentioned picture is also applicable in this country.

From the above findings, as well as from other sources on the significance of work in man's life (Terkel, 1972; Neff, 1977; Baker et al., 1969) the majority of complaints about work revolve around the following factors:

- constant supervision, control and constraint to work;
- lack of diversity and variety in work;
- lack of autonomy and decision-making;
- unchanging and boring work;
- repetitive work;
- meaningless work;
- isolation in the work;
- lack of participation and one's own decision-making in the work.

Things that people most wish to experience in their work, in order of preference, are the following:

- interesting work;
- adequate help and equipment to do the work;
- sufficient information to be able to do the work;
- adequate authority to plan and execute work tasks;
- adequate compensation;
- opportunities to develop specific skills;
- work security;
- to be able to see the results in and of the work.

In conclusion the relationship between work and adjustment is illustrated by Mortimer and Borman (1988) as follows:
Work affects adjustment

- by providing a context in which social support and community feeling are derived;
- by providing a source of material rewards necessary for satisfying physical and social needs;
- by providing a sense of mastering or self-efficiency;
- by providing a sense of self-worth through occupational prestige and fulfilment of a culturally valued 'breadwinner' role;
- by providing a source of identity, a sense of belonging in the social structure;
- by providing a way of making life predictable;
- by providing more meaning to a person's life activities; and
- by contributing to the development of problem-solving abilities and general coping powers that increase the ability to adjust successfully to the environment and to outside demands.

Contrary to the above, however, work can also contribute to psychological maladjustment:

- through unfavourable working circumstances, which may overwhelm a person, thereby undermining his or her sense of mastering;
- by demeaning a person, thereby undermining a sense of self-worth;
- through overloading a person, thus preventing problem-solving abilities and coping powers from being fully developed;
- by demanding obedience to authority and an amorality, so that the person's sense of authority and identity is undermined;
- by exhausting a person to such an extent that he finds himself with little energy to pursue psychic rewards after work;
- by demanding that a person do meaningless tasks, thus giving rise to feelings of cynicism and alienation;
- by encouraging excessive competitiveness and hostility towards others; and
- by failing to provide adequate material rewards, thus creating chronic financial strain for the individual.

9.6 MENTAL HEALTH DEFINED

Unlike physical diseases where the norm for health and indisposition is generally clear, psychology does not always have clear, ideal or generally accepted norms (criteria) or models for adjustment (normality), maladjustment (abnormality) and psychological optimality. In the relevant literature on mental health you will often find definitions, descriptions, explanations and criteria from different and sometimes conflicting viewpoints and theories—even different classification systems.

In the case of psychopathology, however, the well-known DSM-classification of behaviour disorders enjoys reasonable acceptance by most interested parties. As was mentioned earlier the field of occupational mental health still does not have an accepted classification system. This shortcoming has many reasons, one being the lack of research and the minor emphasis on psychological well-being as compared to physical health, industrial hygiene and occupational diseases due to toxic pollution. Only recently, in South

Africa, by way of Government actions and research by Universities and the HSRC as well as a renewed interest in mental health and health psychology, did a new sensitivity to the psychological health of people in the work place appear (Visser, 1990).

As indicated earlier mental health is a broad term for the nature and quality of adjustment (normality), or maladjustment (abnormality) or very good adjustment (optimality), as is indicated in figure 9.2.

FIGURE 9.2

Maladjustment to optimality

negative	average	positive

abnormal	normal	optimal
maladjustment	health	actualized

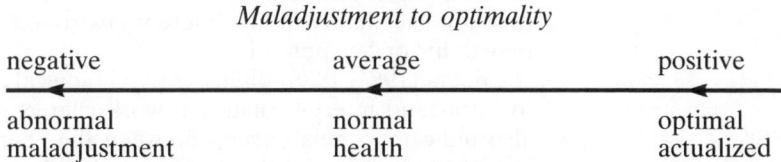

Although the concept and condition of psychological optimality is not defined formally and clearly in the literature, there has recently been a tendency, for example in the so-called growth and health psychology, to move the emphasis away from negative, abnormal behaviour towards the positive, and towards the human motivation to grow and to actualize potential. As a matter of fact, in a lot of personality theories, especially the humanistic and existential ones, one finds concepts that emphasize what is positive and excellent in human functioning. Typical of such personality theories are those of Jung (individualizing), Adler (superiority), Fromm (productivity), Horney (self-realizing), Erikson (emotional integration), Allport (adulthood), Rogers (self-actualization and the fully functional person), Frankl (self-transcendence), Maslow and Perls (self-actualizing), Berne (winners' behaviour), Ardell (high level health) and Carkhuff (wholeness) (Cilliers, 1984). Other approaches that also emphasize optimal functioning are the so-called coping theories. According to these, some people show more resistance to internal and external influences as a result of successful coping behaviour or because of the existence of certain intrinsic personality dispositions (Pearlin and Schooler, 1978; Ashford, 1988; Fisher and Reason, 1988).

Psychological optimality or exceptional functioning is also found in the emphasis on so-called personality or behaviour repertoires. These represent integrated behaviour patterns, cognitions and emotions, which enable the individual to behave effectively in his environment. Kobasa (1979), for instance, makes use of the concept of hardiness, Antonovsky (1987) of the sense of coherence, and Meischenbaum (1977) refers to learned resourcefulness. Rotter's (1966) concept of locus of control and Friedman and Rosen's (1979) well-known A- and B-type personalities can also be viewed as behaviour repertoires. In recent literature, for instance, the A-type behaviour pattern is associated with achievement behaviour and the healthy individual — and not only with stress and proneness to cardiovascular diseases.

The above emphasis on health psychology is perhaps best expressed by Antonovsky's concept of 'solutogenesis' (1984). This concept indicates people's ability to manage stress and stay well, that is, to modify conditions which create stress, modify the meaning of stress factors and methods of coping with stress experiences.

Solutogenesis also implies that we should reconsider existing disease classification practices, reconsidering the idea that stress is only bad and that research on health behaviour should also emphasize positive outcomes of so-called unhealthy lifestyles.

The literature clearly shows that the definition and description for the concept and condition of psychological optimality is still vague and a lot of research must still be done. It is also obvious, however, that psychological optimality is more than the mere absence of symptoms or adjustment. It is a transcending well-being, wholeness or totality in the human psyche, which enables a person to adjust and function excellently in his different environments, to develop and to realize his or her potential.

Cilliers (1984, 1988) discusses psychological optimality with regard to intra- and interpersonal and work characteristics. Cilliers (1984) also indicates a relationship between the characteristics of psychological optimality and those associated with managerial success.

9.6.1 Definitions and descriptions of mental health The World Congress on Mental Health (1948) defined mental health as 'the condition which in a physical, intellectual and emotional respect allows the development of the individual in as far as it is compatible with other individuals' (Ruhmke, 1957, p. 56).

Romano defines it as follows: 'The healthy person is one who is reasonably free from undue pain, discomfort, and disability' (Freedman and Kaplan, 1967).

Geldenhuys (1975) contrasts the 'normal' and the psychologically 'ill' person, and describes a normal person as one with consistent behaviour patterns of openness and readiness for life so that he is relatively free to observe his world as it is and to encounter it meaningfully (p. 39). A mentally disordered person experiences a state in which not only the observation and experience of his world are hampered, but also the consequences for himself (p. 17).

Katz and Thorpe offer a comprehensive definition containing several criteria. A normal person shows no signs of mental disorder, is free of emotional conflicts, has a satisfactory capacity for work, and he is satisfactorily adjusted to the daily requirements of life as far as both he and the community in which he lives are concerned (Le Roux, 1968, p. 19).

Allport (1961) has a very *positive view* of human behaviour. He believes that a healthy or adult person acts rationally and in awareness of himself and his environment, that he is responsible, that he is in control of what happens to him, and that he is self-motivated for growth and development (self-actualization).

Carl Rogers (1961) who, like Allport, has a positive view of human nature, emphasizes that a healthy personality is a process of growth and development. He believes that a 'healthy' personality is a 'fully functioning person' who, in his striving towards self-actualization, experiences congruence between his perception of himself (his self-image), his communication and his experiences with his environment so that he can be himself spontaneously, openly and freely.

In describing the psychopathology of work, Neff (1977) regards the work personality as 'a semi-autonomous area of the general personality' (p. 192). He believes that 'work psychopathology implies some area of deficiency or defect in the development of the work personality' (p. 192). Since a work maladjusted person has not learned *a productive role* through his development and experiences, he displays certain styles of responses that do not satisfy the requirements of the work situation.

Goldenhar (in Carone et al., 1978, p. 146) regards work as an important factor in mental health and defines the 'misfits' in the industry as 'individuals who are devoid of certain qualities and abilities or who have physical or emotional handicaps' (p. 83).

Jay Haley (1963) and interactionalists such as Goffman (1969), Erikson (in Haley, 1967), Van Kessel (1974), Kiesler and Anchin (1982) and Sullivan (1953) describe symptoms of *maladjustment as tactical communication or behaviour styles* in an individual by means of which he defines his interpersonal relationships in specific ways. His objective is to benefit from a situation in a manipulative manner, while pretending not to do it or to be unconscious of acting in such a manner. People like Rogers (1961), Haley (1963) and Rossiter and Barnett Pearce (1975) put special emphasis on congruent communication as the basis of mental health.

In support of them and of the systems theorists, Haley (1963) also asserts that 'the ills of the individual are not really separable from the ills of the social context he creates and inhabits, and one cannot with good conscience pull out the individual from his cultural milieu and label him as sick or well' (p. 2).

Szasz (1966, p. 13) says that when we speak of symptoms we actually refer to 'a patient's communication about himself, others and the world about him'. Kanfer, in Swart and Wiehahn (1979) agrees with Szasz and describes a psychological problem as difficulties in a person's relationships with others, his perception of his environment and his attitude towards himself.

The last two types of definitions emphasize *symptomatic behaviour as interaction, communication or features of a relationship* that have a special significance for an individual in a certain context, for instance in an interpersonal, intrapersonal, cultural and environmental context. In other words, maladjusted behaviour is linked to the individual's present or past multisystems. Writers like Carson (1969), Minuchin (1974), Byng-Hall (1980), Andolfi (1979) and Carson et al. (1988), stress the fact that the *individual is the symptom-bearer* of his greater systems. This emphasis in the work situation is stressed by people like Katz and Kahn (1978), Cummings (1980), Warshaw (1979) and Harrison (in Cooper and Payne, 1978).

If *maladjustment* is described as behaviour that *has meaning for every individual in a specific context*, it seems as though *psychiatric labels*—or even the support of theories of behaviour and techniques for the treatment of conditions—are unnecessary. We can say that the theories and techniques should be applied in a particular setting. One has to take note of the function of the individual's behaviour to determine which interventions will be the most effective for him and by whom they should be made. Your definition of mental health will determine how you define your relationships with others, also when you have to enter into a counselling relationship with a problem worker.

9.6.2 Occupational Occupational mental health is an applied field of clinical and
mental health abnormal psychology. It deals with the adjustment or maladjustment
of individuals and groups in a work and organizational context.

This field of study is also known as industrial or occupational
clinical psychology (Miner, 1966; Manuso, 1983) occupational mental
health (McClean, 1970), industrial mental health (Noland, 1973),
psychopathology of work (Neff, 1977), ineffective work behaviour
(Miner and Brewer, in Dunnette, 1976), and, more recently, as work
stress (McClean, 1979), and occupational health (Levy, et al., 1988).
Terms like work alienation (Kanunga, 1982) and burnout (Muldary,
1983) are sometimes used synonymously with mental health.

It is also obvious that elements of other disciplines—for example
development, personality, career, personnel and organizational
psychology—and related fields such as psychiatry, medical sciences,
anthropology and sociology form part of contemporary literature on
industrial mental health.

In the literature and in practice definitions of and views on
occupational mental health include one or more of the following:

- the problem worker as a psychopathological or psychiatric case,
  (physical health is also taken into consideration)
- the well-adjusted worker whose emotional problems need not
  necessarily have an adverse effect on his work behaviour
- the importance of physical health and health behaviour for
  effective work and managerial behaviour
- the place and role of management in occupational mental health.
  In this regard we can also speak of 'organizational mental health'.
- the functions of the industrial psychologist or other personnel
  specialists in the field of mental health
- the emphasis on work and organizational causality and on the
  individual with his personal and social needs
- occupational mental health as an interdisciplinary field of study
- industrial mental health as an applied field of study

On the other hand McClean (in Noland, 1973, p. 125) defines
industrial mental health from a very *narrow* point of view:

In the narrowest sense, it is concerned solely with the psychiatri-
cally ill worker whose symptoms interfere with his effective
functioning on the job.

This view reflects the emphasis that we still find on the role of
medical science and psychiatry in the treatment of occupational
maladjustment. Causality and symptomatic behaviour is linearly
attributed to the individual.

In a *more comprehensive* view McClean (in Noland, 1973) stresses
that a worker's mental health can refer to thoughts, feelings and
behaviour that may affect work behaviour as well as behaviour away
from the work situation. In this definition McClean refers to mental
health as a more complex condition in which the individual is also
seen in the context of the organization and the environment.
Causality and symptoms are also regarded as system-related. The
definition also implies the responsibility of management and the
implications of its policy on mental health. In this regard you may be
familiar with people like McGregor, Blake and Mouton, and Argyris
(in Cummings, 1980) who maintain that the assumptions of

management about the workers' needs, values, capabilities and expectations will determine the method of management. Conflict between management and workers is often the result of invalid assumptions about human behaviour. Several writers assert that organisational effectiveness and efficienty as well as the health of an organisation are a function of management's constant diagnostic and developmental functions to effect optimum individual-organizational interaction and to adapt to change.

In much of the literature on work stress, such as Cooper and Payne (1978, 1980), Newman and Beehr (1979), McClean (1979) and Warshaw (1979), the emphasis is on the interactive roles of management and the worker, and on coping with, fighting and managing stress problems. The role of management in guidance and therapy is emphasized in recent works such as those of De Board (1983), Manuso (1983), Roseman (1982) and Roberson (1986).

Kornhauser (1965, p. 11) defines occupational mental health as a comprehensive condition that includes adjustment and maladjustment as 'behaviour, attitudes, perceptions and feelings, that determine an individual's overall level of personal effectiveness, success, happiness and excellence of functioning as a person'.

Baker et al. (1969, p. xiv), define mental health problems not only as neuroses and psychoses, but also as a response to work stress, for instance in the form of accidents.

Kutash, Belinson (in Noland, 1973) and Neff (1977) emphasize the *total personality* of the individual, the role of management in the treatment and better utilization of problem or maladjusted workers, and also the role of management in creating a climate for optimum mental health in its personnel and management functions. Kutash (in Noland, 1973, p. 27) refers to the usefulness of problem workers for the industry: 'Not all people with anxieties and emotional disturbances are problem employees, and not all problem employees are emotionally disturbed.'

D'Alonzo and Belinson (Noland, 1973) define the tasks of industrial mental health services (occupational psychiatry) as follows:

- diagnosing and treating the symptoms of workers with emotional conflicts in both serious and less serious cases;
- research on the factors that cause or support emotional maladjustment;
- training medical and personnel workers to manage workers with emotional problems and teaching them how to act towards rehabilitated workers, and training in general health programmes for workers;
- consulting medical services on problem workers;
- advising departments on the selection, placement and rehabilitation of workers with emotional problems or workers who have received treatment;
- consulting management and advising them on matters such as the policy on mental health and methods of coping with individual cases or groups with emotional or behaviour problems.

Cohen, Gordon, Minninger and Meincker (Noland, 1973) support the comprehensive view of mental health and the *interactive roles* of individuals, management and the psychologist (psychiatrist, etc.).

They also maintain, however, that several disciplines play a role in such a comprehensive process of managing mental health.

Occupational maladjustment is defined as work stress by writers like McClean (1974, 1979), Schuler (1980, 1982), Cooper and Marshall (1976), Shirom (1982) and Beehr and Newman (1979). More specifically, work stress is regarded as a field of study dealing with all the factors (stressors) affecting the individual, and with the factors in the work situation, in the organization and in the external environment that create strain in the individual and give rise to specific physical or psychological problems, for instance cardiac diseases and psychopathology, with the resultant work-related symptoms such as absence, accidents, lower production and job dissatisfaction.

It is obvious from these views that a more *comprehensive definition* of occupational mental health is needed.

Occupational mental health is the scientific study of the causes, symptoms and characteristics of individuals and groups, organization and management, the work situation and the external environments that lead to and support various forms of occupational maladjustment, and the study of the treatment, management and utilization of problem or rehabilitated workers.

This definition makes it clear that industrial mental health is an applied field of study that involves several disciplines, which is also obvious from the correlation between this definition and the one on psychopathology. The resemblance between occupational mental health and the study of psychopathology is reflected in the definition offered by Mechanic (in Baker et al., 1969): 'Thus the study of illness behaviour involves the study of attentiveness to pain and symptomatology, the examination of processes affecting how pain and symptoms are defined, accorded significance and socially labelled, and the consideration of the extent to which help is sought, change in life regimen affected and claims on others made.'

When you have completed the course you should be able to compile a list of the contents of the field of industrial mental health.

You should also be able to identify more contemporary problems, such as the following:

- renewed emphasis on the harmful effects of the physical work environment
- greater emphasis on the psychological implications of changing work attitudes and work values
- the progressively growing problems of career development, especially in view of a longer life expectancy in the midst of decreasing job opportunities, increased (sometimes forced) leisure-time activities, earlier retirement and loss of jobs
- the growing involvement of women in the work field, including on management level
- the problems of work role and family role conflicts in dual career couples
- the particular problems of the so-called 'invisible' worker, in other words the growing number of workers who work at home and elsewhere in a process of decreased interaction with management and colleagues

- behaviour phenomena among workers which have been described as 'executive neuroses', 'executive stress', 'executive suicide', 'workaholism', 'burnout', et cetera
- technological unemployment
- the idea that the work organization as a whole can display adjustment problems
- in South Africa, new challenges and problems in the light of changing levels of interaction between groups and individuals amongst fast-changing labour, economical, political and socio-ethical and moral situations
- the adjustment problems and counselling of individuals inflicted with the AIDS virus

9.6.3   Criteria for mental health   Criteria for mental health refer to *standards or characteristics* against which human behaviour is measured or evaluated in order to determine the extent of adjustment or maladjustment.

Your study of various views of mental health and of diagnostic approaches should have made it obvious that criteria for mental health—adjustment and maladjustment—are affected by these approaches. Objections to criteria are based on such matters as their subjectivity or objectivity, their vagueness, ambiguity, their cultural determination, their non-job relatedness, non-measurable criteria, their invalidity, et cetera. People who are in favour of determining criteria maintain that criteria and, hence, classification, are necessary for communication in the subject area and between practitioners, and for the determination of intervention procedures.

We would like to emphasize that a person's behaviour and the meaning of the behaviour have to be compared to certain criteria in the context of his actions.

We refer to only a few classifications of *general criteria*. You can compare the application of the criteria with their incidence in specific problem areas.

Maslow (in Barocas, Reichman and Schwebel, 1983) describes the following characteristics of the self-actualizing (optimalizing) personality as compared with the so-called average (normal) person. The self-actualizing personality:

- has a superior perception of reality
- shows a greater acceptance of the self, others and nature
- shows more spontaneous behaviour
- is problem-orientated, rather than self-centred
- shows more disinvolvement and need for privacy
- is more autonomous and independent
- shows richer emotional reactions—attaches more value to people and things
- has more opportunities for great experiences, for instance mystical and religious experiences, which can lead to transcendence
- is able to show more empathy and understanding
- has deeper, more intimate and more enduring interpersonal relationships
- manifests a more democratic character—that is, respecting and bearing with differences between people without unnecessary dominance

- shows enduring values and is able to distinguish more easily between right and wrong without sacrificing standards in order to gain advantage
- has a philosophical and considerate sense of humour, and does not behave in a hostile and aggressive manner
- has more use of creative sources on a continuous basis
- does not behave in a conformist way and can stick to his own point of view

Van der Schoot's five characteristics of mental health are concerned with the individual:

- sufficient ability to integrate
- the capability of using intellectual abilities freely (not too much anxiety or too many defences)
- a fairly harmonious emotional life
- the ability to fulfil the ordinary demands of life without too much stress
- a commitment to spiritual values (Geldenhuys, 1975).

Suinn (1975) describes the following seven 'normal' characteristics of behaviour:

- effectiveness (instrumental and purposeful behaviour)
- efficiency (the realistic use of energy, acknowledging one's potential and limitations)
- appropriate behaviour (responses to environmental stimuli are determined by age, they are appropriate and realistic)
- flexibility (the ability to use alternative methods in conflict situations)
- the ability to learn from experience
- interpersonal effectiveness
- self-security (self-appreciation, realistic knowledge of oneself).

The classification in Brammer and Schostrom (1982) incorporates basically the therapeutic objectives aimed at development. It is very similar to Rogers' ideas and also contains elements of the ideas put forward by Maslow, Allport, Van der Schoot and Suinn. It includes the following observations, which are relevant to psychological optimality:

- independence from the physical and social environments
- spontaneity towards others and an 'openness' for personal and other experiences
- living in the present (this implies that the individual has the ability of participating wholeheartedly and joyfully in the activities of life without fixating on the past or entertaining fantasies of the future)
- self-confidence, which refers to the individual's confidence in himself as a person, his self-esteem and his acceptance of the validity of his decisions and actions
- self-knowledge, the consciousness that one lives and responds in one's environment and the experiencing and acceptance of every emotion
- honesty or congruency—the individual's ability to be himself, not to hide behind defence mechanisms and to know himself so that he can learn to know others
- responsible activities, which implies conduct that will benefit both himself and others

- effectiveness—the individual's ability to live intentionally because of the aforementioned skills, in other words, to fulfil the requirements of life within the context of and in terms of the level of development

In analysing psychological optimality Cilliers (1988) describes the following characteristics.

Intrapersonal characteristics

These characteristics are related to physical, cognitive, emotional and conative functioning:

- *Physical characteristics*. The optimally functioning individual is physically active, healthy and fit. This provides him with enough energy and stamina to cope effectively with stress. He is realistically aware of his somatic and physical functioning and so is able to accept his condition without preconditions or objection.
- *Cognitive characteristics*. The person uses his cognitive abilities optimally. He experiences his world objectively and rationally; he is also disciplined in his thinking and reasoning is lenient, and makes well-thought through optimistic cognitive assessments and judgements which help him to have insight into the meaning of life.
- *Emotional characteristics*. The optimal-functioning person is open, aware and sensitive to his emotions, feelings and needs, which he can accommodate and verbalize. He also takes responsibility for his emotions which lead to emotional independence, and a rich emotional life. These behaviours lead to self-insight and knowledge, which helps the person to form a realistic self-image with self-valuing, self-respect and self-acceptance. These qualities will decrease anxiety and lead to eustress—a pleasant, exhilarating and facilitating form of stress. The person experiences fulness in life while he continues to explore and grow, rather than a situation of stability.

Interpersonal characteristics

From his own self-acceptance he shows optimistic and unconditional acceptance and respect towards others, a preference for qualitative, deeper and richer interpersonal relationships. This type of relationship is characterized by responsible, spontaneous, natural and open, genuine behaviour according to his own feelings, but the person is also considerate of and in a relationship of love for others.

This type of behaviour in managers also encourages and facilitates similar behaviour on the part of subordinates and colleagues. These characteristics are represented in the so-called person-oriented psychotherapy by four essential conditions for effective interaction. These are:

- respect—a deep recognition, valuing and regard for the self-worth of the other person and his right as a free individual, an unconditional positive care and warmth
- empathy—which indicates the ability to be consciously aware and to feel and understand another person's meaning and deepest feelings from within that person's frame of reference and to communicate this empathy accurately

- honesty (transparency) indicates a congruence between what is said and done and the true meaning of communication
- concreteness—which means that the person makes specific and factual statements rather than vague and general ones

Work characteristics

The psychologically optimal person is totally involved in his or her work. All the intrapersonal and interpersonal characteristics mentioned above are therefore preconditions for optimal work performance.

More specifically, optimal work performance requires purposefulness, productivity, responsibility, motivation, lenience, initiative, concentration, creativity and optimal time management. The person who performs his work best is focused on the here and now, yet is aware of the past without being a victim of his history while also being future directed. Such a person is co-operative, which shows that he is able to transcend opposites and to experience his role in the organization realistically.

The optimal-functioning person's managerial style is based on humanitarian values, and is therefore democratic. He plans and organizes pro-actively by prioritizing his activities and by delegating appropriate tasks. By doing this he creates a safe and permissive climate in which subordinates and colleagues are permitted to develop their own potential and to be more responsible for their own behaviour and the working environment. In this way the subordinate's working behaviour becomes more productive, directed at the organization's working objectives, without denying his own needs. This indicates an authentic working relation in which the manager increases his own and other peoples' awareness and acceptance in such a way that his subordinates are enabled to do the same. In this way choices that are characterized by negative feelings and repressed energy are transformed into positive growth situations, resulting in higher productivity and a better quality of life.

Although the criteria may include adjusted and maladjusted behaviour by implication, some authors supply criteria for the abnormal personality.

Suinn (1975) defines abnormality in terms of four criteria:

- subjective or psychological pain which includes symptoms such as discomfort, stress, conflict and unhappiness
- irrationality or unpredictability, which refers to illogical and bizarre behaviour such as incoherent speech, delusions and hallucinations
- conditions that require psychiatric treatment
- an ipsative definition in which the individual's behaviour patterns are compared

These *criteria* can also be found in literature on *occupational maladjustment*, although most writers add a category to refer to work-related requirements.

French and Kahn discuss criteria for mental health by means of a systems model in which the person-in-the-environment is considered. They point out that the criteria can refer to the person, to the behaviour or to the external physical or psychological environments. Some of the criteria can also refer to the interaction between these variables. Although they use an eclectic integration of the classifications for criteria, they base their classification on the one devised by Jahoda for positive mental health (in Baker et al., 1969).

The following criteria are regarded as general characteristics within which more specific criteria can be set:

- attitudes towards and observations of one's own personality (self), which include accurate observation of one's self-image, attitudes towards one's own personality (self) and an understanding of one's identity
- growth, development and self-actualization, where the level of development and the person's usefulness in a role are evaluated
- integration, which refers to the individual's ability to assimilate and handle influences from the environment
- autonomy, which implies the ability to act effectively by means of internal powers (needs, etc.) without the unnecessary domination of external influences
- the observation of reality, which implies the accurate assessment of the external environment in terms of internal psychological needs
- interpersonal efficiency, which refers to the establishment of interpersonal relationships
- affective conditions, which include emotional manifestations such as manic-depressiveness, anxiety, fear, et cetera
- physiological conditions, which refer to physiological responses to a situation, for instance blood-pressure and heart rate
- specific pathological conditions, both physically and psychologically, for instance schizophrenia, neuroses, brain syndromes, et cetera
- adjustment and adaptability, in other words, the person's ability to meet the demands of the environment in terms of his personal capabilities
- specific criteria for the performance of a task or work, which include standards defined by the organization such as the quantity and quality of production, absence, personnel turnover and job satisfaction

The six characteristics used by Kornhauser (1965) to indicate mental health are based on job satisfaction:

- manifested anxiety and emotional stress
- an index of self-esteem (positive and negative feelings towards the self)
- hostility versus confidence in acceptance of people
- sociability and friendship versus withdrawal
- an index of complete contentment in life
- personal morale versus alienation and despair.

Steinmentz (1969) identifies a poor or underachiever in terms of the following qualities:

- resistance to change
- moodiness
- disorganization
- a feeling of contentedness in the sense that the worker feels himself to be indispensable
- isolation

- the inability to communicate
- no sense of responsibility
- intolerance
- an apologetic attitude
- a highly-strung nature
- unimaginativeness
- a strong tendency to defend oneself against criticism, et cetera.

Kasl divides the characteristics of mental health in the work situation into four categories:

- indexes of functional effectiveness or role behaviour, which refer to the worker's inability to perform his daily task and social activities—including factors like hospitalization, absence, and a change of work
- indexes for general welfare, which refer to emotional conditions (depression, etc.), symptoms such as stress and trembling, and measurements for self-esteem and contentedness (self-evaluation, job satisfaction, contentedness with life and need satisfaction)
- indexes of mastery and efficiency, which include features such as development, self-actualization, efficient performance, the exploitation of abilities and the achievement of predetermined objectives
- psychiatric symptoms such as a reality testing, disorientation, et cetera (in O'Toole (ed.), 1974.)

It must be obvious that not all these criteria are behaviour specific, and that the diagnostician has to convert the general characteristics into observable and appropriate behaviour for every person. This is why people who make interactional analyses are concerned with the meaning of behaviour and not with the category or symptom attributed to the individual.

9.7 AETIOLOGY OR CAUSAL FACTORS IN MENTAL HEALTH PROBLEMS

From your study of the principles of learning theory (stimulus, response, reinforcement, generalization and so forth) you know that the cause-effect relationship of human behaviour is not always logical and clear. From the preceding definitions and criteria, it is also clear that aetiology and problem are not always clearly distinguishable. Although a single factor or *stressor* can often have a dominant influence, mental health can best be understood by considering the continual interaction between a complex number of factors. It is also clear that the same factors or stressors that facilitate healthy adjustment and personality development, can be responsible for maladjustment. In this connection the *systems and interactional theories* especially stress the fact that one should be careful not to try to explain behaviour too simplistically from a linear model. It is necessary to note that the individual himself is a fully fledged system consisting of a number of subsystems (such as body, mind, intelligence, emotions and motivation) which are influenced by and function within many other systems and subsystems for instance political government, nation, culture, work group, religion, family relations and marriage. The interactive and circular influence of factors on the individual and his behaviour and the context of behaviour should always be taken into consideration. For instance a man's alcohol problem could have a specific functional meaning if he achieves something through it or if the family or work group functions according to it. To the outsider however, who does not consider all the implications, it is sometimes easy to say on a linear basis that the man has a drinking problem because he is a weakling and so forth. The result of such a simple explanation could also be less effective as a method of treatment.

In conjunction with the theories of personality and personality development the aetiology of maladjustment can be subdivided into three groups:

- *Physical stress*, which has an organic or biological basis. We are here concerned with the influence of the nervous system, heredity, hormones and neurohormones, physical neurochemistry, nutrition, infections, intoxication, brain injuries and tumours, and degenerative changes in the human body (due to age).
- *Psychological stress*, which is caused by motivation, especially unconscious motivation. Conflict and frustration in, say, the sexual field, aggression, dependence, anxiety, guilt feelings and work stress are studied.
- *Sociocultural influences*, which emanate from culture, family dynamics and the immediate environment, for instance, socio-economic factors, urbanization, religion, ethnic groupings, marital state, educational and social status, and numerous other influences.

This classification also applies when the *factors influencing work adjustment* are considered. There are, however, also more specific classifications such as those by Miner & Brewer in Dunnette, (1976), Neff (1977) and Steinmetz (1969)).

The following classification of aetiological factors is only indicated briefly and includes aspects that relate to psychopathology and work adjustment.

As an introduction to the other causative factors, stress can be viewed as a generic determinant for a lot of adjustment problems.

9.7.1 Stress, conflict and frustration The *stress model* explains mental health (adjustment and maladjustment) as a function of the individual's ability to display effective (or ineffective) *adaptive behaviour* when internal and/or external *stressors* lead to physical and/or psychological *stress*. Stress is a condition which develops when the demands made of the individual exceed his adaptive (coping) abilities. We see from this definition that stress is a complex phenomenon (Hurrell, Souter et al., 1988; Fisher and Reason 1988; Fleming, Baum et al., 1984; Frankenhaeuser and Johansson, 1986; Hobfoll, 1988; Appley and Trumbull, 1986).

In the *first instance*, stress refers to a *specific response* by the individual, for instance a physical reaction such as snatching away the hand when experiencing pain, withdrawal when an unsafe situation is expected, and physical illness. The effects of stress may be slight (e.g. physical exhaustion or fright), moderate (e.g. a physical disease or pain, or feelings of anxiety), or serious (e.g. cardiac diseases, stomach ulcers, neurotic and psychotic conditions, and even death). Added to this, reactions to stress may be purely physical, purely psychological, or psychophysical. An example of the latter is a cardiac disease which is a physical reaction to psychological stress.

Secondly (and following on the explanation of responses), stress can also refer to the individual's *coping behaviour*. Such behaviour in response to stress may be either very direct—for example physical flight, withdrawal, attack, or compromise—or psychological defence mechanisms and techniques such as physical recreation and exercise, diets, and psychological therapy. The individual's adaptive behaviour is always aimed at achieving a state of physical and psychological homeostasis.

Thirdly, stress can act as a *stimulus or stressor*. Internal factors (e.g. needs, physical functions) and external influences (e.g. pressure at work, finances, death in the family, or natural disasters) create a state of tension in the individual. Frustration and conflict are two important sources of stress. Holmes and Rahe (Carson et al., 1988) compiled a list of stressors which make serious or less serious demands on the individual's adaptive ability. In subsequent discussions on the role of aetiological factors in maladjustment you will also come across stressors which largely correspond with Holmes and Rahe's classification. Stressors which continually affect the individual reduce his effective adaptation and resistance, and this in turn may have grave consequences. The effects of stressors, and the individual's response to them, will depend on the following factors which determine the *intensity of stress*:

- the importance, duration and number of demands
- the proximity of the stressor, for instance the death of a close member of the family, or the day before an examination
- the individual's perception of the stressor
- his stress threshold or ability to tolerate frustration, and his adaptive abilities
- his external sources of support, for instance his family, relatives and religion

Hans Selye's *General Adaptation Syndrome* (GAS) model helps to make the above discussion clear and explains how the individual reacts physically and psychologically to stress. It describes how the human body reacts by means of the nervous system and endocrine functions when it experiences stress from internal or external influences.

In the *alarm-and-mobilization phase* the individual prepares to counteract stress and its effects. The functions of the central and autonomous nervous system are especially important in this phase.

TABLE 9.1

The social adjustment scale of Holmes and Rahe

Holmes and his colleagues (Holmes & Holmes, 1970; Holmes & Rahe, 1967; Rahe & Arthur, 1978) have developed the Social Readjustment Rating Scale (SRRS), an objective method for measuring the cumulative stress to which an individual has been exposed over a period of time. This scale measures life stress in terms of 'life change units' (LCU) involving the following events.

Events	Scale of Impact	Events	Scale of Impact
Death of spouse	100	Change in responsibilities at work	29
Divorce	73	Son or daughter leaving home	29
Marital separation	65	Trouble with in-laws	29
Jail term	63	Outstanding personal achievement	28
Death of close family member	63	Wife begins or stops work	26
Personal injury or illness	53	Begin or end school	26
Marriage	50	Change in living conditions	25
Fired at work	47	Revision of personal habits	24
Marital reconciliation	45	Trouble with boss	23
Retirement	45	Change in work hours or conditions	20
Change in health of family member	44	Change in residence	20
Pregnancy	40	Change in schools	20
Sex difficulties	39	Change in recreation	19
Gain of new family member	39	Change in church activities	19
Business readjustment	39	Change in social activities	18
Change in financial state	38	Small mortgage or loan	17
Death of close friend	37	Change in sleeping habits	16
Change to different line of work	36	Change in number of family get-togethers	15
Change in number of arguments with spouse	35	Change in eating habits	15
High mortgage	31	Vacation	13
Foreclosure of mortgage or loan	30	Christmas	12
		Minor violations of the law	11

For persons who had been exposed in recent months to stressful events that added up to an LCU score of 300 or above, these investigators found the risk of developing a major illness within the next two years to be very high, approximately 80 per cent. (From Carson et al., 1988, p. 144.)

At the psychological level the individual will begin to display emotional reactions, experience more stress, be more sensitive, and so forth. Adaptive behaviour may also follow, for instance, flight or withdrawal. Psychological reactions may not be too serious, for instance anxiety or physical reactions such as increased tension and stomach cramps.

The second phase, *resistance*, is also characterized by alarm and mobilization, but the rate of adaptive reactions increases since the endocrine system comes into operation. For instance, the cortex may facilitate the secretion of adrenaline, or hormones may be released into the blood to stimulate blood circulation. At this stage the individual actually experiences the alleviation of stress at the psychological level through effective defensive or genuine problem solving behaviour. On the other hand, the individual's adaptive behaviour may be less successful; there may be more serious physical and psychological problems and his adaptive behaviour makes no progress because he clings to unsuccessful methods of solving problems.

In the third phase of *exhaustion and disintegration* the sustained stress exceeds the individual's capacity for physical and psychological adaptation. Serious physical and psychological symptoms or conditions may follow, for instance metabolic changes, physical diseases, and psychosomatic conditions, such as cardiac or stomach diseases and paralysis. At the psychological level there may be symptoms which indicate the serious decompensation caused by stress. These symptoms include extreme anxiety, phobia, breaking with reality, delusions and hallucinations, thought and speech disorders—in other words, symptoms associated with psychoses—and which can lead to death.

This approach, as well as others such as Pearlin and Lieberman (1981)) and those based on developmental and sociocultural models, are largely responsible for the fact that mental health is now regarded as a process and a function of the interdependence between body, psyche, and social environment. Man does not *have* a body and a spirit; he *is* both and is in constant interaction with a variety of environmental influences.

All stressors can ultimately be grouped together under what is known as frustration and conflict.

Frustration arises when someone is prevented in some way or other from attaining his objectives. The type of reaction or frustration can also be determined by the importance of the objectives, the intensity of the needs for them, the period of frustration and so forth. What is more important however is the individual's *tolerance for frustration*. Tolerance of frustration is, apart from biological determination, largely a function of the individual's learning behaviour—how he learnt to have his needs satisfied.

Conflict is a condition which arises when the person wants to satisfy several needs at the same time. The individual's problems arise from the fact that he then experiences choice anxiety especially if he has strong negative and positive feelings about an objective (approach-avoidance conflict), has to choose between equally attractive objectives (double approach conflict) or has to choose between equally unattractive objectives (double avoidance conflict).

9.7.2 Factors unique to the individual

These influences include a person's *individual or idosyncratic characteristics* resulting from his biological equipment, his development and the learning experiences he brings with him when he enters a job. These features characterize his behaviour, actions, and methods of solving problems in his environment. The following factors are important:

- the individual's intellectual abilities and skills—or the lack of them
- the individual's genetic biological and physical equipment—and possible deficiencies—which may affect his skill in the physical work environment and determine his methods of coping with stress
- typical styles of behaviour and methods of communication and interaction which govern the individual's behaviour towards others and his methods of dealing with and solving problems from the environment
- special needs, attitudes, values, and interests which direct work behaviour
- the individual's motivation—unconscious needs which, though unsatisfied because of repression, still activate and direct

behaviour—or, on the other hand, the individual's lack of motivation for work and achievement

- the individual's occupational concepts, in other words, acquired attitudes to, and values about work and his occupation
- the individual's self-image or ego identity, which includes every thing he knows, learns and feels about himself through learning and experience—problems will develop if his self-image concepts are not confirmed in the work situation
- the individual's perception of his role in the work organization, his understanding of his tasks at work, and his job satisfaction
- possible psychiatric problems, such as neurotic, psychotic and organic conditions, personality disorders, alcoholism, and drug addiction, which have an adverse effect on work adjustment
- work related problems, for instance absenteeism, or accident proneness, which may affect work adjustment
- physical diseases
- influences from the individual's family and other groups, which may affect his work behaviour
- aspects such as sex, race and other group links, which may affect work behaviour
- job alienation, which may be the result of the isolation which often occurs in a large organization and which may affect the worker's psychological adjustment to the work

Some of these aspects will now be discussed in some more detail.

9.7.2.1 Symptomatic behaviour as a function of the environment or context of action Environmental influences, like biological factors, may relate to the quality of the individual's mental health. His dominant interactive, relationship and communication patterns—even if they are limited, restrictive and rigid—are formed through a process of interaction with the *environmental systems and sub-systems*. In this regard the family is of special importance. The family system and extended systems of relatives are the primary groups or models where the individual learns his cultural values, where he learns to evaluate his self-image, to experience career concepts and work attitudes, and where typical repetitive behaviour patterns are formed. The *family system* can be the crucial positive factor in mental health, but it can also reinforce symptomatic behaviour, thus promoting maladjustment.

Because of the close relationship between work and the family, the family often suffers as a result of stress at work, examples being divorce rates and family murders.

9.7.2.2 Mental health problems as a function of social support Recent literature shows that social support is an important positive factor in physical and mental health. Social support has an important mediating or buffering effect between adjustment, health and stress (Cronkite and Moos (1984), Ganster and Victor, 1988). Social support is defined as meaningful relationships with other persons in and outside the work place, for instance colleagues, family, friends and neighbours. Social support can manifest itself as emotional help, such as love, empathy, group involvement and so on; as informational assistance such as opinions, facts and feedback or as other forms of help, such as financial support.

9.7.2.3 Mental health as a function of human development and change

If we consider that individual personalities have similarities and differences and that maladjustment among individuals also has similarities and differences, it appears that physical and *psychological development* plays an important role (Gerdes, 1988). Human development consists of several stages in which a person is exposed to various influences; his later behaviour—whether normal or maladjusted—is frequently a reflection of the entire process of development. Several theorists make provision for personality development as one of the main determinants of healthy functioning and adjustment. It appears as though a healthy personality retains the same qualities throughout the entire process of development. In Carson et al. (1988) the emphasis is on heredity, environment and the formation of the self-image as the fundamental determinants of development and characteristic behaviour patterns. The role of motivation is also strongly emphasized. Career psychological theories on the choice of a career and on work behaviour—for example the theories of Super, Ginzberg and Roe—explain work behaviour in terms of career development. Cooper and Payne (1978), Stout and Slocum (1988) and Warshaw (1979), stress the role of some aspects of career development in job stress. Super's theory of career development assumes that, although counselling has a function of 'fitting' the person and his work, this process will be determined by the qualities and skills the individual has developed so far. Super (1980), Mortimer and Borman (1988) and Super and Bohn (1970), maintain that career development is a lifelong process during which the individual passes through a number of crucial phases and where the acquisition of certain skills and career concepts is essential for the choice of a career, for occupational adjustment and for progress. The focal point in Super's theory of career development is the development of the self-image; this implies that the choices and decisions made by the individual must be congruent with his self-evaluation. The individual's self-concept consists basically of his pattern of attitudes, interests and aspirations that develop and change over time and in different stages and which finally culminate in occupational choices. The task of a counsellor in the choice and development of a career is to help the client to acquire certain basic skills since the client has failed to develop self-concepts and career concepts because of problems in the development of one or more phases.

The theory of Ginzberg (1972) on career development is very similar to Super's theory, except for the fact that the former put much emphasis on the compromise between the individual's personal needs and the demands of the external environment. Roe (1956) asserts that the development of an occupational identity is a lifelong process which is largely affected by the needs that develop as a result of the earlier parent-child relationships. The type of orientation that develops will determine whether the individual wishes to work with people or objects, depending on the needs he would like to satisfy. Roe stresses the fact that occupational adjustment is not based on personality orientation only, but also on the interaction between the individual concerned and external factors. Holland (1973) believes that vocational adjustment is a process of development determined by the congruence between personal traits and environmental requirements. This is why the individual tries to enter into the type of environment that will suit his 'type of personality' and, hence, his characteristic style of personality. In his theory on adjustment to work as a continuous process of development Dawis (in Cull and Hardy, 1973) stresses the individual's efforts 'to achieve and maintain correspondence with his work environment'. This agreement between the individual and his work environment is a function of the individual's skills and needs and of the extent to which these qualities are reinforced or blocked.

When intervention techniques are applied to the individual, to groups or to components of the organization, the developmental stages and crucial events must be taken into account.

Neff (1977) explains the 'work personality' as a process of differentiation and development out of which the 'productive role' grows. This means that the psychopathology of work lies in the successful or unsuccessful 'development of a work personality' (see 9.8.2.3). Recent research emphasizes the effect of some aspects of career development, for instance promotion and status, which could lead to work stress and role conflict if expectations are not fulfilled.

Recently a lot of attention is given to improving the individual's and group's coping skills and to being able to manage change effectively.

9.7.2.4 *Personality types and mental health* This refers to *behaviour patterns where the individual will respond in a particular way* to stimuli; in other words, a *certain style of behaviour* can be a predisposing factor for the response to stimuli. The literature often contains descriptions of these typologies. Horney has differentiated between an orientation towards or away from people. In literature on career psychology we find that Roe and Holland identify different career orientations among people; this enables an individual to make a selective choice so that he and the occupational environment will be as congruent as possible (Holland, 1973; Roe, 1956; Latack, 1981).

Related to these are the 'coping' theories, which hold that people handle or control stress more effectively as a result of certain defence mechanisms, emotional, cognitive and behavioural coping methods or by integrated personality or behavioural dispositions. In this regard a lot of research has been done on the so-called A and B-type behaviour patterns (Ivancevich and Matteson, 1988). A-type behaviour is the type of work behaviour and involvement associated with stress-related problems, such as coronary heart diseases. Other personality dispositions, such as internal or external locus of control, learned resourcefulness, hardiness, sense of coherence, and self-actualizing style, also seem to be related to ways of coping with stress and to general health (Manning, Williams et al., 1988; Hobfoll, 1989; Folkman, 1984).

9.7.2.5 *Styles of interaction, the formation of relationships and communication styles* We have repeatedly showed that the individual learns to *act in his environment*, to *define his relationships* and to *communicate in such a way that he will receive the maximum benefit from a situation and will be in control of himself and his environment.*

Writers like Haley (1963) regard *symptomatic behaviour as relationship behaviour* which originates and exists as tactics or manoeuvres between two or more people. If two individuals meet, their mutual relationship is defined in particular ways right from the start. The behaviour between them is determined by verbal and non-verbal behaviour, which can be either direct or indirect and which can either confirm or contradict the other person's behaviour. The main object of this is to be in control of the situation so as to benefit from it and to cope with the demands of the environment.

Haley (1963) points out that the relationship can be defined as *symmetrical*—which implies constant opposition—as *complementary*—where the two people will display different types of behaviour, for example, leader and follower, aggressive or compliant—or as *parallel*—which implies that the behaviour (and, hence, the control) varies between symmetrical and complementary. The last-mentioned type of relationship (parallel) is regarded as the 'healthiest' style of interaction. A fourth definition of a relationship is when one individual permits the other *metacommunicatively* to be in control of the situation whereas the first individual is in fact in control. Problems occur in relationships when the parties are unable to work out a workable relationship, when behaviour roles are so rigid that one person must always be in control and when one person manipulates the situation by pretending that the other is in control whereas this is not the case at all. Such a problem is exacerbated if the individual denies that he has 'manipulated' the situation or has done it unconsciously.

Haley (1963) explains that the definition of the relationship and of the controlling member is further *qualified or disqualified* by the type of verbal and non-verbal communication. Since man can never 'not communicate', he constantly qualifies his messages in some way. When a person says something (verbal) and his physical reactions (non-verbal) indicate the same, his communication is *congruent* and the recipient will understand exactly what he means. Furthermore, if the *overt content* of his message is qualified by the relational aspect, that is, by metacommunication, the recipient will also understand exactly what is expected of him. The fluency of the communication will obviously be determined by the selectivity with which the recipient is listening. Symptomatic behaviour can be regarded as disturbed communication when the individual's levels of communication are *incongruent* or too rigid so that the recipient does not know whether he will be right or wrong if he should respond in any way. Communication can be so ambiguous or paradoxical that it immobilizes one of the parties so that he does not know how to act. Like a schizophrenic he then has to create his own reality—a world of paradoxes where he need not respond or where he is in control so that others will not know how to respond.

Through the interaction in his various systems the individual may *have learned to act rigidly and incongruently* in his role and communication behaviour (and to retain this behaviour for the system's functioning). He will, however, experience problems if his behaviour is not accepted in certain places. The literature (Carson, 1969; Watzlawick et al., 1967; O'Connell, 1979; and Rossiter and Barnett Pearce, 1975) describes typical styles of interaction or communication which can be regarded as symptomatic in certain situations. This includes managing-autocratic behaviour, responsible-hypernormal behaviour, self-humiliating-masochistic behaviour, rebellious-suspicious behaviour, aggressive-sadistic behaviour and competitive-narcissistic behaviour. We also find references to styles such as the avoider, dependent, denier, pleaser, humiliator, confessor, monopolizer, intellectual, moralizer, one-upper, martyr, blamer, and the dictator. These are all typical ways of defining interaction (see 9.8.2.3).

9.7.2.6 *The individual's career concepts and career development as factors of mental health* Work has a positive value, especially in the Western culture. An *individual's success or failure as a person*, as head of the family, and so on, is measured by criteria such as the fact that he works, his type of job, his training for it and his progress in his job. Work is seen as an anchor in a person's life; it structures time, provides self-esteem, an identity, status and opportunities to satisfy physical, psychological and social needs (Isabella, 1988; Slaney and Russell, 1987; Stout, Slocum, et al., 1988).

Unemployment, for instance as a result of dismissals, economic recessions, physical health problems, et cetera, is perhaps the most dramatic illustration of the psychological significance of work for man. Studies have shown that unemployment has seriously detrimental consequences for the individual's physical, psychic and social well-being. Unemployment gives rise to intense feelings of worthlessness, uselessness, loss of positive evaluation of self-image, marital and family problems and even reactions such as severe depression and suicide (Kahn, 1981; Levitan and Johnson, 1982). The despair of the jobless is illustrated by the following typical reactions from case studies (in Kahn 1981, pp. 80–1): 'I felt like a bomb hit me—no place to go'; 'Pretty damned mad, burned up worked up inside'; 'A heartbroken business just like if my wife died'.

Career maturity refers to the level of an individual's vocational development, his vocational attitudes and his decision or choosing skills at different stages of his life. An individual's career maturity is a function of his particular developmental history, his age, sex, behaviour styles and socio-economic factors. His inability to make a choice or to perform developmental tasks at specific points in his career development may lead to stress and emotional problems. In our culture an individual has to face extremely high expectations as far as his career is concerned. Any inability to develop his career—for example failure to be promoted, indecision and uncertainty in making a choice—is regarded as a problem and as a weakness that must be rectified.

There are many causes for vocational uncertainty, for instance adjustment problems, indecision, incongruence between one's capabilities, one's other qualities and the requirements of the post, behavioural traits such as dependence, choice-anxiety, a lack of information, and intra- and interpersonal conflicts. Vocational uncertainty may also be the manifestation of an uncertain interactional style in the context of the individual's job by means of which he tries to cope with his job.

An individual's career concepts, his attitudes of work and of training, his attitudes towards his employers and the positive or negative view he entertains about his role will determine his attitude and expectations on entering the job, adapting to it and developing in it.

The individual's job satisfaction and adjustment will also be determined by the emphasis his employer puts on career development, and by what happens to the individual in terms of his role fulfilment, task performance, job changes, promotion and status, and by events such as retirement, unemployment and economic recessions.

Isabella (1988) demonstrates that career-stage has a definite influence on the way in which managers perceive, interpret and act on events in the organization. Even the organization's stage of development influences the criteria used to determine organizational and individual effectiveness.

Apart from the influence of choosing an occupation, entering a career and later retiring, the so-called *mid-life crisis* at the age of approximately 30–40 years is regarded as an important period of adjustment for some people. This mid-career crisis is brought about by man's fear of ageing and simultaneous questioning of his self-esteem, the purpose of life, and also uncertainty about future career development. Manifestations of this stage include changing jobs, alcohol abuse, poor interpersonal relations, anxiety, depression, hypochondria, marital problems, adopting a new, sometimes strange lifestyle, problems with physical health and appearance and a decrease in sexual energy (Levinson, 1977; Warshaw, 1979; McClean, 1979). It is therefore not surprising that Constandse (1972) refers to this period in the lives of men as 'the male menopause'. In women this phase is likely to coincide with the menopause and the resultant physical and emotional problems.

Wiener et al. (1981), have found that the individual's feelings of career and job satisfaction are more important for mental health than such aspects of work as job design and supervision, since the first are associated with individual needs, performance and motivation. The authors come to the conclusion that worker attitudes can be moderator variables in the relationship between aspects of work and individual characteristics.

9.7.2.7   Individual differences as an aetiological factor   The individual's self-image and his relationships with others are affected by his potential for achievement in various fields. His negotiations with and his entrance into the organization are usually based on what he can offer the organization in terms of capabilities and qualities such as personal style, interpersonal skills, values, interests, attitudes and motivation. His success, progress and personal efficiency in the job will be evaluated on the basis of these individual skills. It is this uniqueness which causes his response to stressors to be different from the response of any other person. It has been established that individuals respond differently to stressors, partially because of psychological differences, but also because of genetic, physiological, biological and neurological differences. In this regard we have referred to Selye's general adaptation syndrome and to research on 'A' and 'B' types of behaviour in coronary heart diseases.

9.7.3 Factors in the work situation In the previous section you have encountered work-related factors, especially with regard to the individual's experience of them. The next two groups of factors deal with the *structures and processes in the organization* (or place of work) that may affect the quality of individual mental health and, hence, organizational health.

9.7.3.1 The individual's perception of his role in the organization The individual's role in the organization is made up of the position, the behaviour processes, the communication and the expectations that have been defined between himself and the organization, his value for others, and the extent to which his role or roles are interactive with and dependent on those of others. The individual can find the process of defining his role painful, since it involves negotiation and relationships to draw up a contract for control and benefit (Payne, Jabri, et al., 1988).

If an individual experiences *stressors in his role* behaviour—for example role conflict, role ambivalence, little responsibility and participation, and few decision-making powers—it may lead to intense feelings of dissatisfaction, frustration and even more serious conditions of stress that may cause coronary heart problems.

9.7.3.2 Work alienation Alienation in general, including work alienation, is a term that is used in a variety of contexts—often vaguely (Kohn et al., 1983; Kunango, 1982). Work alienation or work estrangement, refers to the worker's emotional and cognitive experience that work has lost its positive value because the worker is no longer part of the work process and work results. It is pointed out that, in the midst of increased industrialization, with phenomena such as automatization, large work organizations, bureaucratization, work specialization and the emphasis on monetary compensation and effectiveness, man's expectations and needs are being frustrated because work has lost its intrinsic meaning (Kanungo, 1982; Neff, 1977; Kornhauser, 1965; Baker et al., 1969; Levitan and Johnson, 1982). The material prosperity brought about by industrial effectiveness has not necessarily resulted in the social and emotional effectiveness of workers.

From a psychological point of view, work alienation in particular is associated with the lack of participation or career involvement and therefore of job satisfaction (Kanungo, 1982; Kakabadse, 1982). As such, work alienation is therefore also an important determinant of poor career- and self-identity and low self-esteem. In this way Jenkins (in Kanungo, 1982) regards alienation as a schizoid condition in which the person develops an unrealistic self-esteem and has to survive in the world by means of defence mechanisms. Physical and psychological reactions to alienation are manifold and virtually all types of psychopathological conditions are mentioned, with specific reference to aggression, alcoholism, drug addiction, depression, underachievement, criminal behaviour and family problems (Kanungo, 1982).

The description of four types of alienation by Seeman (in Kohn et al., 1983) can be regarded as different types of reactions. These four types of reactions, which are often used for the measurement of alienation, are the following:

- *helplessness*—a lack of control and freedom

- *isolation or self-estrangement*—a lack of self-esteem, a feeling of aimlessness and work behaviour which is aimed purely at external factors, for instance money, with little intrinsic value
- *normlessness*, sometimes also referred to as anomie—refers to the experience that existing norms and values are no longer adequate—sometimes foreign, almost negative and unscrupulous methods need to be used to achieve objectives, which may lead to isolation since the individual's own norms are no longer accepted
- *cultural estrangement*—the experience that the individual's objectives, beliefs and values are not accepted, reinforced and rewarded

9.7.3.3 *Organizational and management processes* In our time the work *organization, as a socio-technical system, achieves its objectives by co-ordinating and differentiating human behaviour*. Human behaviour is controlled by means of complex organizational structures and behaviour processes. The individual may sometimes feel that his needs conflict with those of the work environment, or he may want to use the work environment for his own interpersonal objectives and achievement. In the process of forming a relationship or a contract between the organization (with its particular context, culture, structure and processes) and the individual (with his unique qualities as a work personality), a psychological climate will develop that may facilitate the individual's adjustment or maladjustment, and which will finally determine the quality of the organizational health. It is important to realize that the individual moves from more limited primary systems—for example the family—to a greater and frequently more impersonal and bureaucratic organizational system or systems. In a probably impersonal work environment with a large number of people and with technology, automatization and control an individual may develop feelings of alienation. The *crucial element in mental health* is probably the extent to which the individual's needs for care, independence, interpersonal relationships and achievement have been satisfied.

Another important point is that *constant changes and developments* in the organization—for example in interpersonal and intergroup behaviour, leadership, decision-making, problem-solving, objectives and production standards—make special demands of the individual as far as adjustment behaviour is concerned. In other words, the individual and organizational problems can never be separated. *You should take note* of the following organizational and management processes as aetiological factors in mental health problems:

- the structure and size of the organization
- organizational changes and development
- management policy and style
- control and disciplinary measures
- communication structures
- opportunities for development and participation
- personnel functions with regard to
  - selection
  - promotion and transfers
  - training and career development
  - remuneration and other benefits

— motivation

— mental health and welfare services

If the organization is also viewed as a developing system it is easy to grasp that the organizational cycles of development are related to organizational and individual effectiveness and adjustment (Parker, 1983; Krantz, 1985; Schuler, 1980; Quinn and Cameron, 1983).

It should be obvious that there are many other and more specific factors and that they can be classified in other ways, as you can see in the systems model (figure 9.1).

9.7.3.4   *Physical* Work stress is often virtually equated with particular physical
factors in circumstances at work. In this respect a discipline such as ergonomics
work and in makes a study of the interaction between man and the physical place
the work of work. Concepts such as industrial hygiene, occupational safety and
situation occupational diseases are closely linked to the influence of the physical work environment and in particular to the physical and physiological well-being of the worker. Some related issues include pollution by toxic substances, working hours, shift work, noise, lighting, temperature, work design, automatization, work load and mass production.

The following are some physical factors that could be taken into consideration:

- sustained concentration and physical exhaustion;
- a work rate that is too fast or too slow;
- physical dangers in the workplace;
- extreme temperatures;
- toxic conditions and radiation;
- poor ventilation;
- badly designed workplace and equipment.

In South Africa most legislation on occupational health is aimed at industrial hygiene and is administered mainly by the Departments of Manpower and Health. The National Council for Occupational Safety (NCOS) is continually promoting occupational safety and fighting industrial diseases, while the National Centre for Occupational Health is a research body which mainly determines the influence of harmful substances and pollution.

9.7.3.5   *Psycho-* In Western culture work is regarded as essential for healthy
social factors development. People are influenced by their parents and other
in work and people to develop certain attitudes to work and to a career (Neff,
in the work 1977).
situation   It seems as though most people experience work positively and that the productive role of work contributes to healthy adaptation and self-esteem. However, there are individuals (and groups) who do not wish to or who cannot associate themselves with the intrinsic (culturally-defined) values of work, or who do not wish to fulfil a productive role (Jenkins, 1973; Neff, 1977; Terkel, 1972). This different attitude may result from the individual's learning experiences and from the type of productive style he has acquired in his relationships. It may also be the result of changing attitudes to work—for instance the view that vocational mobility and even

unemployment need not necessarily be symptomatic behaviour—or the result of greater freedom in work, for instance demands about the utilization of leisure and shorter hours. Furthermore, relationships in the work situation, characteristics of the place of work, the role of *technology* and automatization, and the worker's perception of the importance and usefulness of his work role may contribute to his or her adjustment and, finally, to the organization's effectiveness.

Note the following influential factors:

- different expectations of the employer and employee, for example, regarding work standards, policies et cetera;
- the congruence between the individual and the work environment;
- relationships in the work situation (social support);
- supervision;
- psychological work load, for example being promoted too early and so on;
- dissatisfaction with one's own work performances;
- no work security;
- change in work demands or being bored as a result of no changes taking place;
- isolation from other colleagues and groups.

9.7.4   External influential factors In the individual's dependence on and interaction with his environment and with *other systems* there are several things that may directly or indirectly affect his adjustment behaviour and hence the interaction between himself and the organization. In the modern world the *rapid changes* that occur in the communications media and in the socio-economic, political and technological spheres make life uncertain and unpredictable, and may be too much for some people.

The organization is also affected through its environmental systems, for instance the type of technological, marketing and production demands it constantly has to face.

Note that many of these external factors have already been discussed in conjunction with the other aetiological factors.

Take note of the following factors:

- Previous experience: If we assume that present behaviour determines the current functioning of the individual or the greater systems, any previous experience—for example the individual's childhood and traumatic events—lie in the past. As we said earlier, the influence of these historical systems should not be underestimated. The organizational culture, which determines the present structures and processes, is in part a function of the organization's history.
- Cultural values and norms.
- Family problems.
- Traumatic events, for example, death, war, economic depression and unemployment.
- Ecological influences such as housing, population, density, pollution and geographical location.
- Political or government influences.
- Trade unions or their influence.

9.8 WORK ADJUSTMENT PROBLEMS

In this section the emphasis is primarily on general adaptive reactions and specific work-related problems. While abnormal psychology or psychopathology is covered elsewhere, references to psychopathological conditions will only cover aspects deemed relevant in the field of occupational mental health. You may note that the study of occupational mental health can be viewed as an applied field of clinical and abnormal psychology. Therefore all psychopathological conditions as discussed in standard textbooks have implications for work behaviour. Up to date no generally accepted classification for a 'psychopathology of work' exist, the most important reasons being the broad scope of possible problems and the recent emphasis on this topic. Some typologies of work adjustment problems, however, have been postulated by inter alia Powles and Ross (in McClean, 1970); Miner (1966); Miner and Brewer (in Dunnette, 1981); Hamburger and Hess (in McClean, 1970); Follman (1978); Steinmetz (1969); Roseman (1982) and Neff (1977). Reading these it becomes evident that criteria for psychopathology and work maladjustment are often also interrelated, again emphasizing the systemic nature of man's behaviour.

9.8.1 Adjustment or adaptive reactions Stress, frustration, conflict and other factors that pressurize the individual physically or psychologically, require some or other form of *adaptive reaction or defence mechanism*. In part of the previous section we pointed out how, according to Selye's general adaptation syndrome, the body reacts as a whole to stress. The single main goal or function of human adjustment reactions is to maintain or acquire *homeostasis* or a condition of equilibrium, whether in biological or psychological behaviour. Although it is possible to single out a number of universally valid kinds of adjustment reactions, it is impossible to describe all the kinds of adjustment, or defence mechanisms. In fact there are as many kinds of adaptive reactions as there are people, situations in which one behaves and ways in which people have learnt to adapt. In a certain sense we can say that all behaviours in our daily comings and goings are based on adaptive reactions. It is also possible to single out certain adaptive or defence reactions in all forms of behavioural disorders (psychopathology). The best known of these are probably the so-called personality disorders where clearly defined defence mechanisms can be identified. This multiplicity of everyday adaptive reactions and the fact that everyone manifests adaptive reactions, make it so much more difficult always to distinguish clearly between adaptive reactions or defences and maladaptive reactions or defences. The difference is probably mostly in the frequency, duration and intensity of certain reactions. For instance ordinary eating habits are essential for life and survival, yet excessive or inadequate eating habits constitute a behavioural disorder with serious biological and psychological implications. It is also accepted that everyone is somewhat disoriented from time to time in terms of time and place, or that we sometimes distrust people's intentions, yet when disorientation of time and place becomes a repetitive pattern and distrust becomes a nagging suspicion towards everything so that daily forms of behaviour are disrupted, we can begin to talk of a certain form of psychological disorder. In the idiom of adjustment literature one speaks in fact of the 'failure to adjust' which actually only refers to what is known as psychopathological conditions or psychological behavioural disorders.

Types of adaptive reactions

Types of defence mechanisms are identified and classified in different ways.

Adjustment and defence

First a distinction is sometimes made between adaptive or adjustment reactions and mechanisms. *Adaptive reactions* refer to everyday forms of behaviour which individuals (children and adults) use to handle everyday problems and crises so as to satisfy possible physical and psychological needs and to alleviate anxiety or stress. Examples are the following:

- touch, for instance the child seeks the protection of the mother's arms;
- music which has a calming effect on many people;
- eating and drinking;
- crying and scolding;
- talking things out and praying;
- work or more work;
- games, recreation, travelling and vacations;
- physical acting out of feelings;
- shopping and buying habits;
- physical habits such as grooming one's hair and nails;
- withdrawal such as developing symptoms of disease;
- purposive relaxation techniques such as progressive relaxation of the body and meditation;
- cognitive adaptive reactions such as reassessment of problems and imaging of problems.

From the above list you can see that many of these forms of behaviour can also form the basis of more serious behavioural disorders. At the same time many of these adjustment reactions also form the basis of techniques and programmes for handling stress, for instance in therapy and vocational guidance.

Defence mechanisms are more comprehensive patterns of behaviour, usually unplanned (automatic) and unconscious, which the individual uses to relieve or avoid emotional conflicts and resultant anxiety and stress. This view of defence mechanisms as intrapsychic, unconscious patterns of behaviour to protect the ego or self against threatening impulses (id impulses such as sexual and aggressive needs) is primarily the Freudian or psychoanalytic view. Conscious defence signifies that the individual consciously and purposively behaves differently or tries to mislead others in order to attain certain objectives. In our discussion of specific types of defence mechanisms we shall stress particularly intrapsychic defence mechanisms.

Direct as opposed to indirect defence mechanisms

This distinction between adaptive reactions is directly related to the above distinction.

With *direct defence reactions* the individual mostly behaves in a conscious and overtly perceptible way to adapt to conflict, frustration, anxiety and stress. Examples of direct behaviour are aggression and withdrawal from a situation. In the case of *aggression* it can be associated with physical attacks, overt rage and violence. Otherwise aggression can occur in a more inhibited way so that rage, for instance, is not as demonstrable. In a case like this aggression is therefore somewhat more internalized and can manifest in somewhat displaced forms, such as verbal sarcasm, refusal to work, strikes and hunger strikes. Although *withdrawal* is mostly reasonably directly observable, behaviour is found in exceptional cases which indicates total inactivity or apathy and depression. In a case like this the person regards his chances of adapting or coping as being so hopeless that he actually stops trying. Examples were observed during wars where soldiers under severe war stress simply stopped fighting and waited to be taken prisoner. Also the post-war stress reactions (the post-traumatic stress reaction) could contain an element of inactivity after severely traumatic experiences or protracted experience of stress.

Another form of direct adaptive reaction, but which manifests in a displaced form are the so-called *symptom-directed* ways of behaviour. Examples are the use of liquor and drugs as well as more acceptable narcotics such as sedatives.

Indirect defence mechanisms refer to the previously mentioned intrapsychic, unconscious adaptive reactions. *Some of the best known will be discussed in more detail.*

- *Repression* implies that the individual seeks to exclude threatening, undesirable and painful impulses, ideas and memories (experiences) from his consciousness. This reaction can also be described as a form of psychological loss of memory (amnesia) where the person uses selective forgetting or in other words, selective remembering. According to Freud repression is the main defence mechanism which is basic to many of the other defence mechanisms. Repression is sometimes regarded as a 'successful' adaptive mechanism because it can provide immediate relief from traumatic events or even for longer periods until the memory of certain ideas or events is safer again, for instance after therapy or as an adult. The disadvantage is that repression does not really solve the problem (for instance guilt feelings), since repressed contents can manifest in disguised or indirect ways, for instance in dreams, fantasies and slips of the tongue. It is also said that in extreme cases the 'repressed' person behaves so defensively and rigidly that he cannot live and experience spontaneously.

  Examples of repression can be the apparent amnesia of a soldier after his friend next to him has been decapitated and the total repression of sexual needs because of traumatic sexual experiences for instance in sexual assaults such as rape and incest. In neurotic personalities (anxiety-based forms of behaviour) the individual may, for instance, forget his date of birth and address or be apparently unable to remember acquaintances. In the work situation repression could manifest in the form of forgetting to perform tasks and forgetting an appointment with the supervisor.

  It is necessary to distinguish between repression and *suppression*. Whereas the first is an unconscious process, suppression is a conscious, rational attempt to keep unpleasant ideas and experiences from the conscious mind. For instance a family could decide deliberately not to speak about a lost member of the family or someone could consciously bear in mind that he finds a task unpleasant.

- *Denial* is related to repression and is based on a total denial of the existence of certain facts or events. In children denial is regarded as a reasonably acceptable defence mechanism because the child's repertoire of problem-solving mechanisms is still limited, for example the boy who denies that his father has left home or the child who denies that he was a baby or is angry. Conversely it is said that in adults a pattern of denial behaviour is based on limited adjustments and problem-solving behaviour, for example the alcoholic or glutton who denies his problem. More extreme cases occur in people who deny that they are seriously ill for instance someone suffering from terminal cancer, or parents who deny that their child is seriously ill or even dead. Protracted denial of reality, for instance someone who denies that she was abused as a child and therefore denies her negative feelings towards her parents, can eventually lead to a schizophrenic reaction. In a work context denial can manifest when someone denies that he was not promoted, has become unemployed and so forth.

  As a very common and simple form of defence denial has the value of relieving the stress of severe trauma. In general however, a protracted pattern of denial can only have detrimental effects for the individual.

- In *projection* the person ascribes his undesirable characteristics, impulses, behaviour, or errors to other people or even inanimate objects. Projection is reasonably common in children in that the child uses all sorts of stories about other children and things to overcome or reduce his own fears. In adults projection is less successful and actually indicates the person's inability to handle his own mistakes, feelings of inferiority and so forth effectively. Examples of projection are seen when someone who experiences strong homosexual impulses then ascribes them to others, the mother with guilt feelings about her early sexual experiences who accuses her young daughter of permissiveness, the worker or student who produces poor work and ascribes his failure to his supervisor's prejudices against him, the tennis player who loses blames his failure on a poor racket, playing surface and so forth. In extreme pathological conditions projection is particularly a characteristic of the paranoid personality and paranoid psychosis. Such people have strongly entrenched ideas that others threaten or persecute them.

- *Reaction formation* involves defence reactions where the person manifests behaviour or attitudes that are the direct opposite of the undesirable impulses. Examples of this are the mother who overprotects the child while she actually harbours feelings of hatred, the apparently self-sacrificing love of a husband for his invalid wife, while he might wish she was dead, someone who over-zealously preserves moral values who is actually defending against his own sexual needs, the boastful Don Juan who is actually secretly afraid of female sexuality and the student who fails and then maintains that he actually does not care whether he passes or not.

- *Regression* refers to a return to earlier or less responsible patterns of behaviour which are inappropriate to the present situation. Regression is common in children, for instance the child who begins wetting the bed again (to gain attention), when a baby arrives in the family. In severe forms of this a continual regression to a narcissistic self-love could inhibit the young child from growing emotionally and socially. Regression is also observed in prisoners who could become so dependent that they cannot think, act or plan for themselves. In everyday life forms of behaviour such as outbursts of rage in the work situation or an inability to complete work, could indicate inappropriate regressive forms of behaviour.

  Fixation is related to regression and implies that with regard to certain behaviours the person's psychological development has progressed only to a certain stage. So mother fixation refers to the fact that a young man could find it difficult to put another woman in his mother's place.

- *Identification* involves the internalization or adoption of the characteristics of another person or even group. Freud regarded the process of identification as an integral part of personality development, particularly the development of cultural values (superego) and the development of sexual identity. According to Freud it is precisely through identification with the father that the boy overcomes his Oedipus complex and concomitant feelings of aggression and fear of the father and male figures. Another extreme case of identification with the strongest person or body was observed in concentration camps where some prisoners tried hard to assume the appearance and behaviour of their oppressors or aggressors. Identification occurs throughout life—in children particularly with hero figures, pop stars, sport stars and so forth and in adults often with leaders and organizations. Although identification has positive aspects, it can also have negative consequences. So aggression and crime could be the outcome of faulty identification. When identification figures are unsuccessful or die the effects are sometimes detrimental. In this connection it is well known that with the death of figures such as Martin Luther King, John F. Kennedy, Elvis Presley and John Lennon some people experienced serious emotional disturbances and even committed suicide.

  When soccer teams lose a match violence often erupts between opposing supporters.

- *Displacement* occurs when someone directs or channelizes intense negative feelings or attitudes away from himself to other people or objects. Some of the best known examples are the displacement of aggressive feelings, for instance the aggression of a high school pupil towards his father is directed at the teacher or school in rebellious behaviour, the worker's aggression towards his supervisor is taken out on the family at home and the childless couple displace their needs by working very hard for child care organizations. Although displacement is an effective form of release for tension and prevents more extreme behaviour, the basic problem however often remains.

According to Freud displacement is a characteristic way of converting unacceptable id impulses (sexual and aggressive drives) into more socially acceptable behaviour. In these ways also, as in identification and sublimation, cultural values are acquired and people can live in greater harmony.

- *Sublimation* is closely related to displacement and is sometimes regarded as a special form of displacement. Sublimation is used to apply the energy of unacceptable sexual and aggressive instincts particularly in such a way as to lead to more acceptable and exemplary behaviour. So it is said in some cases that the vocation of minister or surgeon could be chosen to sublimate aggression, a sexually frustrated woman could become a nurse, a baby might suck his thumb or another object instead of the mother's breast and the schoolgirl could fall in love with her teacher out of admiration for her father. Another good example is the premise that Leonardo da Vinci's preference for painting women (such as the well-known Mona Lisa) arose from an intense longing and need for his mother.

- *Rationalization* consists of a person finding socially acceptable reasons for his behaviour or events while the real reasons are repressed. The person misleads himself (and sometimes others as well) by justifying his behaviour or the course of events. Rationalization is however not necessarily lying behaviour but an attempt to adjust and to alleviate or avoid disappointment or stress. Rationalization is one of the most common forms of defence, also in everyday life. For instance the unsuccessful student could contend after the examination that the paper was in any case unfair or that he did not really learn or want to pass. The worker who is not promoted maintains that he is actually glad to remain in his old post, or that he would actually lose too much by changing jobs. Aesop's fable 'the fox and the grapes' illustrates how the fox when he could not get the delicious bunches of grapes concealed his disappointment by accepting that the grapes were sour—hence the saying 'sour grapes'. Other proverbial rationalizations are expressed in sayings such as 'every dark cloud has a silver lining' or 'tomorrow is another day'.

Negative or very unreasonable rationalizations are illustrated by Hitler's war crimes for instance which he claimed were done for love of the fatherland, or the family murderer who kills his wife and children and claims that he wanted to save them from the suffering of a difficult life on earth.

- *Intellectualization*, also called isolation (or sometimes regarded as a form of isolation) occurs when someone isolates threatening emotional experiences or behaviour or events from himself by speaking about them in an excessively intellectual or rational way. In ordinary life intellectualization often occurs among people in careers where they have to work with human pain and suffering. For instance a medical doctor, nurse and even the commander of soldiers will give intellectual reasons for events. An individual is regarded as an object of study who can be used to save other lives.

When intellectualization becomes so intense however that the individual misleads himself and loses contact with his feelings and therefore has limited emotional experiences, this form of defence becomes maladjustment. For instance a young man could have severe sexual fears. He tries to appear to be 'adjusted' in this respect by philosophizing and speaking rationally about sex, marriage and so forth also in his contacts with women.

Another form of isolation is referred to as *emotional insulation*. In this case the person will begin to behave passively, apathetically and despairingly during or after traumatic events such as unemployment, imprisonment, war or death. Someone like this is however merely hiding behind a protective 'wall of emotionless' behaviour in an attempt to avoid further shocks. Although such behaviour can relieve acute traumas, protracted emotional withdrawal will amount to an isolated and rigid way of experiencing life.

- *Compensation* amounts to protecting the self-image by over-achieving in some or other inadequate or inferior area of behaviour. Direct compensation occurs when an unattractive woman uses too much make-up or follows a mannequin course or when a slightly built man takes up a course in body building. In history people such as the American president, Theodore Rooseveldt, and the Greek orator and statesman, Demosthenes, are cited as examples of cases where compensation for weaknesses lead to great achievements. In the world of sport, also in South Africa, there are many examples of people who have achieved a great deal irrespective of a physical handicap or weakness.

  Indirect compensation is reflected in a different type of behaviour than is indicated by an apparent deficiency. For instance someone who is poor at sport could perform well academically or politically and a slightly built, short person (such as Napoleon) could behave very domineeringly or a young man from a poor family could do well academically or financially to compensate for his family's shortcomings. Even Freud and the musician, Haydn, it is said were outstanding in their fields because they in fact had few opportunities.

- *Fantasy* consists of the fulfilment of unsatisfied needs, wishes and desires through imagination and wishful thinking. In this way the individual creates images of people, things or events in order to try to satisfy needs or as a way of finding a temporary escape from frustration, conflict and tension. Fantasy is mostly not negative and is found particularly among children and often also among adults. In this connection you can note how often adults participate in children's games or television programmes and fairy tales that are actually intended for children. Fantasy is also regarded as an element of creativity. When fantasy becomes pathological, it actually means that the individual cannot handle reality and therefore lives in a naïve or childlike way in a fairytale world of flights of the imagination. Many psychopathological conditions such as schizophrenia and psychopathy contain elements of fantasy in the disordered patterns of behaviour.

The above are the main adaptive and defence mechanisms. As indicated defence mechanisms are a way of coping and sometimes of handling conflicts and tensions. Defence mechanisms entail maladjustment however when they become the only way in which the individual can handle reality, his problems, conflicts and tensions. In such a case the person robs himself of energy, spontaneity and creativity with the result that he cannot experience events, himself and interactions with others fully. Such a person continues to mislead himself and his problems are never really solved.

9.8.2 Psycho-pathological conditions The following is a brief discussion on some psychopathological conditions and their relevance to work behaviour.

9.8.2.1 Stress reactions We have referred to stress as an important aetiological factor in physical and psychological decompensation. Next we shall describe briefly more extreme examples of stress reactions.

- In the so-called *adjustment disorders* the stress reactions are the result of adverse life events (see figure 9.3). The reactions such as depression, anxiety, behavioural disorders, emotional outbursts, loss of work capacity, and withdrawal, can follow acute 'severely traumatic stress' or chronic (protracted) stress. Examples of life events that can lead to adjustment disorders are unemployment, divorce or separation, enforced relocations and loss such as the death of a loved one. Although these types of stress reactions are associated with intense emotions and often progressive phases of reactions (such as shock, rage, denial, withdrawal and acceptance), recovery is usually complete as soon as the stressor has faded or the individual has learnt to adapt.

- *Post-traumatic stress reactions* occur during, immediately or some time after an intense, traumatically acute or chronic stressor. These reactions are more intense than the adjustment reactions, are difficult to diagnose since the condition has diverse symptoms and recovery is more difficult. A distinction is made in post-traumatic stress reactions between *acute* (begins during or within six months of the stressor), *chronic* (lasts longer than six months) and the *delayed reactions* (begins at least six months after the stressor).

In general the post-traumatic stress reactions are characterized by repeated experience of anxiety about the stressor, a lack of responsiveness to the environment (apathy) and a variety of symptoms such as fright reactions, irritation, fatigue, insomnia, intolerance (for instance for noise), nightmares, loss of concentration, memory impairment, depression, heightened aggression and withdrawal. Examples of experiences that can or have evoked post-traumatic stress reactions are catastrophes (such as collisions, floods, earthquakes, fires, explosions and also rape). Wars such as the First and Second World Wars with resultant events such as the atomic bombs on Hiroshima and Nagasaki, the mass deaths of Jews in the Nazi concentration camps, prisoners of war, loss of limbs, as well as wars such as those in Vietnam and the situation in Israel drew renewed attention to the intense influence of traumatic stressors. Concepts such as 'shell shock', 'operational fatigue', 'war neuroses', 'combat exhaustion', and more recently 'burnout' are used to refer to post-traumatic stress reaction. Although a great deal of research is still required about post-traumatic stress reactions, with regard to diagnosis and treatment, particularly delayed reactions in Vietnam veterans and survivors of concentration camps illustrate the protracted and possible irreversible effects of acute and chronic stress. Treatment requires intense medical, psychiatric and psychological intervention and the emphasis recently is on early identification and treatment of potential post-traumatic reactions.

We see in the literature that sustained stress affects the individual's work behaviour at various levels, namely his physical, physiological, emotional, motivational and cognitive functions. In the case of serious decompensation this may lead to psychiatric disorder and even death. Job stress is also associated with emotional disorders such as anxiety, fear, depression, aggression and anger, poor interpersonal relationships, and gives rise to absenteeism, high staff turnover, accidents and underachievement. Role conflicts in the work situation, especially work overload and role ambivalence, are prominent stressors which have been correlated with coronary heart disease. Factors such as status, managerial responsibility, technological change, automatization, shift work and assessment procedures have also been correlated with stress, anxiety and other personality disorders. Physical stressors, such as noise, loss of sleep and extreme temperatures, also have an adverse effect on achievement in work. Temporary conditions of stress in the individual and in his environment—for example, financial problems, the war on the border, the death of a member of the family, rumours about the abolition of posts, changes in the organization or management, or losing a job—may affect work behaviour negatively. This may in turn be manifested in low motivation, anxiety, depression, uncertainty, low productivity, inaccurate work, and higher alcohol and drug intake. In the case of women it has been found that domestic events such as illness, pregnancy, divorce, and marital problems cause job stress and may be directly responsible for high personnel turnover, absenteeism, complaints of illness, and so on. Research also shows a close relationship between job stress and psychosomatic disorders such as stomach ulcers, headaches, hypertension, and cardiac diseases. This costs the industry an enormous amount in terms of lost working time, loss of income, hospital costs, early pensions, not to mention the physical and psychological discomfort experienced by the individual and other persons.

9.8.2.2 *Anxiety-based disorders (neuroses)* Neurotic conditions are characterized by *anxiety and other internal emotions*, which the individual handles by means of adjustment behaviour such as defence mechanisms. The individual's emotional behaviour may lead to an unrealistic evaluation of the demands of reality, which can result in evasive rather than in positive adjustment behaviour. This can have an adverse effect on the general adjustment and work behaviour of an individual with emotional problems. It is wrong to assume that neurotic behaviour immobilizes the individual completely or impairs his effectiveness totally. Brophy and Raubenheimer (1978) have found that, in terms of twelve work criteria, a neurotic worker is not significantly worse than a non-neurotic worker.

In certain cases it in fact appears as if the neurotic worker can have a strong affiliation with work. In the sense that he can satisfy certain needs through work, for instance the need for authority, to achieve, to be accepted and to please others, it does provide him with an outlet for certain fears and anxieties (Freedman and Leary, 1961). This involvement with work for the sake of personal gain can mean that on an interactional level the work situation can actually reinforce and support particular styles of behaviour. This type of interaction with work can possibly also explain the, sometimes almost self-destructive, work behaviour of the so-called workaholic (Muldary, 1983), the A-type personality etcetera.

Neuroses or anxiety-based disorders include anxieties, somatic disorders and dissociative conditions.

The application of work criteria has showed that *neurotic behaviour usually affects work behaviour indirectly* (McClean, 1970). Work behaviour is characterized by lower production, poor motivation, job dissatisfaction, irresolution, poor self-esteem, helplessness, dependence, disturbed interpersonal skills and phenomena such as sick leave, absence, complaints about illness and risky work behaviour that may lead to accidents. Intense anxiety may affect the individual's intellectual functioning, his cognitive judgment, visual perception, accuracy, rate of work and psychomotor activities, and physiological functions such as respiration, heartbeat and muscular tension (McClean, 1970; Miner, 1966; Greenwood and Greenwood, 1979; Follman, 1978).

The general literature indicates that neurotic behaviour—or such aspects of it as anxiety, fear, aggression, depression, uncertainty and feelings of guilt—affects personal and work behaviour. People with this type of emotional complaint probably need help. One should, however, beware of generalization; everyone's problem must be analysed and treated in context. This will make it possible to establish in which spheres of conduct the individual is experiencing problems, where intervention is needed and where he is still productive, in other words, where his skills can be utilized.

9.8.2.3 Personality disorders and criminal behaviour We are here concerned with deviant behaviour that can be described as *characteristic and repetitive behaviour patterns*. The individual observes, defines his relationships and communicates in ways which do not always work for himself and which cause inconvenience to others. This type of symptomatic behaviour is frequently the only behaviour the person is familiar with; he may also be unaware of such behaviour, pretend that he cannot help it or deny that he has acted in a certain way. As in the case of neurosis, such a person may sometimes be very effective in his job, socially and at the interpersonal level. In other words, an individual's 'symptom' must be understood and treated in context.

Textbooks usually differentiates between personality disorders, the antisocial person (psychopath) and criminal behaviour.

Behaviour problems in the work situation frequently coincide with personality disorders, and, together with neurosis, psychosomatic conditions and alcoholism, they constitute the *chief problem in the industry*. The classifications of Leary (in Carson, 1969), Neff (1977) and Steinmetz (1969) are particularly important.

The *classification of vocational maladjustment* made by Neff (1977) must be regarded as a description of ways or *styles of responses in the work*. The styles of responses can be manifested in any worker and need not necessarily be symptoms of psychoses, neuroses, et cetera. This relates to Neff's view that the work personality is a separate aspect of the total personality; in other words, personality problems need not be manifested in every work situation. Neff regards mental health in the work situation as a function of the work personality, which is characterized by a productive role. The productive work personality develops as a process of the normal personality development. This is why people differ in this respect; some cannot be productive since they have not learned to be efficient in their environment and since cultural values determine work motivation. The productive role is not, however, a function of the individual only, but also of the work situation. The development of the work personality is largely a function of competency motivation and of the individual's self-image evaluation. Neff describes the following nosology or classification of occupational maladjustment (the writer has added comments and interpretations to every type):

Persons with poor motivation and a negative role conception of work and of their roles as employees

These are people whose basic personality structure does not contain built-in cultural norms with regard to work, because of their education and background. For them the community, and hence work, pose a threat to their ego; they are against or negative towards the community and work, and they have little or no sense of responsibility. They do not satisfy the basic requirements of the work situation and are ignorant of the meaning of productive role fulfilment. They generally display symptoms such as absence, arriving late, poor production and passive or indifferent attitudes to work. They do not associate work with need satisfaction and their motivation is based on impulsive action such as aggression, theft and dishonesty (immediate need satisfaction). They show little initiative, are inclined to justify their mistakes and defend themselves by always nursing a grudge. Accidents, revolt against authority and even alcoholism and drug addiction are safety valves for their impulsive motivation and inadequacy. The most severe manifestation of these symptoms is found in the sociopath or the psychopath. Their inadequacy in their work is merely an extension of such behaviour in other spheres, for instance in marriage. There is relatively little to be done for these people, since their type of work behaviour is fundamentally an attitude to life. In practice we sometimes make use of group behaviour therapeutic techniques to achieve the long-term objective of changing their attitude.

Individuals who respond to work mainly with fear and anxiety

In this type of person we find that cultural norms with regard to work have been strongly—probably too strongly—impressed upon them, with the result that there is tremendous motivation for achievement. However, the motivation is handicapped by vague or even more serious feelings of anxiety and fear, tenseness, touchiness, discomfort, distress and fear for interpersonal relationships. They doubt their own capabilities, with the result that they are unable to fulfil a productive role.

Other symptoms include varying standards of achievement, poor interpersonal relationships, withdrawal symptoms, depression, absence, self-imposed absence ('sick leave'), little enterprise, an accident record, psychosomatic complaints and a compulsive possessedness with the successful performance of a task, which sometimes succeeds but usually fails. Fears about losing a job and even paranoid traits can be characteristic. People in this category have probably experienced failure in several other spheres, for instance the disappointment of parents and poor achievement at school.

Causes are sought in a too strict upbringing, too high expectations by parents, repeated failures, too high aspirations in comparison with abilities, *and so on*. In other words, work stress is an extension of the individual's personal anxieties. Criticism in the work situation exacerbates the condition, competition is a threat and even group work (co-operation) creates anxiety. Although symptoms of this nature can be manifested generally, they are typical of life stress conditions, neuroses, psychosomatic disorders and depression. In these cases occupational maladjustment is a function of the degree of anxiety that is experienced. What is known as the 'fear of success' in contemporary literature can be regarded as typical of these workers. Corrective procedures based on positive motivation will probably be the best, for instance supportive supervision in workshops where a person will learn to trust his capabilities.

Persons whose chief responses in the work situation are openly hostile and aggressive

Because of possibly negative cultural influences, personal shortcomings and limited abilities people with these types of responses regard work and its requirements as restrictive and as a punishment. The slightest stress and provocation cause aggression where the person is prepared to defend himself and to attack others. These people are moody, frequently cross, negative, inclined to argue and to do things to annoy others, and they are sarcastic and insulting. Accidents may occur because of their impulsiveness. In other words, their energy is used in a constant struggle against their co-workers and against management. Their problem is to keep their jobs and they frequently change jobs because of throwing up their job or because of dismissal. The main reason for their dismissal is their poor human relations. A type described as 'the abrasive personality' by Levinson (*Harvard Business Review*, May/June, 1978) probably falls into this category. If we have to look for psychopathological symptoms or conditions in such a case, we can compare the characteristics of paranoid schizophrenia, paranoid personality, explosive personality and passive-aggressive personality with it. The neurotic who tries to disguise his anxiety through aggressive behaviour may also fall under this category.

Individuals who respond mainly with dependence and immaturity to job requirements

This type of person is uncertain about his own capabilities and retains a childlike need for the help and support of others—an analogy with the child-parent relationship. They are constantly trying to satisfy authority figures, they only work effectively under supervision, and they display little initiative and independence. Because of their search for security and support, these workers are a burden to their fellow-workers and to supervisors, mainly because it is difficult to create a supportive atmosphere in a task-oriented work situation. Certain personality disorders can fall into this category, for instance schizoid symptoms, hysteria and inadequacy. This type of personality can benefit from rehabilitation workshops where independent behaviour is reinforced.

Occupational maladjustment can also be a characteristic of the socially naïve person

Cultural norms about work have not been impressed upon this type of person, since they have never perceived work and work requirements probably because of too little exposure to work or because of insufficient ability. Their responses are based on ignorance rather than on resistance, aggression, et cetera. These workers accept working conditions as they are, they experience little stress and show little initiative. Socially naïve people are unpredictable in their feelings for others, they fail to realize the effect of their behaviour and they are generally ignorant of how to act socially. Overprotected children, for instance, if they had been overprotected because of a physical handicap, may have this type of response. In rehabilitative work situations such a person must be exposed to the work and to work-related requirements.

In 1967 Neff and Kultuv conducted a study of about 100 workers and assessed them on a coping scale. After the study Neff asserted that the above-mentioned typologies are fairly reliable and relatively independent. However, much research is still needed. Neff describes two additional types, namely the *reserved* (apathetic) type and the *self-deprecatory* type. The former type of response is characterized by a lack of vitality, by indifference towards everything, emotional unresponsiveness, non-involvement and nonchalance. The self-deprecatory type is critical towards himself, distrusts himself, his own capabilities and qualities, and likes to talk about his weaknesses (Neff, 1977).

Steinmetz's (1969) *criteria for underachievement* (see 9.6.3) are very similar to Neff's classification. He describes the following additional characteristics of poor achievers: persons who do not wish to discuss their ineffective work behaviour because of their natural reserve or their somatic inadequacy; the formation of cliques in the work situation which leads to 'group defence mechanisms' which, in turn give rise to poor achievement. 'Group resistances' include resistance to small social groups; reactive individualism as a response to the informal group (e.g. keeping information from the group); mutual fault-finding; and self-imposed absence. Steinmetz also describes the following types: the blind spot syndrome which appears in an individual who is ignorant of his limitations; 'a lack of just one more skill type', which applies to the type of worker who attributes poor achievement to the fact that he lacks the capabilities for the job; the 'OK on routine, weak on troubleshooting' type, who easily performs simple tasks but who cannot cope with unusual tasks. The 'tenacious individual syndrome' is characteristic of the hardboiled type of person who always thinks he is right. Steinmetz (1969) describes all these types of responses in terms of the possibilities of behaviour change. He describes other forms of unsatisfactory work achievement in the following typologies: resistance to change; moodiness; disorganization work and work methods; the inability to communicate effectively; the person who rarely takes the initiative; intolerance; the individual who invariably wishes to appear blameless; the emotionally sensitive worker; unimaginativeness; and the worker who is always defensive.

Leary (in Carson, 1969) describes the following types of *interpersonal behaviour styles*, which, if we analyse them, could definitely affect the individual's work behaviour.

Managerial autocratic behaviour

'Behaviour in the managerial-autocratic range is strong, assertive and confidential in tone. It communicates the message, "I am a strong, competent, knowledgeable person on whom you may rely for effective guidance and leadership"' (Carson, 1969, p. 107). It requires that other people be submissive, obedient and respectful. Extreme forms of this behaviour can be dictatorial, pedantic and dogmatic.

Responsible-hypernormal behaviour

Important features include affectionate, friendly, dominant but also supportive behaviour. 'It communicates the message, "I am a strong, competent, emphatic person on whom you may count for understanding and emotional support" and it tends to invite others to respond with dependency and affection' (Carson, 1969, pp. 108–9). Extreme forms of this behaviour may include an overdeveloped sense of responsibility and interference in other people's affairs.

Co-operative excessively conformable behaviour

A typical behaviour style in this case is the passive affiliation with indications of submissiveness, which is an indication of the striving for a compromise and for harmony rather than the clear definition of personal importance. 'It communicates the message, "I am an exceedingly friendly, agreeable, unchallenging person who would like you to like me"' (Carson, 1969, p. 109). This type of behaviour stimulates others to be supportive and friendly. Extreme behaviour includes false heartiness, excessive conformation and the readiness to come to an agreement, even if there are differences.

Obedient-dependent behaviour

This type of behaviour is basically submissive, though friendly. 'It conveys the message, "I am a weak and helpless person in need of your aid and support"' (Carson, 1969, p. 109). Extreme behaviour includes a clinging dependence on others who may find it inconvenient.

Self-deprecatory-masochistic behaviour

This consists of dependent and submissive behaviour, coloured with aggression and hostility. 'It tends to communicate to others the message, "I am a weak, deficient, unworthy person, justly deserving of your domination, rejection and contempt"' (Carson, 1969, p. 110). This type of behaviour stimulates others to be arrogant and cruel, and to exploit the person. The most extreme form of his behaviour can amount to total inadequacy, self-condemnation and depressive responses.

Rebellious-suspicious behaviour

Typical features of this behaviour style are hostility and asocial behaviour in conjunction with passivity and powerlessness. 'This behaviour communicates to others the message, "I reject and mistrust you, for you are, or are certain to become unworthy of my affection and esteem"' (Carson, 1969, p. 110). This behaviour style gives rise to punishment or a disciplinary attitude, to rejection and to indignance in others. In psychiatric terms we refer to these styles of behaviour as 'paranoid' and 'schizophrenic' traits.

Aggressive-sadistic behaviour

This behaviour style consists of the direct expression of hostility and dominance at the verbal and non-verbal levels. 'This category of behaviour communicates the message, "I am a threatening and dangerous person, and you are a suitable target for my wrath"' (Carson, 1969, p. 110). This behaviour gives rise to fear and feelings of guilt in other people. Extreme forms of the behaviour can include cruelty and sadism.

Competitive-narcissistic behaviour

This consists of dominant behaviour, strongly coloured by aggressive qualities. It can be described as 'one-upmanship' and can be aimed at the submission of others. 'I am superior to you, and you being a lesser person, are hardly worthy of my serious consideration' (Carson, 1969, p. 111). This type of behaviour can cause passive aggression and submission in others. Its extreme form can amount to an inflated, a boastful, an exhibitionistic and a rejective attitude.

Other sources of information about the relationship between personality disorders and work behaviour include Kohn et al. (1983), Miner (1966), McClean (1970) and Follman (1978). In this regard reference is often made in literature on work stress to the so-called A and B personality types. These two personality types represent two different ways in which people react in the work situation, perform tasks and cope with stress. Type A is associated with the following behaviour patterns as well as with a high risk factor for coronary heart diseases and other stress-related problems (Price, 1982; Glass and Carver, 1980).

- *Intense aspirational behaviour* and conscientiousness—this style of behaviour is characterized by traits such as high ambition, strict performance criteria, willingness to work hard, suppression of tension, working long hours, displaying very responsible behaviour and linking production to self-esteem, competing even during recreation.
- An irrepressible *tendency towards urgency*, characterized by virtually impossible time limits for the completion of tasks, impatience, restlessness, a feeling and sensation of constantly working under pressure, doing everything quickly, for instance eating, walking and talking fast, quick emotional reactions, attempting to do several things at once and even attempting to project occurrences.

• *Interpersonal relationships* display a lack of caring for other people. Characteristics of this style of behaviour include hostility, sometimes aggression and anger, egotism, difficulty in following someone else and accepting his point of view and often displaying frustrated reactions towards others with less insight, should they receive negative feedback on their interactions.

The Type A personality therefore continually wants to be in control. Sometimes, however, in the midst of unrealistic aspirations, he simply does not command the physical, emotional, cognitive and social adjustment mechanisms, with a resultant loss of control which may lead, inter alia, to total helplessness and stress reactions in the form of coronary heart diseases in particular. Rosenman (1974) points out, however, that the behaviour problems of the Type A person should never be likened to those of the neurotic. Sir Peter Medawar (Nobel Prize winner) describes the Type A person as follows: 'Type A's are without doubt the great doers of the world. Even if Type A's lead shorter lives they live more life while they are living it' (in Friedman and Rosenman, 1974, p. iv).

The Type B personality represents behaviour on the opposite behaviour continuum to that of the Type A. Behaviour is characterized by greater work satisfaction, shorter work hours, satisfaction with less compensation, a more relaxed attitude, less competitiveness, more patience, hard work, but without an intense drive and constraint and they do not set such critical time limits. Type B's like to relax and maintain sound interpersonal relationships (Howard et al., 1977).

9.8.2.4 Psycho-logical factors and physical illness (psychosomatic disorders) These conditions, previously also called psychosomatic disorders, refer to the manifestation of physical symptoms as a result of psychological stress and negative emotions. There is sufficient evidence to prove that negative stress and emotions are harmful to physical health, while positive emotions create an increased ability to counteract physical illnesses. In this connection you are familiar with Selye's stress response syndrome (general adaptation syndrome) where he indicates how the nervous and hormonal systems inter alia affect the body during stress. Moreover he maintains that certain lifestyles such as those filled with stress, those that include rich diets, smoking and drinking and little exercise, are additional contributory factors to psycho-physiological diseases. Although a multitude of psycho-physiological symptoms are reported, particularly stomach ulcers, anorexia nervosa, migraine and tension headaches, hypertension and coronary heart diseases are classic examples.

Stomach ulcers are caused by excessive secretion of acids and digestive juices that damage the stomach or intestinal linings. Although diets and other organic conditions can cause stomach ulcers, they are ascribed particularly to emotions such as worry, rage and anxiety. The problem centres in addition on the fact that the physical symptoms are in turn followed by further emotional reactions.

Coronary heart diseases are probably the most frequently related to negative stress conditions. In this connection the A type person is described as having the kind of personality which entails a high risk of coronary heart disease because of a stressful life-style and over-involvement with work, achievement and time.

Psychosomatic problems are among the major work-related problems encountered among managers. In severe cases these conditions can result in death, early retirement, disability, hospitalization or poor health, which leads to losses for both the individual and the organization. The effect of the stress preceding the final condition is equally serious. Apart from the physical discomfort for the individual, there are also psychological and emotional factors with personal and work-related consequences. The relationship between stressors and work—including those linked with psychosomatic conditions—is extensively described in contemporary literature by people like Miner (1966), McClean (1970, 1979), Cooper and Payne (1978, 1980), and Greenwood and Greenwood (1979) and in several magazine articles (Krantz and Raisen (1988), Booth-Kewley and Friedman (1987), Frankenhaeuser and Johansson (1986).

9.8.2.5 *Narcotics problems: Alcohol and drugs* Narcotics problems are caused by alcohol or drug abuse and by physical and psychological dependence on them. Addictive problems may take the form of behaviour problems because of the use of alcohol or drugs; the problems can also be the *after-effects* of the excessive use of some form of addictive drug. Examples of these are the chronic stage of alcoholism where the individual is unable to function effectively at the personal, social and work levels; psychotic conditions because of alcoholism and drug abuse; physical diseases; intellectual deterioration and even death.

Industry in general acknowledges narcotics problems, especially *alcohol problems*, as a 'disease', it understands the cost implications and it designs intensive internal and external programmes to treat workers with alcohol problems and to re-employ rehabilitated persons. On the other hand, the existence of narcotics problems in the work situation is often denied; insensitive interpersonal and managerial conduct contributes little to the recovery or re-utilization of this type of problem worker.

The main personal problem of the alcoholic—and of the drug addict—lies in his *denial* that he is having difficulties. This is probably a reaction to the condemnation by community systems of these types of problems. Such an attitude can have serious consequences in the work situation, for instance in terms of interpersonal relationships, inaccurate work, unimaginativeness, rigid or compulsive perfectionism, absence, poor quality work, accidents, vocational immobility (e.g. the fact that the person makes no progress or refuses to undergo training), and feelings of uncertainty, dependence, and aggression—all of which makes heavy demands on other workers; there are also financial and material losses (Miner and Brewer, in Dunnette, 1976; McClean, 1970; and Miner, 1966). The same inefficient action and interaction occur outside the work situation too, for instance in family and marital problems, financial problems, clashes with the law and traffic offences which, in turn, affect work behaviour.

Different types of *drugs* have different effects. As far as work is concerned the general effect of the abuse of and the dependence on drugs is the same as the effect of alcoholism. However, the excessive use of certain drugs may have even more drastic psychological and physical consequences than in the case of alcohol. Figure 9.3

FIGURE 9.3

Alcoholism: Employee behavioral pattern chart

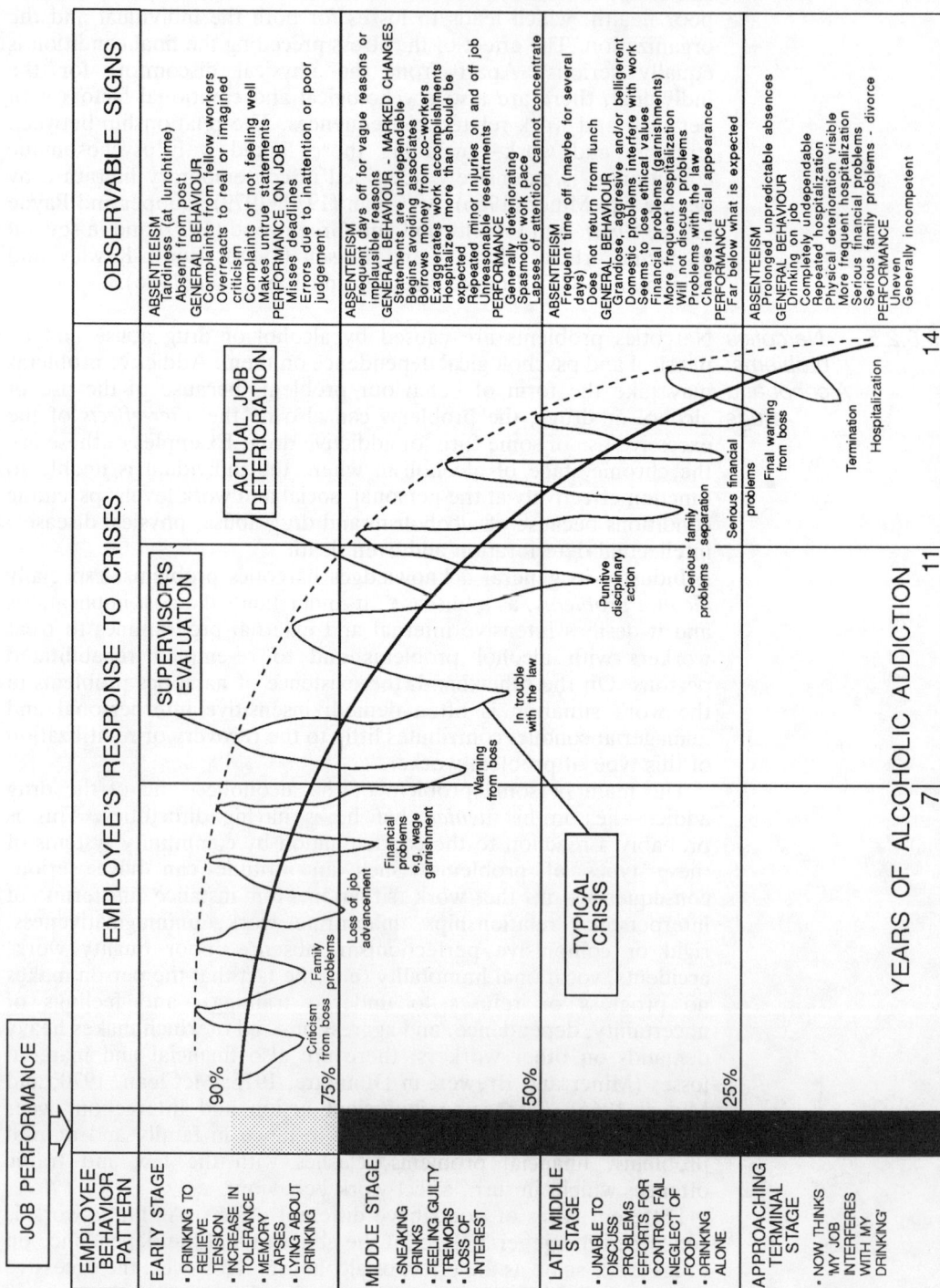

JOB PERFORMANCE

EMPLOYEE BEHAVIOR PATTERN	EMPLOYEE'S RESPONSE TO CRISES	OBSERVABLE SIGNS
EARLY STAGE • DRINKING TO RELIEVE TENSION • INCREASE IN TOLERANCE • MEMORY LAPSES • LYING ABOUT DRINKING	90% Criticism from boss Family problems 75%	**ABSENTEEISM** Tardiness (at lunchtime) Absent from post **GENERAL BEHAVIOUR** Complaints from fellow workers Overreacts to real or imagined criticism Complaints of not feeling well Makes untrue statements **PERFORMANCE ON JOB** Misses deadlines Errors due to inattention or poor judgement
MIDDLE STAGE • SNEAKING DRINKS • FEELING GUILTY • TREMORS • LOSS OF INTEREST	Loss of job advancement Financial problems e.g. wage garnishment Warning from boss	**ABSENTEEISM** Frequent days off for vague reasons or implausible reasons **GENERAL BEHAVIOUR - MARKED CHANGES** Statements are undependable Begins avoiding associates Borrows money from co-workers Exaggerates work accomplishments Hospitalized more than should be expected Repeated minor injuries on and off job Unreasonable resentments **PERFORMANCE** Generally deteriorating Spasmodic work pace Lapses of attention, cannot concentrate
LATE MIDDLE STAGE • UNABLE TO DISCUSS PROBLEMS • EFFORTS FOR CONTROL FAIL • NEGLECT OF FOOD • DRINKING ALONE	50% In trouble with the law Punitive disciplinary action	**ABSENTEEISM** Frequent time off (maybe for several days) Does not return from lunch **GENERAL BEHAVIOUR** Grandiose, aggressive and/or belligerent Domestic problems interfere with work Seems to lose ethical values Financial problems (garnishments) More frequent hospitalization Will not discuss problems Problems with the law Changes in facial appearance **PERFORMANCE** Far below what is expected
APPROACHING TERMINAL STAGE • NOW THINKS 'MY JOB INTERFERES WITH MY DRINKING'	25% Serious family problems - separation Serious financial problems Final warning from boss Termination Hospitalization	**ABSENTEEISM** Prolonged unpredictable absences **GENERAL BEHAVIOUR** Drinking on job Completely undependable Repeated hospitalization Physical deterioration visible More frequent hospitalization Serious financial problems Serious family problems - divorce **PERFORMANCE** Uneven Generally incompetent

ACTUAL JOB DETERIORATION

SUPERVISOR'S EVALUATION

TYPICAL CRISIS

YEARS OF ALCOHOLIC ADDICTION

7   11   14

illustrates the progressive reactions and work behaviour during the different stages of alcohol addiction.

The chart in figure 9.3 depicts the working life of an employee in his chosen field of endeavour after the point of addiction. Compiled from 230 case studies in the aerospace industry, the findings correlate with the studies made by Dr Milton Maxwell of Rutgers University.

The job efficiency per centage rating decreases in direct proportion to the number of years of addiction if a company does not have an Employee Assistance Programme.

Detecting work-performance deterioration is extremely difficult during the first seven years of addiction. Any referrals in this area would be mostly self-referrals.

The area of greatest cover-up is in the seventh to eleventh year of addiction. This is where *early identification* by means of proper documentation and a control programme is most effective because the greatest number of employed alcoholics fall into this category.

As the disease progresses beyond the eleventh year, the alcoholic is no longer able to conceal his illness and he finds work is interfering with his drinking. This also is the area where the employee shows up in the Medical Department with clinically detectable symptoms, and where many valuable employees are dismissed or resign to take up work that is less demanding.

On the right side of the chart you will note the general deterioration pattern that takes place which is *documentable*, such as absenteeism, excessive sick leave, general work performance, attitude and general behaviour.

9.8.2.6   *Organic* In these conditions, which are also known as organic psychoses, the
conditions emphasis is on *biological aetiology*, particularly on the *functioning of*
and mental *the brain*. Treatment is usually based on a medical model, although
retardation coherent behaviour problems and rehabilitation for work definitely belong to psychological and related disciplines. *Organic brain syndromes are characterized by brain damage*, which affects intellectual capabilities and the associated functions either completely or partially. *Mental retardation is characterized by underdeveloped intellectual functioning*. In both cases there are emotional and physical problems apart from the intellectual impediment.

Because of the nature of these conditions, serious problems can make the individual totally *unsuitable for work* in the ordinary labour market. Special posts have to be created for these people, or they can work in sheltered working places during and after rehabilitation. The place of work must often be designed to suit the worker's physical handicap.

The *age psychoses*, where there may be serious or less serious brain dysfunctioning because of physical and psychic processes of change, constitute a special problem area. The problems of older or retired persons are of particular importance for the industry. *Work problems* in this case are due partly to cultural norms, namely that 'old people' are dependent and no longer able to play a productive role, and partly to the individual's subjective feelings about retirement, age and uselessness. Research—for example by Brewer and Miner (in Dunnette, 1976), Eaton (1969) and Welford (1976)—has proved that older workers, although slower from a motor point of view, are still able to work accurately. They may, however, experience problems with memory processes, with the physical demands of the job and with complex abstract intellectual tasks. Perceptual and motor retardation may also be a safety factor, and physical health may be a problem. On the other hand, the writers point out that the older worker can offer better integrated knowledge, greater responsibility, positive work attitudes and management skills. Eaton (1969) refers to the increasing stressors the older manager has to face.

In South Africa the Departments of Health and of Manpower Utilization do much for the mental health and occupational situation of the intellectually handicapped person and worker. Much has been written about these matters in the journal *Rehabilitation in South Africa*. As in the case of other conditions, we find that not all brain dysfunctions make the individual useless for work. In cases where there are specific and localized brain dysfunctions the persons may be fully trainable and capable of occupying a position.

9.8.3 Specific work-related problems We have referred time and again to the influence of stress and other psychological disorders on behaviour at work. The following discussion involves a number of specific work-related adjustment problems which can manifest themselves because of work-related factors or even because of psychological disorders. These difficulties can in turn lead to other problems.

9.8.3.1 Personnel turnover According to Miner and Brewer (in Dunnette, 1976) personnel turnover relates to general *job satisfaction* with regard to organizational and industrial variables. The variables include work attitudes towards managerial practices, the quality and nature of working conditions, remuneration, the worker's feelings on the question of whether management is treating them fairly, and work group attitudes. *Emotional conditions* such as anxiety, depression, neuroses, personality problems, alcohol and drug addiction, physical diseases and age can contribute to personnel turnover.

Personnel turnover is an *expensive* industrial phenomenon. Dalton, Krackhardt and Porter (1981) maintain that it can also be beneficial for the organization. *Functional personnel turnover* comes into question when the organization summarily allows the individual with a negative evaluation to leave. *Dysfunctional turnover* comes into question when the organization allows an individual to go without trying to stop him, although it would like to retain his services. Dalton et al. (1981) point out that this category, together with voluntary, non-voluntary, unavoidable and controllable desertion, has to be taken into account to establish the true effect of personnel turnover.

9.8.3.2 Absenteeism Absence from work is one of the *main indications of organizational stress*, and it involves great costs, especially with regard to the loss of productivity. *Illness*, especially respiratory problems, stomach disorders, gynaecological problems (menstruation, menopause, spontaneous abortions), and stress conditions such as headaches, insomnia, fatigue, heart problems and endocrinal disorders are responsible for most absences. *Other factors* that contribute to absence include dissatisfaction with organizational and work factors, for instance insufficient training and supervision, disturbed work relationships, poor work group cohesion and morale, and the physical job design. Follman (1978) refers to the psychological determinants of absence by describing the following characteristics of persons with an extensive record of absences: uncertainty, stress, self-pity, anxiety, the incidence of compulsive tendencies and phobia, paranoid and schizophrenic qualities, conversion hysteria, neurosis, alcoholism, broken marriages, behaviour that indicates defence, suspicion, unhappiness, the inability to make friends easily, dissatisfaction, hostility and resistance to change.

The problems surrounding personnel turnover and absence from work are further complicated by contemporary issues such as more leisure time and the so-called 'invisible worker', that is, people working from locations away from the work place.

From the literature it also becomes clear that personnel turnover and absence are complex problems and are also closely related. In order to determine effectively in what way these forms of behaviour affect the individual and the organization, more accurate assessment procedures are necessary. There should be a clearer distinction between types of personnel turnover and also different forms of absenteeism in order to plan a more effective course of action.

9.8.3.3 *Industrial* Industrial accidents refer to occurrences in the work place and work
accidents behaviour which may give rise to unsafe working conditions, injuries, death and loss to the worker, his colleagues and the work organization. Research has revealed a strong connection between situational factors and worker behaviour which leads to either the prevention or the occurrence of industrial accidents.

There is the well-known theory of *accident proneness which emphasizes* that particular human characteristics will lead to accidents, no matter how safe the working conditions are. Although this theory also has its followers, people such as Muchinsky (1983) points out that such an assumption is invalid, especially in the light of factors such as intrinsically dangerous work and the influence of factors such as fatigue, alcohol abuse, drug addiction, et cetera. Workers are often also inclined to ignore their safety requirements in order to satisfy other needs. Another factor these days may be that the training of workers, particularly in respect of perception and motor skills, no longer keeps track of the technology of modern work environments. In this respect it has also long since been found that physical work design and equipment can contribute to accidents— especially when physical and psychological fatigue and the time of occurrence is taken into account.

Work situations and organization factors which are associated with accidents include, for instance poor physical working conditions such as lighting and noise, obsolete and unsafe equipment and high-risk tasks, while work attitudes and attitudes towards the organization and management can contribute towards accident-prone behaviour.

Another explanation for the occurrence of accidents is that *particular individual characteristics*, in some situations in particular, may be a *predisposition* for accidents, as is indicated by the following research findings: repetition of accidents take place mainly in the age group seventeen to twenty-eight years, after which it progressively decreases. Older employers may, especially in the light of the decline in perceptual and motor activities, pose a risk as far as work safety is concerned. Miner and Brewer (in Dunnette, 1976) consequently maintain that 'accident proneness' should preferably be interpreted on the basis of temporary personality disorders—particularly at the age of about 30 years. This period in life, for some people perhaps the start of the mid-career crisis, may be accompanied by emotional lability, risky behaviour, and so forth. Hirschfeld and Behan (1963) and also Hill and Trist (1962) have already argued that accidents may be motivated behaviour, for instance self-destructive needs and an attempt to withdraw from the work situation. The combination of specific personality traits and situations which repeatedly lead to accidents, could rather be described as *accident repetitive behaviour*, according to McCormick (1981). Other personality traits which may be associated with industrial accidents are expressed by Miner and Brewer (in Dunnette, 1976) and Miner (1966) as follows: physical handicaps and inefficient task skills; inadequate training; feelings of hate, aggression, et cetera, towards management; depressive and self-destructive tendencies; negative work attitudes; characteristics such as impulsiveness, tenseness, immaturity, social irresponsibility and lack of intimate interpersonal relationships.

Selzer, Rogers and Kern (1968) have found that *stress effects and psychopathology* occur more frequently among drivers who have caused fatal accidents. These psychological problems have been identified as paranoid characteristics, inclinations towards suicide, depression, violent action, social stress (e.g. personal problems and finances), upsetting experiences some time before the accident, and a history of accidents. As far as the last aspect is concerned there is much research that indicates a pattern of repetitive accidents (Miner and Brewer, in Dunnette, 1976).

A so-called theory of *biorhythms* explains industrial accidents on the basis of the interaction between the individual's physical, emotional and cognitive functions. When one of these aspects reaches a low, such as poor cognitive judgement or emotional tension, accidents can occur. Investigations by Carvey and Nibler (1977) and Wolcott et al. (1977) could not confirm this theory.

In respect of the management of and actions regarding industrial accidents, the astronomical costs incurred through bad accident reporting and inadequate criteria are often pointed out. Better selection procedures, more systematic training and improved work design are recommended as possible areas of improvement as regards accident prevention.

9.8.3.4   *Physical* Physical handicaps—caused by factors such as organic brain damage,
           disability accidents, toxic and nutritional influences, and including disabled limbs, blindness, deafness, epilepsy and paralysis—are health problems which may make an individual's general work adjustment very difficult. The problems are partly due to community or 'traditional' *attitudes towards the 'differentness' of a handicapped person*. There are so many prejudices and stereotyped views about handicapped people in the labour market, that we can practically

speak of job reservation for them; they do not have a free choice of vocation. This is contrary to present and past examples of handicapped individuals—for example, blind, deaf, epileptic and crippled people—who have been very successful as people and as professional persons (Miner and Brewer, in Dunnette, 1981). Much progress has been made with *job design* for handicapped persons; this underlines the fact that there should not be unrealistic expectations and demands with regard to competent handicapped workers, even though they display a positive attitude to work. At the employment of a handicapped person, his problems should be evaluated in context, his capabilities and skills have to be considered and he must be utilized optimally, also in terms of job requirements and practical considerations, for instance the safety of the worker and that of other people (Noel, 1990).

According to Anglin (in Dunnette, 1976) orthopaedically handicapped and deaf people have the best *work adjustment*, whereas epileptic cases are the least able to adjust. Miner (1966) points out that any physical disease or ailment—for example, an injury—may have an important effect on a worker's performance. Because of the close relationship between physical and emotional aspects, even temporary physical handicaps may have an intensive emotional effect on the worker. Generally speaking the work adjustment of physically handicapped people is good—better than that of emotionally handicapped people. Absences and accidents do not necessarily occur more often than among other workers, and the personnel turnover is in fact lower than in the case of other groups (Miner, 1966). These findings agree with research in the RSA, as has been reported in several editions of *Rehabilitation in South Africa*.

9.8.3.5 Under-achievement Although divergent criteria make it difficult to define underachievement, it can be manifested as any *behaviour* by an individual who *does not satisfy job requirements and expected standards* in terms of his skills. Underachievement in the job can be caused by all the aetiological factors in an individual, by the organization and the work situation, also by external factors and by the incidence of any of the emotional behaviour problems and psychopathology dealt with in this chapter.

9.8.3.6 Change and work alienation In views on work alienation the emphasis is on the *negative effect of the modern work environment* on the individual. Man, with his need for care, relationships and self-esteem, is increasingly being isolated from meaningful contact with others, and work has lost its intrinsic value for the individual. In the overall process of bureaucratic macro-organizations the individual loses his self-esteem, he feels that he is worth little, and he finds that his physical, social and emotional needs are being sacrificed for the sake of organizational and community objectives. The main reason why some individuals continue to work is because the consequences of unemployment are less pleasant than work. The *reasons* put forward for work alienation include technology, automatization, poor working conditions and managerial practices.

One of the main causes of work alienation and the concomitant stress and psychiatric problems is *changes in the work situation*. These include changes in the physical job design, new management and management processes, technological change, promotion, transferences, change of work, mid-career crisis and the prospect of unemployment.

9.8.3.7 *Work motivation and work attitudes* These two determinants are *mutually inclusive and interactive*. The extent to which the individual's needs have been satisfied determines his inputs in the work and, hence, his attitudes towards the organization and place of work.

Job satisfaction can be a function of the need for achievement, recognition, responsibility, interpersonal relationships and of the physical aspects of the job. Taveggia and Hedley (1976) have found that job specialization may contribute to job dissatisfaction. Other *causative factors* include organization and management processes, supervision, salary and working conditions.

Job dissatisfaction is associated with responses such as physical illness, stress problems such as cardiac diseases, frustration, accidents, absence, change of work, the fear of failure, lower standards of performance and practices that have little connection with the tasks of the job in question.

The individual's job satisfaction and work attitudes—for example, loyalty—can also be a function of the *work group's cohesion and morale*. The individual may find the type of psychological climate in the group which confirms his self-esteem and contributes to behaviour which will promote his own objectives and those of the group. Individual complaints and symptomatic behaviour may be merely the manifestation of the fact that the work group is experiencing stress Payne and Jahbri et al., 1988).

9.8.3.8 *Managerial stress and 'organizational pathology'* We have often referred to the *contextual meaning of mental health*, for instance that the symptom-bearer can have a function for and inside the system. The system, in turn, experiences problems in its interaction with sub-systems and environmental systems.

The *manager* of our present-day large industrial organizations *probably experiences more stressors* than the workers. The *causative factors* can once again be divided into the characteristics of the individual, physical and social work factors and external factors. Intense stress effects are attributed to the manager's position, his roles and the expectations linked to all these factors. Since he is decision-maker, innovator, co-ordinator and risk-taker, the slightest stress may affect his behaviour and, if it is noticeable, it will lead to further stress. Moreover, the manager's work behaviour is usually achievement-oriented, an 'A' type of behaviour which is an indication of the incidence of cardiac diseases (Raelin, 1984).

Eaton (1969) mentions *five factors* which cause problems, especially in *older managers*:

- the realization of limited possibilities for progress;
- the achievement of a long-expected or idealized career objective;
- increasing isolation and narrowing interest;

- the realization of their approaching retirement; and
- the early incidence of emotional and psychiatric symptoms associated with a high age.

The manager finds himself in the position where the climate for the incidence of emotional stress, physical and even psychiatric problems is optimal. Because of the manager's qualities, his adjustment mechanisms operate well initially, but he is inclined to overtax these mechanisms. Consequently any warnings usually appear too late.

The organization is also subject to the influences and changes affecting the individual. The complex structures and processes in the organization are frequently the reason why it cannot adjust rapidly enough to change. In other words, its regulating and retentive functions may be the cause of its downfall (Parker and De Cottiis, 1983; Krantz, 1985).

According to Herman (1963) and Krantz (1985) the *organization in conflict*—and its management—experiences the following organizational and individual problems:

- an increase in withdrawal behaviour (dissatisfaction, low production, absence and personnel turnover);
- an increase in and an intensification of conflict situations;
- fewer communication channels;
- an increase in authority structures, so that only a few people take part in decision-making;
- greater stress for authority figures as the authority becomes more centralized;
- authority figures evade responsibilities as the stress increases;
- a decline in standards because of the stress effects on authority figures;
- the further reduction of communication channels;
- increasing conflict between management and other units in the organization;
- more people withdraw from tasks and activities because of the increasing conflict;
- fewer communication channels for the collection and distribution of information as the conflict and problems increase;
- the further increase of conflicts and withdrawal behaviour as organizational standards become even lower;
- the reduction of specific communication will lead to further withdrawal and less available information; and
- the withdrawal of any section will cause even fewer communication channels.

These sequential crisis factors illustrate that *organizational and individual problems are interrelated* and that diagnosis and intervention have to take both into account.

Finally you should note that the above-mentioned problem areas are not the only ones. Aspects such as guest labourers' problems (culturally-strange people), the problems of women in the labour market, older and new workers can constitute separate fields of study. Other aspects that can be discussed as problem areas include managerial policy, management functions and technology, mentioned earlier as aetiology.

9.8.4 **Other problem areas**

The following phenomena are discussed because of the recent emphasis on these in recent scientific and popular literature.

9.8.4.1 Workaholism

Like the phenomena of work alienation, burnout and the Type A personality, workaholism also refers to a *particular type of involvement* with work. Like the others, the term 'workaholism' is also still only vaguely and indistinctly defined and, like them, the existence of this behaviour manifestation is accepted by some authors while others dismiss workaholism as a socially fabricated symptom (Machlowitz, 1978). Both Kahn (1981) and Oates (1971), for instance, associate workaholism with work addiction, namely a compulsion or irrepressible need to work continually. Kahn (1981), however, distinguishes between workaholism and work addiction in the sense that he argues that where the work addict enjoys his work, the workaholic is totally unable to manage his work time effectively. Gherman (1981) also describes workaholism as a stress reaction under pressure of time and also as a defence mechanism that is employed in an attempt to associate work overload with success, while it is in fact a withdrawal reaction, for instance to unpleasant domestic problems or an inability to relax. Gherman portrays the workaholic's actions as aimless toil and labour, since the workaholic never really masters his work. Machlowitz (1978), perhaps one of the few experts in this field, differs from those who over-emphasize the time factor. According to her the nature of the workaholic's actions is such that time, and more specifically uninterrupted time, is hard to determine. The workaholic should rather be recognized by his relationship with work, namely by the fact that the workaholic works more than is in any way necessary. The workaholic's work load never decreases. Machlowitz (1978) outlines the following characteristics of the workaholic:

Workaholics

- are intense, energetic, competitive and drive themselves—the motivation for this is not necessarily financial gain, it can also be knowledge or purely competition;
- seriously doubt their own abilities—hard work can be an attempt to compensate for inabilities, often in spite of an apparent attitude of self-confidence and arrogance;
- prefer work to relaxation—they hate being away from work, find weekends and holidays depressing and fear the day of retirement—the workaholic will use any place to work;
- use their time efficiently—sleep no more than six hours, often combine meals with work, try to save time, for instance they do not easily wait for elevators, use note books, computers, et cetera, to organize their work and time;
- draw no clear distinction between their work and recreation activities; if they do have hobbies or take part in activities such as jogging, it is carried out with the same intensity as their work.

In order to determine what the consequences of workaholism are for the individual's physical and psychological wellbeing will still require much research. According to Machlowitz (1978) the workaholic does not work purely and simply for a particular compensation and is not necessarily a very successful worker. It becomes evident that the workaholic will doubtlessly experience interpersonal problems—at home as a result of the fact that he neglects his family and cannot participate in leisure activities, while the workaholic, as a result of his full work programme, also has little time for friends. Workaholism is also described as a life-long, virtually unchangeable phenomenon. If we should believe in Selye's general adaptation syndrome and in addition compare the workaholic with the Type A personality, it appears indisputable that the workaholic must be subjected to immense physical and psychological stress reactions.

9.8.4.2 *Burnout* In respect of work behaviour the meanings given to this term are at present still controversial as well as vague and varied (Muldary, 1983), Odendaal and Van Wyk (1988), Eisenstat and Felna (1984), Jones (1982). In the field of clinical psychology the term 'burnt child syndrome', for instance, refers to previous intense emotional experiences, with the result that the child—and later the adult—reacts with great difficulty to any emotional stimuli, such as affection (Klopfer et al., 1954).

As initially defined by Freudenberger (1974) and confirmed by later research, burnout refers to work overload which influences the work behaviour and physical and mental health of workers. This was found particularly in the case of people-oriented groups such as medical practitioners, nurses, psychologists and attorneys. Maslach's definition (in Muldary, 1983, p. 11) of this phenomenon shows that a combination of symptoms, behaviour and attitudes can be involved. 'The loss of concern for the people with whom one is working include physical exhaustion and characterized by an emotional exhaustion in which the professional no longer has any positive feelings, sympathy, or respect for clients or patients.'

The definition of Muldary (1983, p. 12), as well as that of Veninga and Spradley, Edelwich and Brodsky and that of Cherniss (in Muldary, 1983) all contain aspects of the above definition, namely physical, psychological and social exhaustion or burnout, which influence physical and mental health.

It also becomes clear from the literature that burnout and work stress are not synonymous; admittedly burnout can be a symptom of stress, although stress need not necessarily result in burnout.

Table 9.2 (from Muldary, 1983, p. 6) illustrates the wide range of physical, psychological and behaviour problems that can be associated with burnout.

Gherman (1981) also discusses burnout as a more general condition when management and the organization are no longer effective. In the individual this incapacity at work can lead to increased use of alcohol and drugs, as well as deterioration of cognitive, emotional and social skills and difficulties with co-workers and marital conflicts.

TABLE 9.2

Signs and symptoms of burnout

PHYSICAL	PSYCHOLOGICAL	BEHAVIOURAL
Fatigue	Feelings:	Dehumanization of patients
Sleep disturbances:	Anger	Victimization of patients
Difficulty sleeping	Boredom	Fault finding
Difficulty in getting up	Frustration	Blaming others
	Depression	Defensiveness
Stomach ailments	Discouragement	Impersonal, stereotyped communication with patients
Tension headaches	Disillusionment	
Migraine headaches	Despair	Applying derogatory labels to patients
Gastrointestinal problems	Apathy	
	Guilt	Physical distancing from patients and others
Frequent colds	Anxiety	
Lingering colds	Suspicion/Paranoia	Withdrawal
Frequent bouts of flu	Helplessness	Isolation
Backaches	Pessimism	Stereotyping patients
Nausea	Irritability	Postponing patient contacts
Muscle tension	Resentment	Going increasingly by the book
Shortness of breath	Hopelessness	Clock watching
Malaise	Attitudes	Living for breaks
Frequent injuries	Cynicism	Absenteeism
Weight loss	Indifference	Making little mistakes
Weight gain	Resignation	Unnecessary risk taking
Stooped shoulders	Self-doubt	Use of drugs and alcohol
Weakness	Other	Marital and family conflict
Change of eating habits	Loss of empathy	Conflict with co-workers
	Difficulty concentrating	Workaholism and obsessiveness
		Use of humour as a buffer from emotions
	Difficulty attending efficiency	Decreased job efficiency
	Moodiness	Suicide
	Decreased sense of self-worth	Overcommitment or undercommitment

Gherman (1981, p. 41) also gives a description of organizational burnout which is particularly characterized by the following symptoms:

- high personnel turnover;
- increased absenteeism;
- scapegoats are often looked for;
- a style of dependence which manifests as anger towards supervision and feelings of helplessness and despair;

- group conflicts and group coalitions;
- critical attitudes towards co-workers;
- lack of co-operation between workers;
- a lack of initiative;
- increased job dissatisfaction;
- negativism in respect of the role of work groups.

9.8.4.3 Women at work and dual career couples The role of women at work, in the midst of themes such as the dualistic role of the women as mother and worker, discrimination against women in the work situation, women's liberation movements, et cetera, always has been and still is a controversial issue. An important point of criticism is that women at work are repeatedly and often studied on the basis of research which has been carried out on the world of the male worker and comparisons are made with male workers . A further controversy exists because female work roles are often tinged by the cultural definition of the woman as in the first place being a mother and then being a worker. Many of the stereotypes of the female work-force, compensation and entry into certain professions as well as conflicts and adjustment problems of women in the work situation can be traced back to the above-mentioned two issues. It has, for instance, been argued that women who have a fear of success, are not sufficiently task-orientated and are not work motivated. Although greater parity is at present being reached, remuneration for women in equivalent posts to men is still often unequal and particular work problems such as higher personnel turnover, absenteeism, physical illness and problems with relation-ships (for example the phenomenon of 'sexual harassment') are still being dealt with in terms of the woman's particular roles and characteristics.

The tremendous increase of the number of women in the work place, in a large number of posts including management positions, is a reality which from its very nature brings its own problems and also requires a changed philosophy and poses new research challenges. Levitan and Johnson (1982) calculate that in 1981 approximately 70 million women were working, as against a mere ten million in 1900. Carone (1978) already indicated at the time that in the USA alone about 27 600 000 children under the age of eighteen were growing up in households where both parents worked. The more significant presence of the woman in the work place also raises questions on other levels. The man may experience greater tension, amongst others as a result of compulsory early retirement. On the other hand the woman has the task of holding her own at home and at work, and then there is increased tension brought about by competing on an equal footing, learning new skills, for example on management level, et cetera. In his book 'Women at work', Joseph (1983) deals with specific problems which the working woman experiences, including the following, which arise particularly as a result of the traditional role that has been assigned to the woman:

- inability to give orders
- fear of risky behaviour
- passivity—waiting for someone else to do things for her
- inability to deal with rejection

- fear of authority
- fear of competition
- confusion in respect of sexuality and the role it plays in the work place
- inability to utilize criticism to her own advantage
- the need to take care of and be available at all times
- the inability to comprehend the art of delegating and team work

The woman's active role at work, together with all the accompanying health and mental health risks, is also likely to give rise to increases in the so-called 'stress diseases', such as heart problems, increased addictive habits, for example smoking, alcohol and drugs; marital and family problems, depression and suicide.

The increasing phenomenon of dual career couples, either in professional groups or other income types, also creates special adjustment problems. Stress is created by work overload and conflict between work roles and family roles and responsibilities. In our times there is a need for counselling such couples to restructure expectations and roles in order to create better work and life satisfaction for all parties involved.

9.9 MANAGING WORK ADJUSTMENT

In practice, also in scientific and popular literature, work adjustment problems are too often only coupled to stress management. Although such programmes are important, it is not the only method and can be an over-simplification of mental health management.

For the purposes of this chapter the *management of mental health refers to* the whole process of preventing problems and of the treatment and the utilization or re-utilization of the worker, the problem worker or the individual suffering from the effects of stress or some form of diagnosed psychopathological symptom. In a more restricted sense it can refer specifically to the management of the problem worker, in which case we are more concerned with corrective action. *Behaviour change* is used as a blanket term to refer to any technique or approach (intervention) for the influencing (rehabilitation or treatment) of people exhibiting symptomatic behaviour so that the behaviour of the individual or the group will change and their functioning become more effective. *Manpower utilization* is a process associated with behaviour change functions. It can either be part of the functions or include specific methods to improve, for instance, the utilization of the problem worker's potential in his situation.

There are *various approaches* to the management of mental health, for instance the preventive, diagnostic and remedial (or corrective) approaches. Some authors differentiate between primary, secondary and tertiary functions in the remedial approach. Steinmetz (1969) differentiates between preventive, therapeutic, self-development and disciplinary measures in the management of the problem worker. Newman and Beehr (1979) differentiate between personal, organizational and external procedures for the management of work stress. In this regard also take note of the classifications by Cooper and Payne (1978, 1980), Warshaw (1979), Greenwood and Greenwood (1979) and McClean (1979). In their systems model for the management of work stress Greenwood and Greenwood emphasize that the individual, the organization and the community all play a role at the different levels of mental health management.

You will find that although the principles, techniques and objectives may differ, it is not always possible or necessary to differentiate between, say, preventive or corrective interventions—either of them implies the other too.

9.9.1 Personal or self-management strategies These coping mechanisms are integrated, in modern literature, into the so-called 'coping' theories. According to these theories the individual has different intrinsic and extrinsic coping resources to handle stress and hindrances. These resources include personality dispositions as well as cognitive, emotional and direct and indirect coping behaviour (Pearlin and Schooler, 1978; Folkman, 1984; Ashford, 1988).

We have pointed out that if we believe the individual to be capable of development, he is also *capable of helping himself if he knows himself*, his body and his psychological responses. The individual must be given responsibility, and experience for himself that change is possible or that it is taking place in himself or in his systems. Personal coping mechanisms are the individual's skills in handling responses or behaviour which change, evade or channel the effect of either the factors within himself (internally) or external stressors, so that their effect will be more beneficial to himself and his environment. These adjustment mechanisms can include the following:

- The individual must have an understanding of aetiological factors (stressors) in himself, the organization and the external environment.
- The individual must know himself and his physical and psychological responses to stressors. According to Greenwood and Greenwood (1979) this means that the individual must know and experience the pros and cons of stress. In other words, he has to understand Hans Selye's general adaptation syndrome so that he will be able to monitor his psychophysical responses.
- The individual can take steps to identify his strong and weak points, for instance by means of medical examinations, psychological evaluation, therapeutic procedures and self-analysis.
- On the basis of these evaluation processes the individual can plan his daily objectives and activities, for instance his rate of activities, his social activities, the people whom he wishes to associate with, and financial affairs. His planning amounts to the determination of needs (e.g. in terms of Maslow's hierarchy) so that he can arrange his activities in order of priority.

Personal strategies to manage psychological stressors or their effects could include the following:

- He could work toward the acquisition or improvement of *interpersonal skills* in order to make interaction with people more effective. This can include the clear expression of feelings, frank and open communication, self-assertive action, sensitivity (warmth, empathy and congruence) towards personal and other people's behaviour, decision-making, and the handling of conflict. The individual can reinforce these social skills by being aware of his conduct, by participating in development groups and by working on it in individual conversations (e.g. therapy).

- *Physical and psychological adjustment techniques* which the individual can easily teach himself. The techniques include progressive relaxation (Jacobson), autogenetic training (Schultz), self-oriented relaxation (Fink, in Greenwood and Greenwood, 1979), and physical exercises, controlled breathing, positive thinking, meditation, self-hypnosis and physical therapy.
- *Biological feedback processes*, which include steps by which the individual can determine how his body responds to stress or how it has already responded. It can take the form of an ordinary medical examination, or techniques such as training in biological feedback by means of feedback thermometers, the electromyograph, the electroencephalograph, the psychogalvanometer, et cetera.
- The *avoidance and control of stressors* or environments which the individual knows will cause stress.
- *Counselling or therapeutic techniques*, which can be valuable for the individual. By learning the principles of therapeutic approaches—for example, consciousness of his own and other people's transactions and interactions, self-assertion, responsibility, relaxing techniques, psychological desensitization, and listening and response skills—the individual can learn to help himself, especially by responding to the reactions or problems of others.

In most of the literature we find particular applications of self-help programmes which include certain aspects of the individual or personal strategies mentioned above. The purpose of the 'Self Directed Search' described by Holland (1973) is a personal vocational and self-evaluation by the individual. Suinn (1976) has designed a behaviour modification programme for 'A' type of behaviour (coronary heart diseases), and Gavin (1977) regards self-help programmes for the management of stress as an excellent management technique.

The purpose of personal or self-management programmes should be the optimal functioning of the individual in order to actualize his or her potential and overcome obstacles in life more effectively.

There are also other techniques that can produce positive results for the personal management of stress. They include diets, a change of environment (e.g. changing one's job), training, a change in work methods, better sleeping habits, holidays, and even increased stress, such as more work or exercise.

9.9.2 Behaviour change in the work situation: Organizational strategies As we said earlier, occupational mental health includes a management policy or philosophy about the responsibility for occupational adjustment and action. Thus the emphasis here is on steps that will make the interaction between individual and organization or the resemblance between individual and work optimal or congruent. Miner and Brewer (in Dunnette, 1981) refer to this as a *control model* which they base on the setting of criteria for measuring (identifying) occupational maladjustment so as to permit corrective interventions in the workers' conduct. The authors describe four steps of a programme for the *reduction of ineffective work behaviour*, namely:

- the selection of people for employment in whom the risk of failure is low
- the determination of work standards so that poor achievement will not occur easily
- the identification of causative factors and the immediate implementation of corrective procedures
- the dismissal of poor achievers as soon as they have been identified

Steinmetz (1969) regards the management of occupational maladjustment (underachievement) as a planning function which forms part of the management policy. He uses the term 'management by objectives' for the identification of underachievers. This implies that the *worker's objectives have to be included* in the organizational policy and objectives, and that management plays an important role in the achievement and evaluation of these objectives. We briefly summarize the steps described by Steinmetz:

- Define the organizational requirements and objectives.
- Make the worker's responsibilities with regard to the organizational objectives clear.
- There must be consensus between employer and employee about the latter's objectives in relation to the global organizational objectives.
- This means that the employee has certainty about what he should do to perform satisfactorily, and that management has a definite structure for evaluating the worker's achievements.
- Management must support the worker in his endeavour to satisfy the predetermined criteria for achievement.
- The worker's achievements must be compared with his objectives.
- Management has to discuss the worker's achievements with him.

Steinmetz believes that, as far as underachievement is concerned, management by objectives has the advantage that management is actively involved and that the worker fulfils a *self-therapeutic role*, as it were. In other words, it is an approach by which conflicts between organization and worker can be reduced, since not only the organization's production objectives, but also the individual's needs are recognized (Steinmetz, 1969).

The planning, policy and management with regard to occupational mental health are increasingly regarded as an integral part of modern management in the organization as a socio-technical system. In this regard you should establish in your studies on health disciplines the extent to which this thesis is true, in South Africa as well; you should also determine what the extent of your involvement as a health worker should be.

Greenwood and Greenwood (1979) mention the following principles which relate to the systems approach:

- the impossibility (uselessness) of working with isolated symptoms in the organization and not considering their effect on the whole system

- the necessity of knowing, in terms of diagnostic functions, what is presently happening in the organization before interventions are undertaken
- the noting by management of an organization of the nature of every organizational system, sub-system and system element, and of the circular nature of interaction and feedback in the relationships between these

In other words, the *effective management of mental health and positive work adjustment, high achievement and organizational success are functions of effective organizational functioning*. This means that vocational maladjustment will be minimized if optimum use is made of the individual by means of the normal personnel and management functions, and if his adjustment to particular work environments is optimal. In other words, many of the staff and organizational functions are nothing less than preventive and even corrective methods to combat occupational maladjustment. Many writers refer to the change or revision of personnel and organizational processes, structures, policies and programmes in order to create a better climate for work adjustment (Newman & Beehr, 1979; Cooper & Payne, 1978, 1980; Warshaw, 1979; McClean, 1979; Greenwood & Greenwood, 1979; Schafer, 1987; Murphy, 1984; Rinas and Clyne-Jackson, 1988).

Meltzer and Wickert (in Newman and Beehr, 1979) believe that, despite many efforts to establish good management techniques, organizations (and probably the larger community) are still 'dehumanizing' (p. 35), and thus responsible for a major part of the individual's stress.

We can make the following classification of organizational strategies that involve individual and organizational functioning, which can be preventive, remedial and rehabilitative, and which apply to the management of mental health in the work, the biological and the psychosocial context:

Organizational and work structures and processes

Evaluation and employment procedures

These procedures are used to *place the right person in the right post* by means of man and job descriptions. An effective employment policy provides for task and worker specifications, determines minimum cut-off points and considers the applicant's early work history so as to predict or identify the potential for successful work behaviour or for problems. Further requirements include familiarity with the diagnostic symptoms of psychopathology or underachievement, and a sound training in diagnostic measuring instruments. Through ineffective selection a certain type of person may be placed in a post which requirements will precipitate underlying psychopathology. Effective employment procedures must include a *policy* on such matters as promotion, transference and job rotation. Caplan et al. (in Newman and Beehr, 1979) feel that it is essential for organizations to have identification programmes by which stress and other mental health problems can be identified at an early stage. Such a programme should also include the OD-techniques, according to which the physical and social job design can be changed. In all cases the complete and accurate 'diagnosis' of problems is essential for the planning of effective and appropriate interventions. Gowler and Legge (in Cooper and Payne, 1980) maintain that *evaluation processes can also constitute stressors*, since the individual is weighed against success or efficiency criteria to which he tries to adjust. This means that his failures and shortcomings may be pointed out to him from an external source, which obviously causes anxiety, frustration and aggression.

Training and development

Training and development programmes can have a major preventive function. As we explained individual traits and capabilities can be important factors in maladjustment. The worker who is incapable of fulfilling the task requirements may defend himself by means of typical responses such as anxiety and aggression, which, in turn, give rise to symptoms such as absences and accidents. A sound management policy makes provision for definite training requirements at different levels so that the worker will be familiar with all the work requirements, both physically and psychologically. In the section on aetiology we referred to the negative effect of such things as role overload, role conflict, role ambivalence, and few opportunities for participation and decision-making. In organizational development functions we must constantly take note of the possibilities for *job expansion and enrichment* so as to offer the worker sufficient opportunities. Few organizations have specific training programmes for underachievers or vocationally maladjusted workers. If there are such programmes, they are frequently based on the same principles as ordinary training programmes. In many organizations, however, there are specific programmes for certain problem areas, for instance for physically and culturally deprived persons and for alcoholics. It frequently happens that organizations co-operate with external bodies in this regard, for instance with institutions for the treatment of alcoholics and sheltered work environments for emotionally and physically handicapped persons. This type of training borders on (or may actually be) clinical-therapeutic. A major problem when such rehabilitated persons are re-employed is that they have acquired their experience in a simulated situation, with the result that their chances of adjusting to the realistic work environment are slight.

The matter of *career development* is an important aspect of training and development. Much of the recent literature (Leibowitz and Schlossberg, 1981; Meckel, 1981); Hill (1981); Sussal and Djakian (1988); Reddy (1987), emphasize the therapeutic role of the manager in personnel counselling and career development. In this regard preparation for the problems of management, working at an advanced age, and retirement is essential. A particular emphasis within the career developmental approach is the so-called self-management approach. On the practical level the emphasis is on the worker's ability to take control of his own occupational progress, thereby being able to handle greater responsibility and change and to cope with more stress more easily.

From the viewpoint of an optimalization model it is also possible to reason that for excellent functioning the worker must be supported if he is to actualize his potential even better. In this regard Cilliers

(1984) has developed a managerial development programme based on the forming of more sensitive relationships, a dimension of psychological optimality.

Training in health and aspects of mental health

The training of management, workers and everyone else in health and aspects of mental health is probably the most important element of any mental health programme. Such an *educational programme must contain information about possible general causes, symptoms and effects and about the nature of particular conditions such as alcoholism, drug addiction and accidents. It must also be aimed at the attitudes of management, the worker and other people involved, for instance workers' unions. Training in interpersonal and communication skills* and factors such as *self-assertive behaviour* and the *handling of conflict* and stress management can be very valuable for every worker and especially for management in personal adjustment behaviour and in the handling of problems. If a better understanding of, and more sensitivity towards, mental health problems can be created, these factors will perform a therapeutic role.

In this regard the use of group techniques such as T-groups, and sensitivity training can be mentioned as methods of improving mutual understanding in relationships. This type of training has the advantage that management, for instance supervisors, are better able to handle problem cases, which implies that the stressors in the individual's social work roles are reduced.

Change in the physical and social work environment

Change in the worker's physical and social work environment can contribute to *greater congruence between the individual and his work*. According to Herzberg, physical and social working conditions can easily lead to dissatisfaction. Unless management makes changes, the individual will respond with absences, work errors, accidents, resignations and negative attitudes.

As far as possible, the *physical work environment must be ergonomically designed* to suit capabilities of the individual, the physically sound or the physically handicapped worker. To further prevent physical and psychic fatigue, matters such as lighting, noise, pollution, safety, work methods, rest periods, shift work and flexitime—apart from the best fit between man and machine—must be carefully considered.

Changes in the *social design of the work* can include matters such as supervisor-worker interaction, the consideration of the workers' preferences in physical job design, opportunities for decision-making and participation, job expansion and enrichment, and recognition of and awards for achievements and services rendered.

Health and mental health facilities

In most work organizations the *medical staff* play an important role. Their services vary from medical examinations for selection, medical guidance and treatment for physical ailments to chemotherapy for stress conditions. Some organizations have *internal health facilities* such as clinics, rehabilitation centres, workshops for sheltered labour and placement services. Organizations frequently follow *a team approach* in which medical, psychological, psychiatric, nursing, social and other services are offered. Apart from *therapeutic services*, preventive services such as *health education* may also be offered. In most cases, however, organizations make use of *external* social health services and of the services of private organizations and persons. Private persons are frequently used in the case of severe psychopathology where the patients are *referred* to them or placed with them for rehabilitation. These services should be extended to include matters such as recreation and physical health programmes, as well as training in and educational programmes on relevant health affairs. The systemic nature of behaviour influencing frequently makes it imperative to involve the worker's other systems in the rehabilitation programmes, for instance his family, spouse or relatives.

In recent times, also in South Africa, much emphasis is placed on the so-called employee assistance programmes. In these multi-disciplinary programmes the emphasis is on health and to assist the problem employee to stay productive in his work situation, without unnecessarily leaving the work place (Dickman, Challenger et al., 1988).

Labour relations for health care management

Industrial psychology and existing organizational theories emphasize the interaction between employer and employee in terms of roles, mainly, then expectations, abilities, objectives and needs in the process of achieving personal and business objectives. Modern organizational theory still does not provide for an employer-employee interaction based on mutual rights (Keeley, 1988). This results in the employer, but more so the individual employee, often being at a disadvantage, for example, in cases of work loss, poor production and bargaining sessions. For protection and his own well-being the employee therefore joins a union and thereby ensures that his rights and relationships are determined and managed in a fair and orderly way.

Labour relationships, as part of more extensive industrial relations, aims at labour peace by maintaining co-operative relationships between employer, employee or unions and Government. Such beneficial relationships or interaction, which also includes physical and psychological well-being, is maintained by certain rules and regulations, for example during resolution of conflict or differences. Handling of grievances or conflict between employees, unions and employers is managed by a negotiation process known as collective bargaining. Labour relations—influencing factors, legal aspects, grievance procedures, conflict management, etc.—is a separate field of study and cannot be dealt with in full in this chapter. Suffice it to say that labour relations and their management by the different parties has important implications for the quality of work life and the employee's general well-being.

As indicated in 9.5 employees have certain needs. As individuals, being contracted to work in a certain capacity, they have the right to such physical, social and psychological working conditions which will enhance an optimal quality of work life. Such expectations might be:

- fair and humane treatment

- adequate compensation
- reasonable leave benefits
- safe physical working conditions
- challenging and interesting work
- freedom of speech and participation
- opportunities for growth and development
- access to management

Coupled to such needs it is also recognized internationally that employees have certain rights, for instance the rights to work, to be trained, to enjoy protection, freedom of association, to negotiate and the right to strike. By the same token the employer also enjoys certain rights which must also be respected by the employee or union. These may be:

- determining of policy and procedures
- determining of pay structures
- setting of work standards
- setting organizational objectives
- management of the organization;
- providing and changing of facilities.

The management of labour relations and the part played by unions especially has particular implications for organizational management for instance on employment practices, supervising, training, assessment of workers, communication structures, remuneration policies, promotion and disciplinary procedures. The quality of labour relations in an organization has definite influences on productivity, motivation, work satisfaction, personnel turnover, absenteeism, feelings of loyalty, security, etc. The costs of physical damages, loss of work hours, injuries and even deaths can be calculated, but the costs and hardships of psychological pain (fear, anxiety, depression, etc.) can never be assessed, sometimes having continuous and long-lasting effects.

It is essential for health care workers and management to be able to identify and handle conflict, thus utilizing it constructively and avoiding the destructive powers of conflict. It is a fact that the cornerstones of creativity and productivity can be in the constructive use of conflict and differences. According to Robbins (1989) symptoms of conflict can be as follows:

- counter productive acts such as strikes and stay-aways
- verbal and physical aggression
- continuous grievances
- poor communication
- high absenteeism
- many industrial accidents and even sabotage
- poor motivation and work attitudes
- high personnel turnover
- low productivity
- more trespassing and disciplinary cases
- mutual strife and rigid attitudes

A further input from management could be the establishment of proper grievance procedures and policies thereby ensuring that all parties at least know how to act technically correctly in such cases.

The influence of unions on health care organizations is now a reality and will increase. Being labour intensive, human resources managers of health care institutions will have to be more effective, especially in the field of labour relations. For this reason more research on the relationship between labour forces and health care management is essential (Huszczo and Fried, 1988).

9.9.3 Therapeutic or counselling approaches In relevant sources you will find that there are *various approaches* to psychotherapy or counselling. This implies that the interventions of helpers will be based on different assumptions and on different evaluation techniques. You will find applications for the various types of therapeutic techniques in the chapters on specific problem areas.

The fact that a therapist supports a specific approach or technique may cause him to be a *rigid* helper and the therapy to be a closed system. *It is impossible to use the same approach or technique for all the clients or symptoms.* One has to realize that every person's problems or symptoms manifest themselves in a unique manner and that they have a particular function in the context of his conduct, for instance in the family, towards his wife, the supervisor or in the work group. The aim of therapeutic or counselling techniques should be to plan appropriate and *purposeful intervention* and to implement it consistently, always in terms of the client's (individual's, work group's) behaviour, its context and its meaning. In a more specific sense we can say that one *has to determine what type of intervention at what time* (crucial point for a change) *and place by which 'helper' will be the most effective for a particular client.*

Irrespective of the therapist's premiss, effective *therapy* in practice is always based—to a greater or lesser extent—on the following *principles*:

- Therapy is a process of events through the medium of the interpersonal relationship that can be defined between therapist and client.
- The relationship between therapist (helper) and client(s) can be regarded as a therapeutic system with all the special systemic qualities. The nature of the processes in this system can determine the client's development and the therapist's effectiveness.
- The therapist-client relationship should create a psychological climate in which the therapist acts in such a way that the client will experience and recognize his self-esteem, that he will be able to speak about the things that are important to him, and that he will experience the possibility and reality of change.
- The essential conditions for an optimal psychological climate can be described as follows:
  - acceptance of and respect for the client as a person without prejudices and external frames of reference
  - positive esteem for the client's positive mental health—in other words, for the fact that the client has potential that can be developed and which he can personally help to develop
  - empathetic understanding for the client's verbal and non-verbal behaviour and the ability to communicate the empathy to the client, also with regard to what is happening in the therapeutic situation

— honesty and congruence, which implies that the therapist can be spontaneous, genuine and transparent (open) about himself and in his relationship with the client, without the facade of defences or a 'therapeutic' role, so that the client will also be able to act congruently

— concreteness, which is the helper's skill in transmitting his messages clearly, specifically and unambiguously so that the client will understand exactly what he means

— a facilitating by the therapist of the therapeutic process intentionally and purposefully, so that the behaviour will develop in the direction of the therapeutic—and, hence the client's—objectives

• Skilled use by the therapist of interpersonal and other skills purposefully and strategically to achieve the objectives of the therapy.

• All the above-mentioned points presuppose that the therapist has certain interpersonal and communication skills. They include accommodation or the creation of rapport, skills to initiate a relationship and to obtain credit from the client, listening, verbal and non-verbal responsive skills, skills to structure the therapy, confrontation and diagnostic skills, and skills to terminate therapy. Note that these skills are not propagated for clinical psychologists only. People like Neff (1977), Steinmetz (1969), Leibowitz and Schlossberg (1981), and Meckel (1981) maintain that these and other therapeutic skills are essential for effective personnel counselling and communication.

With all this information in mind, we can compile the following *definition of therapy*:

Therapy is the process (system) of purposeful reciprocal communication in the interpersonal relationship between two or more persons. Therapy or counselling takes place through verbal and non-verbal interactions during which the helper collects, exchanges and evaluates certain information under certain essential conditions by means of purposeful and planned interpersonal strategies and techniques in order to facilitate optimal behaviour and attitude changes in the client.

The writer believes that although counselling may have other fields of application, and perhaps another type of client, the underlying processes and principles are exactly the same as for therapy. At this stage we can hardly differentiate between therapy and counselling, especially if we consider the fact that in most of the so-called counselling problems—for example vocational uncertainty and mid-life crises—the real problem is emotional and not a simple matter of information or a lack of information. Furthermore, any vocational problem requires the individual to have certain choice, decision-making and other relational skills. If he has failed to acquire them over a long period, if he has learned them wrongly, or if he does not have these skills at all, he will have problems in his present interactions.

To a greater or lesser extent the health worker (if he wishes to become involved in the management of mental health as a helper) and the vocational, career and rehabilitation counsellor need the same skills as the therapist. As we said earlier, everyone in the work situation, but especially the supervisor, the personnel officer and the manager, play an important 'therapeutic role'. There should be training in therapeutic skills—or at least in more effective interviewing skills—at every level.

The necessity of counselling and therapeutic facilities for the worker is emphasized by writers like Sternhagen (1969), Berg (1970), Green (1974), Neff (1977), Bolton and Jaques (1978), Noland (1973) and Follman (1978). The need for these services is strong in the case of psychopathological and adjustment problems, but also in matters such as the collection of information, career progress and development, performance assessment counselling, exit interviews, group conflicts and financial counselling. Some writers emphasize the importance of mental health and rehabilitation programmes with a multi-disciplinary approach, and also the mutual responsibility and participation of all parties—the worker, the supervisor, management, work unions and the community (Noland, 1973; Kane, 1975; Bolton and Jaques, 1978).

Apparently individual and group therapeutic work is rarely done in the work situation, except in a few organizations where clinical, counselling or therapeutic psychologists have been appointed. In most cases individuals are *referred* to outside organizations, or psychologists are appointed internally on a session basis. There are many reasons for there being so few therapeutic facilities, for instance: there are people who perform therapeutic functions without realizing it or who are unaware of the effect of their interventions; there is a shortage of trained psychologists or people with therapeutic skills; the belief that therapy applies only to severe cases—that is, to psychiatric cases—which rarely occur in the work situation; people fail to realize the development functions of therapy or counselling; and the fact that management frequently fails to regard the workers' mental health as part of their responsibility and to include it in personnel policy.

In terms of principles and processes, counselling or therapy in the industry should be the same as that offered by a therapeutic psychologist in his consulting rooms, or as described in textbooks. We may assert that therapy in industrial practice is more counselling-oriented, as pointed out by Brammer and Shostrom (1982); 'Counselling, therefore, stresses more rational planning, problem-solving, decision-making, intentionality, prevention of severe adjustment problems and support for situational pressures arising in the everyday lives of normal people' (p. 8). Both Steinmetz (1969) and Neff (1977) stress the more *client-centred therapeutic approaches* (all approaches should be like this!) in which the client receives the opportunity of participating in the helping process, to assume responsibility, to explore feelings, to set objectives, and to evaluate alternatives—thus actualizing his potential. In the practical situation the industrial psychologist and health care worker work sometimes has to work on the adjustment problems of people with severe emotional and physical handicaps.

Apart from the individual counselling techniques mentioned above, we also find various types of *group techniques* in practice (Neff, 1977; Noland, 1973; Bolton and Jaques, 1978). Not only therapeutic groups are used in the industry, but also T-groups—especially for training purposes—which have strong underlying therapeutic power factors. The group leader must have the same skills as those applying to individual therapy or counselling. The effectiveness of group work lies in the group dynamic processes, in other words, in the 'helping' or 'curative' factors facilitated by group activities and interactions. Yalom (1975) describes the *power factors* as follows: the perception of similarity between group members (universality); group members care for one another (altruism); group members find it easy to speak of feelings or experiences (catharsis); group members identify the group leader and other group members in 'family roles' (the group as the second family, etc.); in the group the members easily become aware of their personal feelings and of verbal and non-verbal behaviour; group members are involved with one another (group cohesion); group members learn from one another and from the leaders (modelling); group members believe that the group process will work (trust); and group members help and support one another (support).

Because of the complexity of groups (e.g. work groups, families and relatives), group skills—such as accommodation, activation, intervention, diagnosis and evaluation—are difficult to acquire and require intensive training. Most writers acknowledge the positive effect of group workers (Rogers, 1961; Yalom, 1975), but they also warn against the emotional damage that may be caused by unscientific, unplanned and uncontrolled group influences (Kagan, 1970; Yalom, et al., 1971 in Brammer and Shostrom, 1982).

Neff (1977) asserts that the conversational technique of psychological therapy or the chemotherapy of the biological approach may be too narrow for some people. Furthermore, the rehabilitation of the problem worker often takes place away from the work situation where there is no task-oriented or work-related reality testing. The *rehabilitation workshop* is oriented towards placing the individual in the work situation or in simulated work situations (including sheltered work situations) where he can experience practically and non-verbally what the return or the adjustment to the real situation will mean. The maladjusted or rehabilitated worker has to experience the demands of *productive role fulfilment* both physically and psychologically. The requirements of the real situation should be duplicated in the simulated situation as far as it is possible to do so. The role of the supervisor varies from task leader to 'therapist', and conditions in the workshop could be varied to achieve certain effects. The workshop also provides the opportunity for supportive group and individual conversational interventions. In practice the workshop technique is frequently used for the rehabilitation of physically and emotionally handicapped people.

You will see from the literature that therapeutic or rehabilitation programmes—consisting of various and combined therapeutic techniques—are used in the following problem areas: absence and personnel turnover; alcoholism and drug problems; stress problems, for instance coronary heart diseases; mental retardation; physical handicaps such as blindness, deafness and epilepsy; people whose culture differs from that of most of their fellow-workers; group conflicts; training in interpersonal skills; the prisoner-client; illiterates; people with brain injuries; tuberculosis; diabetics; old people and haemophiliacs.

9.9.4 **Crisis** A crisis can be defined as a situation that has reached a critical phase, **intervention** a 'turning point for better or worse' (Fink, 1986, p. 15).

From a business or service-oriented point of view a crisis is any situation that runs the risk of:
- escalating in intensity
- coming under close media or Government (authority) scrutiny
- interfering with the normal operations of business or services
- damaging the image which a company enjoyed
- damaging or interfering with the company's basic objectives— e.g. income, training, etc.

From a behavioural perspective a crisis may be 'a state of disorganization in which helpees face frustration of important life goals or profound disruption of their life cycles and methods of coping with stressors. The term crisis usually refers to the helpee's feelings of fear, shock, and distress about the disruption, not the disruption itself' (Brammer, 1985).

For the health care worker, the helpee and all parties involved in dealing with a crisis calls for crisis intervention techniques that are flexible and rapid and which will offer alternatives and new goals to the stressed person in such a way that he/she can be functional again as soon as possible.

The skills for crisis intervention calls for coping skills which must be learned like any effective intervention method. Although it is more complex crisis intervention or management comes down to:
- identifying the crisis and its causes quickly
- isolating the crisis and its manifestations quickly
- managing the crisis quickly

Referring to Brammer (1985, p. 19) in more detail, these coping skills for crisis intervention entails the following:
- perceptual skills (seeing problematic situations clearly, as challenging or dangerous, and as solvable)
- cognitive change skills (restructuring thoughts and altering self-defeating thinking)
- support networking skills (assessing, strengthening, and diversifying external sources of support)
- stress management and wellness skills (reducing tensions through environmental and self-management)
- problem-solving skills (increasing problem-solving competence through applying models to diverse problems)
- description and expression of feelings (accurate apprehension and articulation of anger, fear, guilt, love, depression, and joy)

In a way crisis intervention or management really involves the managing of decision-making. A lot will depend on how accurately and swiftly decisions are made and applied.

Only some hints or aspects concerning crisis intervention will be discussed further.

The *causes* for crisis may be complex but may generally relate to the following which will also indicate the type of crisis dealt with:

- *severe loss* (bereavement, divorce, unemployment, disaster, imprisonment)
- *internal distress* (hopelessness, despair, fatigue, drug taking, suicidal attempts, depression)
- *life transitions* (job change, pregnancy, relocation, new family member, job choice, family conflict, illness).

In this regard, Holmes and Rahe's social adjustment events apply (Table 9.1).

For identifying the crisis it is also necessary to recognize the phase of crisis development. Generally a crisis may progress through the following stages which are similar to Selye's GAS model (see 9.7.1).

- During the *prodromal crisis stage* the initial tension is experienced and may be accompanied by warning signs and habitual adaptive responses.
- The *acute crisis stage* is marked by increased tension, marked by lack of success in coping and efforts to reduce tension. Frustration is increased by feelings of inefficiency and distress.
- The *chronic crisis stage* is marked by events that are beyond turning point in cases, tension increases and some release may only be experienced because emergency internal and external resources are mobilized. Certain damage may have been caused, such as behaviour dysfunctions and loss of emotional control.
- The *crisis resolution stage* when healing starts under the influence of self-management skills or the influence of external interventions.

In more detail and in behaviour terms, typical reactions in crisis situations may be as follows:

- shock and disorganization
- expression of anguish and/or relief
- experience of denial and minimization of the loss
- sadness and lowered self-esteem
- taking hold of a new way of life and letting go of the past
- final acceptance of change and planning for the future
- reflections on learning from the transition experience

(Brammer, 1985, p. 93).

Although simplified, the following clues for crisis intervention or management skills might be useful. Suffice to say that in-depth training in certain of these aspects is necessary.

In very general terms crisis intervention might be helpful by following the steps below:

- liberal use of emotional support through close contact, reassurance and listening to feelings
- changing of the helpee's environment such as ensuring a safe place and understanding people
- starting to change or influence the helpee's perceptions about his crisis situation.

Specific crisis intervention techniques can be many and may involve some of the health management methods discussed in this chapter. As was said, the process of crisis intervention entails firstly the accurate appraisal of the situation and/or the person involved and the options which are available, followed by a decision on the type of help and available resources; the third step consists of concrete and purposeful acts of help, followed by resolution of the crisis in which the person and/or situation once again experiences some balance and calm.

The following strategies are mentioned only briefly:

- Multiple impact support strategy involves a combined effort of several disciplines to ease distress—for example in a family crisis the family as a whole will be intervened on in an intensive two day round the clock programme, preferably away from the familiar environment.
- Individual or group counselling or therapeutic interventions must be based on building and maintaining hope and attempts to foster renewal and growth. These objectives will only be achieved if the helper is trained in using acknowledged therapeutic skills as described under 9.9.3.
- Creating or renewing a helpee's support systems involves identifying people, places and things which may be physically and emotionally helpful to the person.
- Referral skills involve the helper being informed about community and other resources in times of crisis.

In conclusion it is necessary to observe that crises cause stress and without some stress life will be sterile. Uncontrolled stress, such as in acute and chronic crises stages, however, may be damaging. On the positive side, stress and crises may have productive and creative outcomes. A prerequisite for these positive outcomes will, however, be determined by our ability to manage our decisions when intervening in crisis situations.

9.9.5 Community mental health and research Although there is a universal desire for intellectual, economic and political security, most people fail to achieve these. There should probably be more emphasis on the *close relationships* between human emotional security and mental health as prerequisites for the other qualities. This requires a shift in emphasis from the individual as 'sick' to the individual as the symptom-bearer of his environment. In this light the emphasis on family and marriage therapy and on therapies such as group work, rehabilitation programmes, and diagnostic and development strategies in the organization are hopeful signs. Training and educational programmes which disseminate information about health and mental health all over the world by means of various media, and the involvement of the community in the accommodation and employment of physically and emotionally handicapped people underline a concept that is gradually gaining acceptance. In the work organization this requires the continued influencing of management and managerial practices, so that man and his behaviour become the focal point, in place of the over-emphasis on 'hard criteria', namely technology, production, economy, etc.

The best method for the effective management of mental health will be based on research into the matters mentioned above, that is, into aetiology, specific mental health problems, better evaluation methods, the relationship between work behaviour and mental health problems, and the success of preventive and corrective action.

Newman and Beehr (1979) and Beehr and Newman (1978) refer to the necessity for systematic evaluative research on the effectiveness of managing managerial stress. For a long time now, clinical and therapeutic psychologists have been worried about the factors determining the effectiveness of interventions, since *every intervention has a definite effect*. Much research has been done about this matter, since it is essential to know whether these influences are helpful, whether they cause change or whether they are detrimental (Truax and Carkhuff, 1967; Garfield, 1981; Lazarus, 1980; Kirsch and Kroll, 1980; Smith and Glass, 1977).

In recent times the professional helper and legal aspects in terms of ethics and conduct with a view to the client and the professional have become important and will have even more important implications in future (Rinas and Clyne-Jackson, 1988).

9.11 BIBLIOGRAPHY

Allport, G. W. (1961). *Pattern and growth in personality*. New York: Holt, Rinehart and Winston.

Andolfi, M. (1979). *Family therapy: An interactional approach*. New York: Plenum Press.

Annual Reports (1981/82). *Department of Health and Health Development*. Pretoria.

Antonovsky, A. (1984). A call for a new question—salutogenesis—and a proposed answer—the sense of coherence. *Journal of Preventive Psychiatry*, 2, 1–13.

Antonovsky, A. (1987). *Unravelling the mystery of health: How people manage stress and stay well*. San Francisco: Jossey-Bass.

Appley, M. H. and Trumbull, R. (eds.) (1986). *Dynamics of stress: physiological, psychological, and social perspectives*. New York: Plenum Press.

Ashford, S. J. (1988). Individual strategies for coping with stress during organizational transitions. *The Journal of Applied Behavioral Science*, 24(1), 19–36.

Baker, F., McEwan, P. J. M. et al. (1969). Industrial organizations and health. Vol. 1. *Selected readings*. London: Tavistock.

Barocas et al. (1983). *Personal adjustment and growth: A life span approach*. New York: St. Martinis Press.

Berg, I. A. (1970). Employee counselling in a well-rounded personnel programme. *Public Personnel Review*, 31(3), 185–9.

Bolton, B. and Jaques, M. E. (1978). *Rehabilitation counselling: theory and practice*. Baltimore: University Park Press.

Booth-Kewley, S. and Friedman, H. S. (1987). Psychological predictors of heart disease: A quantitative review. *Psychological Bulletin*, 101, 343–62.

Brammer, L. M. (1985). *The helping relationship: Process and Skills*. New Jersey: Prentice-Hall.

Brammer, L. M. and Shostrom, E. L. (1982). *Therapeutic psychology*. New Jersey: Prentice-Hall.

Brophy, R. H. and Raubenheimer, J. van W. (1978). The effectiveness of neurotics as workers compared to non-neurotics. *Perspektiewe in die Bedryfsielkunde*, 4(3), 1–16.

Byang-Hall, J. (1980). Symptom bearer as marital regulator: clinical implications. *Family Process*, 19(4), 355–65.

Carone, P. A., Kiefer, S. M. et al. (eds.) (1978). *Misfits in industry*. New York: S. P. Medical and Scientific Books.

Carson, R. C. (1969). *Interaction concepts of personality*. Chicago: Aldine.

Carson, R. C., Butcher, J. N. and Coleman, J. C. (1988). *Abnormal Psychology and modern life*. (8th ed.) Glenview, Illinois: Foresman & Co.

Carvey, D. W. and Nibler, R. G. (1977). Biorhythmic cycles and the incidence of industrial accidents. *Personnel Psychology*, 30, 447–54.

Chimezie, A. B. and Osigweh, Y. G. (1988). The challenge of responsibilities: confronting the revolution in workplace rights in modern organizations. *Employee Responsibilities and Rights Journal*, 1(1), 5–23.

Cilliers, F. v N. (1984). 'n Ontwikkelingsprogram in sensitiewe relasievorming as bestuursdimensie. Proefskrif, D.Phil. Potchefstroom: PU vir CHO.

Cilliers, F. v N. (1988). Die konsep sielkundige optimaliteit in bestuur. *IPB–Joernaal*, 7(5), 15–18.

Cooper, C. L. and Marshall, J. (1975). The management of stress. *Personnel Review*, 4, 27–31.

Cooper, C. L. Payne, R. (eds.) (1978). *Stress at work*. Chichester: John Wiley.

Cronkite, R. C. and Moos, R. H. (1984). The role of predisposing and moderating factors in the stress-illness relationship. *Journal of Health and Social Behavior*, 25, 372–93.

Cull, J. G. and Hardy, R. E. (1973). *Adjustment to work*. Springfield: G. C. Thomas Publishers.

Cummings, T. G. (ed.) (1980). *Systems theory for organization development*. Chichester: Wiley.

Dalton, D. R., Krackhardt, D. M. and Porter, L. W. (1980). Functional turnover: an empirical assessment. *Journal of Applied Psychology*, 66(6), 716–21.

De Board, R. C. (1983). *Counselling people at work*. Aldershot: Gower.

Dickman, F., Challenger, B. R., Emener, W. G. and Hutchison, J. R. (1988). *Employee assistance programs: a basic text*. Springfield: Charles C. Thomas.

Dunnette, M. D. (1976, 1981). *Handbook of Industrial and organizational psychology*. Chicago: Rand McNally.

Eaton, M. T. (1969). The mental health of the older executive. *Geriatrics*, May, 126–34.

Eisenstat, R. A. and Felner, R. D. (1984). Toward a differentiated view of burnout: Personal and organizational mediators of job satisfaction and stress. *American Journal of Community Psychology*, 12, 411–30.

Fink, S. (1986). *Crisis management: Planning for the inevitable*. New York: AMACOM.

Fisher, S. and Reason, J. C. (eds.) (1988). *Handbook of life stress, cognition and health*. Chichester: Wiley & Sons.

Fleming, R., Baum, A. and Singer, J. E. (1984). Toward an integrative approach to the study of stress. *Journal of Personality and Social Psychology*, 46(4), 939–49.

Folkman, S. (1984). Personal control and stress and coping processes: A Theoretical analysis. *Journal of Personality and Social Psychology*, 46(4), 839–52.

Follman, J. F. (1978). *Helping the troubled employee*. New York: AMACOM.

Forbes, R. (1979). *Corporate stress*. Garden City, New York: Doubleday.

Frankenhaeuser, M. and Johansson, G. (1986). Stress at work: psychobiological and psychosocial aspects. *International Review of Applied Psychology*, 35, 287–99.

Freedman, A. M. and Caplan, H. I. (1967). *Comprehensive textbook of psychiatry* Baltimore: Williams & Wilkens.

Freedman, L. Z. and Leary, S. A. (1961). Psychopathology and occupation: work and competition. *Occupational Psychology*, 35, 93–110.

Freudenberger, H. J. (1974). Staff Burnout. *Journal of Social Issues*, 30, 159–65.

Friedman, M. and Rosen, R. H. (1974). *Type A behavior and your heart.* London: Wildworld House.

Furnham, A. (1984). The protestant work ethic: A review of the psychological literature. *European Journal of Social Psychology*, 14, 87–109.

Ganster, D. C. and Victor, B. C. (1988). The impact of social support on mental and physical health. *British Journal of Medical Psychology*, 61, 17–36.

Garfield, S. L. (1981). Evaluating the psychotherapics. *Behavior Therapy*, 12, 295–307.

Gavin, J. F. (1977). Occupational Mental Health focus and trends. *Personnel Journal*, 4, 198–201.

Gechman, A. S. (1974). Without work life goes. *Journal of Occupational Medicine*, 16(11), 749–51.

Geldenhuys, B. P. and Du Toit, S. I. (1975). *Psigopatologie.* Kaapstad: Academia.

Gerdes, L. C. (1988). *The developing adult.* Durban: Butterworths.

Gherman, E. M. (1981). Stress and the bottom line. New York: Amacom.

Ginzberg, E. (1972). Toward a theory of occupational choice: a restatement. *Vocational Guidance Quarterly*, 20, 169–76.

Glass, D. C. and Carver, G. D. (1980). Helplessness and the coronary-prone personality. In J. Garber and M. E. P. Seligman (eds.) *Human helplessness: Theory and applications.* New York: Academic Press.

Green, M. (1974). Counselling for employees. *Personnel Practice Bulletin*, 30(3), 234–43.

Greenwood, J. W. and Greenwood, J. W. (1979). *Managing executive stress.* New York: Wiley.

Haley, J. (1963). Strategies of Psychotherapy. New York: Grune & Stratton.

Haley, J. (1967). Milton H. Erickson: *Advanced techniques of hypnosis and therapy.* New York: Grune & Stratton.

Healy, C. C. (1982). *Career development: counselling through the life stages.* Boston: Allyn & Bacon.

Herman, C. F. (1963). Some consequences of crisis which limit the viability of organizations. *Administrative Science Quarterly*, 8, 61–82.

Hill, N. C. (1981). *Counselling at the workplace.* New York: McGraw-Hill.

Hirschfield, A. H. and Behan, R. C. (1963). The accident process: Ethological considerations of industrial injuries. *The Journal of the American Association*, 186, 193–9.

Hobfoll, S. E. (1988). *The ecology of stress.* New York: Hemisphere Publishing Co.

Hobfoll, S. E. (1989). Conservation of Resources: a new attempt at conceptualizing stress. *American Psychologist*, 44(3), 513–24.

Holland, J. L. (1973). *Making Vocational choices: a theory of careers.* Engelwood Cliffs: Prentice-Hall.

Howard, J. H., Cunningham, D. A. and Rechnitzer, P. A. (1977). Work patterns associated with type A behaviour. *Human Relations*, 30, 825–36.

Hurrell, J. J., Murphy, R. L. R., Sauter, S. L. and Cooper, C. L. (1988). *Occupational stress: Issues and developments in research.* New York: Taylor & Francis.

Huszczo, G. E. and Fried, B. J. (1988). A labour relations research agenda for health care settings. *Employee Responsibilities and Rights Journal*, 1(1), 69–84.

Isaacson, L. E. (1985). *Basics of career counselling.* Boston: Allyn & Bacon.

Isabella, L. A. (1988). The effect of career stage on the meaning of key organizational events. *Journal of Organizational Behaviour*, 9, 345–58.

Ivancevich, J. M. and Matteson, M. T. (1988). Type A-behaviour and the healthy individual. *British Journal of Medical Psychology*, 61, 37–56.

Jones, J. W. (1982). *The Burnout syndrome: current research, theory, interventions*. Illinois: London House Press.

Joseph, A. (1983). *Women at work*. Oxford: Allen.

Kahn, R. L. (1981). *Work and health*. New York: Wiley & Son.

Kakabadse, A. (1982). *People and organizations*. Aldershot: Gower.

Kane, K. W. (1975). Corporate responsibility in the area of alcoholism. *Personnel Psychology*, 54(7), 380–4.

Kanunga, R. N. (1982). *Work alienation: An integrative approach*. New York: Praeger.

Kaplan, H. B. (ed.) (1983). *Psychosocial stress: Trends in theory and research*. New York: Academic Press.

Katz, D. & Kahn, R. L. (1978). *The social psychology of organizations*. New York: Wiley.

Keeley, M. (1988). Individual rights and organizational theory. *Employee Responsibilities and Rights Journal*, 1(1), 25–38.

Kiesler, D. J. & Annchin, J. C. (1982). *Handbook of interpersonal therapy*. New York: Pergamon.

Kirsch, J. & Kroll, J. (1980). Meaningfulness versus effectiveness: paradoxical implications in the evaluation of psychotherapy. *Psychotherapy: theory and practice*, 17(4), 401–13.

Klopfer, B., Ainsworth, M. D. et al. (1954). *The Rorschach Technique*. New York: Harcourt Brace.

Kobassa, S. C. (1979). Stressful life events, personality, and health: An inquiry into hardiness. *Journal of Personality and Social Psychology*, 37(1), 1–11.

Kohn, M. L. and Schooler, C. (1983). *Work and personality*. New York: Ablex.

Kornhauser, A. (1965). *Mental health of the industrial worker*. New York: Wiley.

Krantz, D. S. & Raisen, S. E. (1988). Environmental stress, reactivity and ischaemic heart disease. *British Journal of Medical Psychology*, 61, 3–16.

Krantz, J. (1985). Group process under conditions of organizational decline. *Journal of Applied Behavioural Science*, 21(1), 1–17.

Latack, J. C. (1981). Person/role conflict: Holland's model extended to role-stress research, stress management, and career development. *Academy of Management Review*, 6(1), 89–103.

Lazarus, R. S. (1980). *Patterns of adjustment*. Tokyo: McGraw-Hill.

Leibowitz, Z. B. and Schlossberg, N. K. (1981). Training managers for their role in a career development system. *Training and Development Journal*, July, 72–9.

Le Roux, A. G. (1968). *Inleiding tot psigopatologie*. Pretoria: Van Schaik.

Levi, L. (1984). *Stress in Industry: causes, effects and prevention*. Geneva: International Labour Office.

Levinson, H. (1975). On executive suicide. *Harvard Business Review*, 53, 118–22.

Levitan, S. A. and Johnson, C. M. (1982). *Second thoughts on work*. Michigan: Upjohn Institute for unemployment research.

Levy, B. S. and Wegman, D. H. (1988). *Occupational health: recognizing and preventing work related disease*. Boston: Little, Brown Co.

Louw, D. A. (ed.) (1989). *Suid-Afrikaanse Handboek van Abnormale Gedrag*. Johannesburg: Southern.

Louw, E. F. (1974). Alcoholism and the employer. *Rehabilitation in S.A.*, 18, 75–9.

Machlowitz, N. H. (1978). *Determining the effects of workaholism*. Ann Arbor: Yale University.

Manning, M. R., Williams, R. F. and Wolfe, D. M. (1988). Hardiness and the relationship between stressors and outcomes. *Work and Stress*, 2(3), 205–16.

Manuso, J. S. T. (1983). *Occupational Clinical Psychology*. New York: Praeger.

McClean, A. (1970). *Mental health and work organizations*. Chicago: Rand McNally.

McClean, A. A. (1979). *Work stress*. Reading, Massachusetts: Addison-Wesley.

McCormick, E. J. and Ilgen, D. R. (1981). *Industrial Psychology*. London: George Allen.

Meckel, N. T. (1981). The manager as career counsellor. *Training and Development Journal*, July, 65–9.

Meichenbaum, D. (1977). *Cognitive behaviour modification. An integrative approach*. New York: Plenum.

Miner, J. B. (1966). *Introduction to industrial clinical psychology*. New York: McGraw-Hill.

Minuchin, S. (1974). *Families and family therapy*. Cambridge, Massachusetts: Harvard University Press.

Mortimer, J. T. and Borman, K. M. (1988). *Work experience and psychological development through the life span*. Colorado: Westview Press Inc.

Muchinsky, P. M. (1983). *Psychology applied to work*. Homewood, Illinois: Dorsey Press.

Muldary, T. W. (1983). *Burnout and health professionals: Manifestations and management*. Norwalk: Appleton-Century-Crofts.

Murphy, L. C. (1984). Occupational stress management: A review and appraisal. *Journal of Occupational Psychology*, 57, 1–15.

Neff, W. S. (1977). *Work and human behaviour*. Chicago: Aldine.

Newman, T. E. and Beehr, T. A. C. (1979). Personal and organizational strategies for handling job stress: A review of research and opinion. *Personnel Psychology*, 32, 1–43.

Noel, R. (1990). Employing the disabled: A how and why approach. *Training and Development Journal*, 44(8), 26–32.

Noland, R. L. (1973). *Industrial mental health and employee counselling*. New York: Behaviour Publications.

Oates, W. E. (1971). *Confessions of a workaholic*. New York: Abingdon Press.

O'Connell, M. J. (1976). The effects of environmental information and decision unit structure on felt tension. *Journal of Applied Psychology*, 4, 493–500.

Odendaal, F. J. and Van Wyk, J. D. (1988). Die taksering van die sindroom uitbranding. *Suid-Afrikaanse tydskrif vir sielkunde*, 18(2), 4–49.

O'Meara, J. R. (1977). Retirement. *Across the Board*, January, 4–9.

O'Toole, J. (1974). *Work and the quality of life*. Cambridge: M.I.T. Press.

Parker, D. F. and DeCotiis, T. (1983). Organizational determinants of job stress. *Organizational Behaviour and Human Performance*, 32(2), 166–79.

Payne, R. L., Jabri, M. M. and Pearson, A. W. (1988). On the importance of knowing the affective meaning of job demands. *Journal of Organizational Behaviour*, 9, 149–58.

Pearlin, L. I. and Schooler, L. (1978). The structure of coping. *Journal of Health and Social Behaviours*, 19, 2–21.

Pearlin, L. I., Lieberman, M. A. et al. (1981). The Stress Process. *Journal of Health and Social Behaviour*, 22, 337–56.

Price, V. A. (1982). What is type A? A cognitive social learning model. *Journal of Occupational Behaviour*, 3, 109–29.

Quinn, R. E. and Cameron, K. (1983). Organizational life cycles and shifting criteria of effectiveness: some preliminary evidence. *Management Science*, 29(1), 33–51.

Raelin, J. (1984). An examination of deviant/adaptive behaviours in the organizational careers of professionals. *Academy of Management Review*, 9(3), 413–27.

Reddy, M. (1987). *The manager's guide to counselling at work*. London: Methuen.

Rinas, J. and Clyne-Jackson, S. (1988). *Professional conduct and legal concerns in mental health practice*. Norwalk: Appleton & Lange.

Robbins, S. P. (1989). *Organizational behaviour: concepts, controversies and applications*. New Jersey: Prentice-Hall.

Roberson, C. (1986). *Preventing employee misconduct: A self-defense manual for business*. Massachusetts: Lexicon Books.

Roe, A. (1956). *The psychology of occupations*. New York: Wiley.

Rogers, L. R. (1961). *On becoming a person: a therapist view of psychotherapy*. Boston: Houghton Mifflin.

Roseman, E. (1982). *Managing the problem employee*. New York: AMACOM.

Ross, E., Powles, W. and Winslow, W. (1965). Secondary prevention of job disruption in industry. *Journal of Occupational Medicine*, 7, 3–4.

Rossiter, C. M. and Barnette Pearce, W. (1975). *Communicating personally*. Indianapolis: Bobbs-Merrill.

Rotter, J. B. (1966). Generalized expectancies for internal versus external control of reinforcement. *Psychological Monographs*, 80(1), Whole No. 609.

Rühmke, H. C. (1957). *Psychiatrie*. Amsterdam: Scheltema & Hakema.

Schafer, W. (1987). *Stress Management for Wellness*. New York: Holt, Rinehart and Winston. Inc.

Schuler, R. (1982). An integrative transactional process model of stress in organizations. *Journal of Occupational Behaviour*, 3, 5–19.

Selzer, M. L., Rogers, I. E. and Kern, S. (1968). Fatal accidents: the role of psychopathology, social stress, and acute disturbance. *American Journal of Psychiatry*, 124(8), 1028(46)–1036(54).

Sharit, J. and Salvendy, G. (1982). Occupational Stress: Review and reappraisal. *Human factors*, 24(2), 129–62.

Shirom, A. (1982). What is organizational stress? A facet analytic conceptualization. *Journal of Occupational Behaviour*, 3, 21–37.

Slaney, R. B. and Russell, J. C. (1987). Perspectives on Vocational Behaviour, 1986: A Review. *Journal of Vocational Behaviour*, 31, 111–173.

Smith, M. L. and Glass, G. V. (1977). Mieta-analysis of psychotherapy outcome studies. *American Psychologist*, 32, 752–60.

Steinmetz, L. L. (1969). *Human relations: people and work*. New York: Harper & Row.

Sternhagen, C. J. (1969). Medicine's role in reducing absenteeism. *Personnel*, 46(6), 28–38.

Stout, S. K., Slocum, J. W. and Cron, W. L. (1988). Dynamics of the career plateauing process. *Journal of Vocational Behaviour*, 32, 74–91.

Stumpf, S. A. and Rabinowitz, S. (1981). Career stage as a moderator of performance relationships with facets of job satisfaction and role perceptions. *Journal of Vocational Behaviour*, 18, 202–18.

Suinn, R. M. (1975). *Fundamentals of behaviour pathology*. New York: Wiley.

Sullivan, H. S. (1953). *The interpersonal theory of psychiatry*. New York: Norton.

Super, D. E. (1980). A life span, life space approach to career development. *Journal of Vocational Behaviour*, 16, 282–98.

Super, D. E. and Bohn, M. J. (1970). *Occupational Psychology*. Monteray: Brooks-Cole.

Sussal, C. M. and Ojakian, E. (1988). Crisis intervention in the workplace. *Employee assistance Quarterly*, 4(1), 71–85.

Swart, N. and Wiehahn, G. (1979). *Interpersonal manoeuvres and behaviour change*. Pretoria: H & R. Academia.

Szasz, T. S. (1966). *The myth of mental illness*. New York: Norton.

Taveggia, T. C. and Hedley, R. A. (1976). Job Specialization, work values and worker dissatisfaction. *Journal of Vocational Behaviour*, 9, 293–309.

Terkel, S. (1972). *Working*. New York: Pantheon Books.

Truax, C. B. and Carkhuff, R. R. (1967). *Toward effective counselling and psychotherapy*. Chicago: Aldine.

Van Kessel, W. and Van der Linden, P. (1974). *Een interactioneel model voor gestoord gedrag en voor psychotherapie*. Unpublished lectures. Instituut voor clinische en Industriële Psychologie: Utrecht.

Visser, M. (ed.) (1990) *Health in South Africa*. Pretoria: RGN.

Vlok, A. (1971). Die probleemdrinker en sy werkgewer. In Blignaut, F. W. (red.) Verslag van die projek alkoholisme: die persoonlikheid en behandeling van die alkoholis in Suid-Afrika, Deel iv, Pretoria: RGN.

Vlok, A. (1981). *Notes on occupational maladjustment and managerial response in 36 large South African enterprises*. Department of Industrial Psychology, Unisa, Pretoria.

Warshaw, L. J. (1979). *Managing stress*. Reading: Addison-Wesley.

Watzlawick, O. and Beavin, J. H. (eds.) (1977). *The interactional view*. New York: Norton.

Watzlawick, P., Beavin, J. H. and Jackson, D. D. (1967). *Pragmatics of human communication*. New York: Norton.

Welford, A. T. (1976). Thirty years of psychological research on age and work. *Journal of Occupational Psychology*, 49, 129–38.

Wiener, Y. et al. (1981). Anticedents of employee's mental health—the role of career and work satisfaction. *Journal of Vocational Behaviour*, 19, 50–60.

Wolcott, A., McKeeton, R. et al. (1977). Correlation of general aviation accidents with biorhythm theory. *Human Factors*, 19, 283–4.

Yalom, I. D. (1975). *The theory and practice of group psychotherapy*. New York: Basic Books.

Chapter 10: Health Promotion at Work

by A. J. Kotze

10.1 INTRODUCTION

Health services are not synonymous with good health. We are increasingly realizing that many hereditary, personal and environmental factors in our lives play a major role in the quality of health in our lives. It follows that the promotion of health can play an important role in preserving whatever good health we experience.

If a more positive attitude can be created to enable people to take an increased interest in and responsibility for their own health, society as a whole can benefit. Health promotion programmes, with the emphasis on disease prevention, and the promotion of positive health, can contribute to the total health of communities.

As most people spend the larger part of their lives in employment, the workplace may be considered a suitable place to introduce health promotion programmes. The financial benefits of health promotion and the resulting improvement in health behaviour cannot be overemphasized.

10.2 LEARNING OBJECTIVES

After studying this chapter, the reader should be able to:
* identify healthy lifestyles
* describe the importance of health promotion
* identify the components of a health promotion programme
* plan and implement specific programmes for health promotion

10.3 HEALTHY LIFESTYLES

Human behaviour is affected by many factors. Promotion pro-grammes aimed at changing behaviour should address as many of these factors as possible. Motivation has always been considered an important factor in the changing of human behaviour and may be used effectively (Girdano, 1986: 7). Girdano gives two essential ingredients for behaviour change:
* a reason to change (motivation)
* the knowledge to know when, where, and how to take action (1986: 7).

In our multicultural society being healthy may mean many different things to different people. To those experiencing socio-economic deprivation, health may not seem as important as food, clothing and shelter; to affluent members of society, factors contributing to an unhealthy lifestyle such as stress, overeating and the lack of exercise may cause ill health, and be a motivation to change behaviour.

Girdano (1986: 9) says that in order to be healthy one must recognize and change unhealthy behaviour. At a general level this involves:
* an ability to recognize imbalance and the behaviours that promote it
* the creation of an environment which supports balance
* the ability to satisfy health-related needs with behaviour that promotes good health, rather than detracts from it
* living in such a way that one's life is balanced, healthy and there are few episodes of imbalance.

10.4 OCCUPATIONAL HEALTH PROMOTION

The idea of prevention of disease and promotion of positive health is not a new one and in many ancient civilizations, such as the Chinese and the Greek, health was seen as something which had to be nurtured and protected (Girdano, 1986: 11).

In our own society, some form of environmental health and health education forms part of the school curriculum from a very early age. Today we realize that these programmes cannot be incidental. They must be planned efficiently and offered effectively, if we are to combat the many threats to human health.

Programmes must be continuous and cover the whole span of human development—childhood, adolescence, adulthood and old age. The workplace can be a natural and potentially effective setting for health promotion programmes, for a number of reasons:

- the workforce is increasing in numbers, and this provides a readily available target group
- people tend to make better use of programmes offered at work
- a part of the workforce is stable and this allows for long-term intervention and evaluation
- high health care costs and a loss in productivity may act as a motivation for industry to become involved in programmes for health promotion
- the family of the worker can also be affected positively by programmes offered to the worker.

Occupational health promotion relies heavily upon the positive attitudes of both the worker and the employer towards promotion programmes. I would go so far as to say that the input of the employer is the major factor which will determine the success of such a programme, as this input is more concrete in terms of facilities, financial contribution, personnel and all the other facets of the planning and implementation of such a programme. At present there is no legal provision to enforce such a programme, and it would therefore depend entirely upon the philosophy of the employer towards the value of such a programme.

Some firms have shown how much they value the health of their employers by instituting some form of health promotion programmes, whilst others still have to follow. Examples of elements of these programmes are:

- health education
- recreational facilities
- opportunities for social interaction
- employer assistance programmes.

Some form of evaluation of these programmes should take place. This can be done by regular health screening for risk factors e.g. high blood-pressure, or by documenting the level of participation in programmes, and finally by assessing positive behavioural changes.

10.5 COMPONENTS OF A SUCCESSFUL OCCUPATIONAL HEALTH PROMOTION PROGRAMME

Girdano quotes Collings and says that 'the ideal health promotion programme is one that identifies target subpopulations with precision, intervening in those populations with selectivity based on carefully selected outcomes, modifies and tailors each intervention to maximize its individual effectiveness and delivers the programme with maximum cost-efficiency' (Girdano, 1986: 21).

The following components are essential for a promotion programme—

10.5.1   Policy A policy should be characterized by the willingness of management to commit itself. Once commitment is guaranteed, involvement of management in the programmes can have an important effect on the presentation of a positive role-model.

10.5.2   Planning A well-prepared programme will be preceded by all the steps of the planning process which may be—

10.5.2.1   Estab- The philosophy of a health promotion programme may be:
lishing a
philosophy
- to create an awareness and responsibility for one's own and the health of one's family
- to establish positive health behaviour
- to change health damaging behaviour to that which may enhance good health
- to obtain maximum participation in health promotion programmes.

10.5.2.2   Formu- These may include long and short-term objectives, stated in
lating measurable terms:
objectives for
the
programme
- the identification of high risk populations
- establishing the interest of employees to assess needs
- determining the kind of programmes required and their implementation
- setting targets for employee participation in programmes
- determining expected outcomes of programmes
- compiling a data-bank with information relevant to programmes
- deciding upon methods of evaluation to determine the effectiveness of the programme.

10.5.2.3   Pro- Objectives can be achieved by applying the following methods—
gramme content

Well person screening

This term is used to describe the process of 'sorting through' a group to identify individuals who may show early signs of the condition under study, or be vulnerable to a disease (Schilling, 1973: 121). Screening can involve high costs and specialized technology, and does not end with screening, but needs to be supported by a follow-up and treatment programme.

In developing countries it seems possible that multiphasic screening could do much to identify vulnerable people and raise the standard of general fitness of the community (Schilling, 1973: 133).

Tailoring to the participants

It has been proved that in more successful programmes, participants are able to choose the type and form of health promotion they prefer. Girdano says that this enhances individual autonomy, increases self-esteem and the likelihood of behaviour change (1986: 24).

A comprehensive programme

The decision whether to plan a single focus or comprehensive programme depends on company policy, finances, resources and facilities available. A comprehensive programme that approaches employees in totality is more desirable.

A multidimensional programme offers more flexibility to the health team and more freedom of choice to the employer. Which components to include in a programme will depend on many factors such as the needs of employees, the results of screening, and the motivation of employees to participate in programmes.

Examples of components of a programme which prove to be popular are:

- first-aid and accident prevention, cardio-pulmonary resuscitation;
- stress management
- mental health
- substance abuse prevention and rehabilitation
- recreation and fitness, and weight control
- prevention of and coping with chronic illness.

10.5.2.4 Adminis- The health promotion programmes cannot be offered without there
trative being an administrative support system available. Girdano says that
structure in-house or in-house personnel with the aid of outside consultants, or outside companies could be contracted to offer the programme (1986: 25). Programmes which are administered internally can be incorporated within the existing administrative structure.

10.5.3 Educational This needs to be decided during the planning phase. The strategies
approach used and techniques applied should be tried and tested beforehand.

In general, principles of good health care or education should be applied and regularly adapted as the programme develops and new or changed needs arise.

10.5.4 Continuous During the planning phase attention must be given to methods to
participation motivate participants to continue taking part in programmes. Various methods can be followed, such as:

- communication, progress reports and incentives to the participants of the programme
- involvement of employee dependants in the programme
- encouragement of employers to be responsible for healthy behaviour; inclusion of methods of self-evaluation in the programme
- use of social support systems to enhance positive behaviour
- ensuring a safe and healthy work environment to emphasise that the efforts of the employer in health promotion are credible.

10.5.5 Evaluation General rules of evaluation in educational settings should be applied to this programme. Evaluation should be part of the planning phase and methods of evaluation to determine the effectiveness of the programme must form part of the programme.

10.6 SOME EXAMPLES OF HEALTH PROMOTION PROGRAMMES

10.6.1 Promoting The large number of women of childbearing age in the work-force
maternal- make issues such as pregnancy and child health important. Preventive
child well- health programmes at work for women and children can eventually
being in the ensure numerous advantages to the employer in the form of a healthy
workplace work-force.

Working mothers are faced with problems among which breast feeding, childhood and other child diseases, illnesses during pregnancy, and child support systems are but a few. They can lead to a high rate of absenteeism in the workforce. If these are addressed by well organized preventative and health support programmes, high employee morale, work retention and good quality work is possible.

Contents of this programme

After assessing the needs of the target group you are dealing with, the contents of the programme is decided upon. This may include aspects of:

- pre-natal care
- counselling and supervision of high risk groups, e.g. H.I.V. positive mothers, single parents and mothers with chronic diseases
- nutrition, exercise and recreation
- caring for an infant
- dealing with childhood diseases effectively
- the provision and supervision of child care facilities
- flexitime facilities for nurturing mothers.

These are a few examples of programmes which can be offered.

10.6.2 The prevention of AIDS (Acquired Immune Deficiency Syndrome) Communities should be well informed about all the aspects of this disease. The employer and the occupational health team has a specific responsibility and role to play in creating knowledge about the condition and promoting positive behaviour to prevent this condition. For the person who has already contracted AIDS, effective health supervision, counselling and management by health personnel with empathy and understanding are required. It is also the duty of the employer to protect other workers and personnel from high risk behaviour, as far as this disease is concerned. An informed community can be a great asset in the prevention of AIDS.

Content of the programme

The content of this programme will be divided into two main sections:

- Health promotion measures to create an awareness of the disease and to prevent the spreading of the condition:
  - promoting responsible relationships
  - promoting protected sexual behaviour
  - AIDS information groups
  - screening programmes.
- Health measures to promote the health of the AIDS sufferer and the carriers of the disease:
  - general health promotion programmes, e.g. nutrition and recreation
  - specific health education related to the problems experienced by the sufferer
  - safe sexual behaviour aimed at protecting partners, the family and the community
  - health maintenance and surveillance
  - health support during periods of illness
  - counselling of contacts, family and employers.

10.6.3 Hypertension screening programmes According to South African statistics for 1986, the total death rate per 100 000 of the population due to hypertensive disease was 59, but the estimated number of people suffering from hypertension runs into thousands more. In America it is estimated that 15 per cent or roughly 37 million people are thought to have hypertension (Girdano, 1986: 168).

Blood-pressure screening programmes can be educational and promote compliance with treatment for those who have been treated, but may also identify high risk populations. The very many conditions of which high blood-pressure is merely a symptom may be prevented, treated and controlled. Many lost workdays and resulting loss in production and finances may be prevented with such a programme.

A successful programme for blood-pressure screening should include elements such as:

- detection
- referral
- diagnosis
- follow-up
- long-term maintenance
- education
- evaluation.

(Girdano, 1986: 171.)

The workplace has been identified as being a suitable site for the initiation, monitoring and the maintenance of treatment of hypertension.

10.7 SUMMARY

Health promotion programmes can save the employer and the community many millions of rands in health care costs, but in a country where occupational health is still not as readily accepted as in first world countries, a lot of work has still to be done. Primary health care features prominently in our present-day health care planning, and this may be the ideal opportunity to introduce health promotion as a component of preventative health care programmes.

10.8 BIBLIOGRAPHY

Gates, D. M. and O'Neill, N. J. *Promoting Maternal-Child Wellness in the Workplace*. American Association for Occupational Health Nurses Journal, June 1990. Vol. 38, No. 6.

Girdano, D. A. 1986. *Occupational Health Promotion*. New York: Macmillan Publishing Company.

Health Trends in South Africa, 1989. Department of National Health and Population Development.

Schilling, R. S. F. 1973. *Occupational Health Practice*. London: Butterworths & Company (Publishers) Ltd.

Index